D0889780

Statistics for Biology and Health

Series Editors:
M. Gail, K. Krickeberg, J. Samet, A. Tsiatis, W. Wong

Statistics for Biology and Health

Antonella Bacchieri Giovanni Della Cioppa

Fundamentals
of Clinical Research

Bridging Medicine, Statistics and Operations

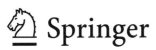 Springer

Antonella Bacchieri
Head, Department of Biostatistics
   and Data Management
Research & Development
Sigma-tau, Pomezia, Rome (Italy)

Giovanni Della Cioppa
Head, Department of Methodology and
   Innovation
Pharma Development
Novartis, Basel (Switzerland)

Series Editors:

M. Gail
National Cancer Institute
Rockville, MD 20892
USA

K. Krickeberg
Le Chatelet
F-63270 Manglieu
France

J. Samet
Deparment of Epidemiology
School of Public Health
Johns Hopkins University
615 Wolfe Street
Baltimore, MD 21205-2103
USA

A. Tsiatis
Department of Statistics
North Carolina State University
Raleigh, NC 27695
USA

W. Wong
Sequoia Hall
Department of Statistics
Stanford University
390 Serra Mall
Stanford, CA 94305-4065
USA

Originally published in Italian: Fondamenti di ricerca clinica, A. Bacchieri - G. Della Cioppa.
© Springer-Verlag Italia, Milano 2004 - Translated by the Authors in cooperation with Maria
Marrapodi and Richard J. Vernell

Library of Congress Control Number: 2006938039

ISBN-13 978-88-470-0491-7

Springer is a part of Springer Science+Business Media
springer.com
© Springer-Verlag Italia, Milano 2007

Typesetting: Compostudio, Cernusco sul Naviglio (MI)
Printing and Binding: Signum, Bollate (MI)
Printed in Italy
Springer-Verlag Italia
Via Decembrio 28
20133 Milano, Italy

To our parents, in particular in memory of Antonio Bacchieri
In memory of Tiziana Mistrali

Foreword

Statistical methodology is an essential component of clinical (and biological) research. Therefore it is not surprising that many textbooks aiming at "explaining" statistical methods to researchers have been published and continue to appear in print. The complexity of the basic issue, that of communication between statisticians and researchers, is illustrated and discussed very well by the authors of this book in their Introduction. Thus it would be of no benefit to dwell further on this theme and on the difficulty of producing truly effective material.

I prefer to start from a personal episode. Way back in 1959, a freshman of the faculty of Statistical Sciences, I found by chance on a stand, the book "Metodi statistici ad uso dei ricercatori", which was the Italian translation of the famous book by RA Fisher. The textbook for the first course of statistics used that year at of our University had left me perplexed. A student like myself, with a good high school scientific education, was fascinated by the wealth of real life examples, but was unable to reconstruct the thread of logical-mathematical reasoning, especially the inductive one. The unexpected access to Fisher's legendary book raised my hopes that I could finally get to the heart of the matter. However, after several attempts at reading it, I reached the conclusion that experimental statistics required first and foremost a spirit of obedience: one was to use formulae which were incomprehensible, but justified by some higher authority. Especially mysterious was the frequently appearing concept of "degrees of freedom", a number which seemed to be reachable only through vague analogical reasoning. Fortunately, my conclusion was a temporary one, because, while still a student, I had the fortune of being exposed to much more constructive critical approaches. But what could be the reaction of the researcher, in principle the target of the book? Most likely that of accepting statistics as a price to pay to make his/her research publishable, definitely not as an important conceptual tool to understand problems and define useful strategies for the gaining of knowledge. RA Fisher's forward reads: *"The author was impressed with the practical importance of many recent mathematical advances, which to others seemed to be merely academic refinements. He felt sure, too, that workers with research experience would appreciate a book which, without entering into the mathematical theory of statistical methods, should embody the latest results of that theory, presenting them in the form of practical procedures appropriate to those types of data with which research workers are actually concerned. The practical application of general theorems is a different art from their establishment by mathematical proof. It requires fully as deep an understanding of their meaning, and is, moreover, useful to many to whom the other is unnecessary"*. In other words: the recent developments in mathematics, which are truly revolutionary as they allow experimental results to be looked at in a totally new way, are the theoretical results obtained by Fisher himself. The methods derived from them should be used by researchers without worrying too much as to their meaning. I do want to emphasize that I am fully convinced of RA Fisher's scientific greatness, but I do find it essential that the above mentioned "results" (which basically are the use of the sample distribution and the theory of pure significance) be accompanied by a crisp explanation of the general context, as the one presented in the following book "Statistical Methods and Scientific Inference" (1956) in which the meaning and the use of the likelihood function are masterfully explained and the limits of the theory of significance are at least partially described. A curious detail is that the second book is reasonably clear and does not hide anything relevant to the reader, whilst leaving several problems open, including some interpretative ones. However it is not meant for researchers…

The pedagogic idea underlying the book "Statistical Methods for Research Workers" is certainly extreme, whereas recent didactic literature usually seeks a compromise. It cannot be denied, however, that sometimes the suggestion to operate without wasting time to give thought to the useless theory does reappear, in the most diverse contexts. This theme could also be discussed with reference to the possible interpretations of recent reforms of the Italian university system, but then we would definitely wander from the subject.

I can now get to the point. The basic idea behind this book is happily at the opposite pole. The Authors, deliberately, intend to explain *everything*. In particular, they try to prevent bio-medical researchers from accepting and applying statistical procedures without understanding their meaning and therefore without applying a critical control, made possible by the subject matter knowledge which typically the statistician does not have. Obviously, the theoretical discussions have to be limited, but everything essential from a logical point of view can indeed be explained and, with some effort, understood, even using only high school level mathematics. In this respect, and also in that of trying to avoid any jargon of obscure logical roots, the book that I have the pleasure of presenting is a proposal of great interest and usefulness. Also, it must be stressed that this book goes well beyond the typical presentations of statistical methods (although this is the aspect on which I am more inclined to comment). The practice of applied research is analyzed and discussed in its complexity, including of course ethical aspects, as well as financial, organizational ones, and so on.

My involvement in clinical research is related to my interest in applications of statistical methods of so called "Bayesian" approach, which are still not fully accepted as standards. So, such methods pose a double challenge: for a comparison between methodologies to have a true meaning, the logic behind both must be clear to the reader, otherwise all one achieves is to propose to replace one blind obedience with another blind obedience. The careful reader of this book will not feel pushed toward the Bayesian approach. Instead, the reader is given the tools to reason and, after an appropriate comparative discussion, is in a position to give his/her "informed consent" to one or the other "school" (or to recognize the merits of both). In fact, the important thing is to understand the general sense of the issue, without giving the illusion (never favoured by the Authors) that statistical methodology is established once and for all. Only with such an open attitude, in my view, can statistical education play a constructive role and not become a boring ritual.

Therefore, I do hope that this book will have the fortune it deserves and that it will stimulate many bright minds to reflect further on important aspects of the methodology of research.

Ludovico Piccinato
La Sapienza University, Rome

Acknowledgements

Writing this book has taken us several years of early mornings (GDC), late nights (AB) and weekends (GDC and AB). We are indebted to all those to whom we denied our time.

A special thank you from both of us goes to:

- Alfredo Ardia for guiding us through the first steps in this profession, teaching us creativity in reasoning and staying our friend for all these years.
- Adelchi Azzalini, Paolo Bruzzi and Ludovico Piccinato for pushing us in the adventure of writing this book, supporting us, and finding the time and energy to comment our draft. Many of their suggestions set us on the right path. Some we ignored. The heavy responsibility of such choices we accept.
- Lidia Merli and Silva Tommasini, for their help with the graphs.
- Our friends, especially those of the "Associazione Laboratorio Nuovo Alfabeto" for supporting us in our effort at intellectual honesty, reminding us how important this is in every "public act", even the very small one of writing a book on the methodology of clinical research.

A special thank you from AB goes to:

Marco Corsi, who has always supported my academic activities and has taught me a great deal on how to build constructive peer-relationships between statisticians and physicians

Finally, a special thank you from GDC goes to:

- Stephen Senn, who has shown me that rigorous thinking and discipline can coexist with fun and a sense of humor.
- James Shannon, who, over the years, with little talk and much example, has taught me many things essential to the practice of clinical research: focus on the essential, calm under pressure, logical thinking and much more.

English is a language of multiple layers of complexity. The task of translating a book like this was daunting. We are deeply grateful to Elaine Hopper for giving us many hours of her time before and after work to review the translation. Any remaining errors are, of course, ours.

Septemper 2006
The authors

Contents

Introduction

In recent years many introductory textbooks on clinical trial methodology have been published, some of which are excellent, in addition to a very extensive specialist literature. Nevertheless, we decided to embark on the adventure of writing together a new book on methods and issues in clinical research. The objectives we set for ourselves, which we hope will justify our effort, can be summarized in three points.

1. Integrate medical and statistical components of clinical research. This is the primary objective of the book. The authors are a statistician (AB) and a physician (GDC) with years of experience in multidisciplinary project teams. In a clinical study (and any biomedical experiment) collaboration between representatives of the "biological" disciplines (physician, biologist, pharmacologist, etc.) and representatives of the "mathematical" disciplines (statistician, data management specialist, etc.) must be continuous and include absolutely all aspects of the planning and implementation of the study and of the analysis, interpretation and publication of results. The more troublesome this collaboration, the more at risk are the ultimate goals of our work as researchers, i.e. to ask relevant questions and provide scientifically sound answers. Unfortunately, however, there is often a complex communication problem between disciplines of biological and mathematical orientation, which can express itself at different levels.

A first, and in our opinion crucial, level of miscommunication is one of language. It is striking to note how frequently many of us make use of jargon, behind which we usually hide relatively simple and accessible concepts. This coded language is often an insurmountable wall for colleagues from different backgrounds. What depths of mathematical reasoning lie behind the term "statistical model"? In fact, the term is often generically used to mean "approach". What complex medical concept is hidden in the expression "differential hematological count"? It quite simply means type and number of cells in the blood.

A second level concerns the necessity to "divulge" (etymologically, to "make accessible to the people"). In order to communicate between different disciplines, it is necessary to simplify and, to some extent, trivialize concepts which are complex and rich with nuance (and fascinating to us for these very reasons). Specialists often have an inborn aversion toward divulging specialist knowledge. We subconsciously perceive it as a form of humiliation, as giving up the depth of knowledge and insight we acquired from years of study and experience. A genuine attitude toward disclosure and simplification is a welcome but rare quality, which requires profound knowledge combined with didactic intuition and empathy with the audience. We strongly believe that such an attitude is absolutely indispensable in order to accomplish interdisciplinary collaboration. We are convinced that the main reason for the limited success of some techniques and methods lie in the impossibility (rarely) or incapability (frequently) of making them accessible to a public of non-specialists. The Bayesian statistical methods are a case in point.

A third level that complicates communication between different disciplines is somewhat philosophical in nature and concerns the very way individuals from different backgrounds think. What is essential for one person may be trivial for another. The statistician often considers the "mechanistic obsession" of the biomedical researcher ridiculous: any result gets immediately fitted (or forced) into a plausible biological explanation, and so does any result reaching opposite conclusions. On the other hand, the statistician's attention to the assumptions behind a certain method is often considered pedantic by the physician/biologist. Understandably, but mistakenly, we tend to think that "our" discipline is slightly closer to the "truth" than any other.

We hope that, through this book, we have made a small step in the right direction. Each and every medical term and concept had to pass the test of a non-physician. Likewise, each formula, statistical term and argument had to be understood and accepted by a non-statistician with only basic mathematical knowledge. Most importantly, the logical flow of each chapter had to make sense to both authors. This was achieved through endless debates and multiple rewrites of almost all chapters (some of which have been completely undone and redone four or five times). The logic behind the methods used in clinical research is the center of this book, not computational procedures or mathematical demonstrations, nor specialist medical or biological issues. Such logic must be equally accessible, through a common language, to the physician/biologist and to the statistician/data manager.

2. Do justice to the operational and practical requirements of clinical research. The decisions on the sample size, the choice of the dose(s) to be used in large phase III studies, the type and number of outcome variables, the degree of blinding of treatments, are just a few examples where operational and practical requirements are of such importance as to prevail at times over the methodological ones.

How often do non-statistical considerations, such as the prevalence of the disease, the geographical distribution of researchers or financial constraints influence the sample size of a study? Isn't it true that in these situations we tend to give a "statistical" justification to a sample size selected on practical grounds? To this end, we initiate a sterile retrospective process and screen the literature for any paper which could help us to justify our magic number; we inflate or deflate the magnitude of the "clinically significant difference" with the same aim, etcetera. Wouldn't it be better to acknowledge the practical limitations and to estimate the power of the study for a range of differences, given the achievable number of patients?

The choice of the highest dose to be used in dose-response studies is frequently dictated not by pharmacological or toxicological considerations, but by limitations in pharmaceutical formulation technology or by the outcome of market research.

When choosing the number of measurements and end-points of a clinical study, a statistically pure, extremely restrictive approach to the problem of multiple comparisons fails to take into account the practical consideration that large clinical trials take years to complete, cost a fortune and very often represent unique opportunities to obtain essential information.

It is a common occurrence that scientifically impeccable protocols demand the impossible of patients and research staff: very frequent visit schedules, measurements taking many hours, repeated invasive procedures, "double-dummy" blinding solutions with dangerously complex dosing regimens. How many researchers seriously stop to consider whether all this truly contributes to improving the quality of data?

A competent researcher must not belittle "non-scientific" issues to the level of bothersome hurdles that get in the way of the perfect experiment, to be delegated to others (the "operational" staff). The real skill of a bio-medical researcher resides in designing a methodologically valid study that gives due consideration to real life and its many limitations. In this book we endeavored to elevate the operational aspects of clinical research to the level of importance they deserve.

3. Give space to the ethical implications of methodological issues in clinical research. Considerable progress has been made in the field of clinical research ethics in recent years. The dignity and rights of patients undergoing experimental procedures are sanctioned and regulated by international as well as national guidelines and regulations (e.g. the Declaration of Helsinki [106]). Ethics Committees (also known as Institutional Review Boards) are now operating almost everywhere. Fraud in research is a recognized problem that is policed both by the institutions where research is conducted (universities, hospitals, pharmaceutical industry) and by the institutions where research is evalu-

ated and regulated (FDA, other National Health Authorities, EMEA). However, a more insidious dimension of the ethical problem exists, which is very close to every researcher: the devious use of techniques and methods. Although this component of the ethical problem is well known to Health Authorities, researchers often ignore it. Whereas the fabrication of data is abhorred by the great majority of researchers, the fabrication of results from real data through incorrect use of methodological and statistical techniques is often considered no big deal and is unfortunately common practice. "After the fact" ("post hoc") selection of objectives based on results, poor use and interpretation of significance testing, subgroup analyses that prevail over the primary ones, statistical analyses that do not take into account the distribution of data nor attempt to verify the basic assumptions, preferential publication of "positive" data over "negative" ones. These are just some of the many ways in which results may be fabricated from real data. Is there such a big difference between fabrication of data and fabrication of results through incorrect methods? We are convinced that the answer is no. Inappropriate use of techniques and methods is immoral, as immoral as the fabrication of data and mistreatment of patients. The damage is just slower in manifesting itself, more difficult to identify and easier to justify with convoluted argumentation. Throughout this book we try to do justice to the ethical implications of poor research methodology. Clearly, the ethics of clinical research is a much larger subject, which goes far beyond the boundaries of our book.

On several occasions, we make reference to the thorny problem of conflicts of interest. Conflicts of interest are everywhere and we must acknowledge this fact. Researchers in academia must publish to obtain grants and to progress in their careers. Scientific journals benefit from new, surprising and unexpected results more than from results confirming previous research or "negative" results. The pharmaceutical industry is centered on financial profit and each company tries to "demonstrate" the advantages of its drugs and the disadvantages of the drugs of others. The large universities and teaching hospitals are most likely to support projects of great public awareness, not necessarily on scientific grounds (obviously to the disadvantage of other projects), in order to attract students and patients. How can research bear scientifically valid fruit in this jungle of conflicting interests? We believe there is no single answer or solution. A large component of the answer lies in the conscience and conscientiousness of researchers. However, much of the answer also lies in the mutual control, critical examination of publications, and repetition of experiments by different groups in diverse professional, cultural and social contexts, and in the use of methodologically correct techniques in the context of a truly interdisciplinary collaboration between researchers of different backgrounds and complementary skills.

At the end of this introduction, we wish to quote one of the reviewers of the English edition of our book, who, in our view, has captured very well its overall strengths and limits. "The authors have a great deal of practical experience and this experience gives the book an authority that is sadly lacking in some other texts. [...] However, a weakness is that, however much experience the authors may have in writing and publishing articles on the results of clinical research, they have not really contributed to the methodological literature themselves. [...] This means that what one has, in my opinion, is a series of well-meditated reflections grounded in experience on methodological arguments and positions that have been expounded or developed by others". The assessment is spot on and we gratefully accept it.

General Outline of the Book

The scope of clinical research is to evaluate the effect of a treatment on the evolution of a disease in the human species.

The treatment can be pharmacological, surgical, psychological/behavioral or organizational/logistic. The disease, intended as an impairment of a state of well-being or a condition capable of provoking such impairment over time, can be universally accepted as such (e.g. a cancer or a bone fracture) or perceived as such only by limited groups of individuals in a given cultural context (e.g. hair loss or weight gain). The course of the disease that one wishes to change can be the one with no intervention or, more frequently, the one observed with the available treatment.

The evaluation of the effect of a treatment on the course of a disease is a lengthy process, which progresses in increasingly complex stages.

As we will see in chapter 12, the clinical development of a pharmacological agent is conventionally broken down into four phases. Phase I (typically lasting six months to 1 year), generally carried out on healthy volunteers, has as its main goals the evaluation of the tolerability of increasing doses of the compound and the definition of its pharmacokinetic profile. The main goals of phase II (duration: ~1-2 years), carried out on selected groups of patients, are the proof of the pharmacodynamic activity and the selection of the dose(s) to test in the following phase. Phase III (duration: ~2-5 years), carried out on hundreds or even thousands of patients who (as a group) are to be as representative as possible of the general patient population, comprises the so-called pivotal studies, which are designed to demonstrate the therapeutic efficacy, tolerability, safety and at times also the socio-economic value of the compound. Finally, phase IV encompasses all the studies conducted after regulatory approval and marketing of the compound, within the approved indication(s). For non-pharmacological treatments the sequence of phases is generally less standardized.

The assessment of the effect of a treatment is a conceptually and methodologically complex process. It is useful to begin this book by asking ourselves why this may be the case. Why isn't it enough to administer the treatment to one subject and then document the outcome?

The basis of this complexity resides in the ever-present variability of all biological phenomena, at times partially predictable, but often totally unpredictable. It represents the "background noise" that must be overcome to recognize and measure the "signal" resulting from the treatment. In fact, clinical research can also be defined as a series of techniques and procedures aimed at separating the signal from the background noise, in order to decide if a change observed after a treatment belongs to the latter or to the former. The sources of biological and measurement-related variability are covered in chapter 1.

In order to separate the signal from the background noise, the clinical researcher can decide to conduct an experiment. What is an experiment? What are its characterizing elements that distinguish it from other forms of scientific investigation? Chapter 2 is dedicated to the characteristics that define a clinical experiment and to the fundamental distinction between observational and experimental studies (the latter typically referred to as clinical trials or clinical studies). Chapter 3 provides a brief introduction to observational studies. This chapter stands somewhat alone compared to the rest of the book. Nevertheless, we decided to include it for completeness and in order to better illustrate to the reader the differences between clinical and observational studies.

A key aspect of any experiment is that it must be carefully planned. The planning process must be complete before the experiment begins. Changes after the start of the experiment are indeed sometimes necessary, but must be the exception, not the rule, because they are complex to implement, have statistical consequences requiring careful consideration, and may have an impact on the credibility of results, as it is difficult to prove that a change has not been made to favor the results hoped for by researchers. The study plan must be documented in detail in the so-called study protocol, a document that requires many months to complete. First and foremost, a clear objective must be defined. Thereafter, a useful approach is to organize the planning of the experiment (and the writing of the study protocol) into six "blocks".

- Definition and quantification of the treatment effect(s): what measurements should be carried out and how many; how to summarize them within each study subject (end-point); how to summarize the end-point within each treatment group (group indicator); how to express the overall effect in comparative terms between groups (signal); what is the minimum magnitude of the signal that must be shown to declare success of one treatment over another.
- Definition of the group of subjects on which the experiment is to be conducted: what features should they have and how many should they be.
- Definition of the experimental and concomitant treatments.
- Definition of the experimental design.
- Definition of the procedures for assessing results (statistical analysis and decision-making rules).
- Definition of logistic, administrative and legal issues.

Chapters 4, 5, 6 and 7 are dedicated to the definition and quantification of the treatment effects being studied, to the logical foundations of the statistical analysis, to the study sample and to the study treatments, respectively. Chapters 8, 9, 10 and 11 give an overview of the most common experimental designs, with emphasis on common methodological errors.

A detailed coverage of the logistic, administrative and legal aspects of clinical research is outside the scope of this book. However, throughout the book we keep reminding the reader of these aspects because, as already mentioned, we firmly believe they have a crucial role in determining the success of a study. The history of clinical research is paved with relics of studies started with great pomp, riding great ideas and great hopes, which drowned miserably because of inadequate logistical preparation. In our experience, the excessive complexity of a clinical trial is the single most frequent cause of failure: the study is perfect on paper, but impossible to implement by patients and staff alike. The distance between the principal investigators and the reality of clinical research in its day-to-day practice is often the main cause of such disasters. We warmly encourage everyone involved in clinical research to get involved in the logistics of a study, learning from colleagues responsible for its practical conduct (clinical research associates, data managers, etc.) and to take part, in person, in the practical implementation of a trial before attempting to design a study protocol.

The book ends with chapter 12, devoted to a brief description of the drug development process and to the phases of clinical development.

The Authors' views expressed in this book do not necessarily reflect those of their employers.

Linguistic and Editorial Conventions

Each term included in the analytical index is highlighted in bold in the chapter where it is most extensively covered (in the index all terms appear as singular and, when necessary, have in parenthesis explanatory words which do not appear in the text). Sentences in bold and italics font are used to separate the longer sections into sub-sections. In formulae, the sign "x" is used to indicate multiplication, but omitted when it is obvious that a multiplication is being carried out.

1
Viability of Biological Phenomena and Measurement Errors

The variability of biological phenomena, as we perceive them, can be divided into three main components: phenotypic, temporal and measurement-related. Measurement-related variability includes every source of variation that occurs as a consequence of measurements and interpretation of results.

Phenotypic and temporal variability refer to true differences, whereas variability associated with measurements refers to errors. The term error in this context is not synonymous with "mistake", but has a technical meaning that we will explain in section 2.1. Measurement errors are an integral part of the variability of biological phenomena, as we perceive them.

1.1. Phenotypic Variability

If we select a group of individuals at random and evaluate a given characteristic (**phenotype**), almost inevitably we will observe heterogeneity for the characteristic examined. This is due partly to differences in the genetic profile (**genotype**) of the individuals and partly to the influence of environmental factors. Let us consider height as an example. It is a fact that some individuals are "tall" and others are "short" (relative to a hypothetical height considered "typical" by the observer, see below). The height of an individual depends on age, sex, race, height of parents and ancestors, nutritional state, medical history and so on. However, it is also influenced by other unknown factors. In fact, even if we were to select our group of individuals, not at random, but from a single family with parents and ancestors of the same race, and if we were to restrict further our choice within that family to the adult males with no relevant disease (current or past), still the individuals included in our sample would have different heights. It is likely that their heights would be more homogenous compared to those of a group selected at random, but differences would persist. Moreover, it would not be unusual for one individual to be phenotypically atypical, that is, much taller or much shorter than the rest of the group, for reasons completely unknown. The same phenotypic variability applies to diseases. As an example, let us consider Parkinson's disease, a neurological disorder characterized by difficulty of movements and tremor. First of all, in any group of individuals at a given moment, some will be affected by the disease and some will not. Furthermore, among those affected, we will find heterogeneity with regard to disease severity, age of onset, and the spectrum of symptoms displayed. Again, only part of the observed phenotypic variability is explainable based on our knowledge of the condition, while the remaining part, erratic and unpredictable, is of unknown origin.

1.2. Temporal Variability

In the previous section we considered biological variability at a given moment in time. In fact, biological phenomena have a temporal course: a beginning, a sequence of intermediate stages and an end. Sometimes the sequence is repetitive, i.e. cyclical. The variability of the temporal course, which we refer to as temporal variability, represents the second major component of biological variability. It can be further divided into two components: one linked to biological rhythms, the other unrelated to them.

Biological rhythms. Many biological phenomena follow an ordered temporal course, that is, change over time in steps that are always the same in their sequence and characteristics. For example, in the human species, height generally increases slowly in childhood, faster during puberty, stops increasing around 18-20 years of age and eventually decreases with advanced age. **Biological rhythms** are often cyclical, i.e. follow a repetitive sequence. The duration of a cycle can be of the order of seconds or fractions of a second (for example, the phases of the cardiac muscle's contraction as shown by the electrocardiogram, or the inspiration-expiration cycle), minutes/hours (e.g. the sleeping-waking cycle or the secretion of some hormones), weeks/months (e.g. the menstrual cycle), seasons (e.g. flares of allergic rhinitis during the pollen season). Biological rhythms are relatively constant, both qualitatively and quantitatively. Yet, superimposed on these patterns, a physiological variability, both qualitative and quantitative, always exists that is compatible with the normal functioning of a given organ or body system. Going back to the electrocardiogram, the QT interval, for example, is approximately 0.45 seconds, but values between 0.43 and 0.47 seconds are perfectly compatible with the normal functioning of the heart. Disease is associated with a departure of biological rhythms from the limits compatible with normal function, or with a disruption of physiological rhythms, replaced by rhythms characteristic of a diseased organ or system.

Temporal variability beyond biological rhythms. It is common knowledge that many phenomena are subject to temporal changes that are completely unpredictable. A sudden increase in emergency room admittance (perhaps related to road construction at a dangerous crossing), the abrupt appearance or worsening of depression in the absence of obvious triggers, the sudden improvement of advanced cancer are just a few examples.

1.3. Measurement-Related Variability

External phenomena exist for us only to the extent they are detected by our senses and understood by our intellect. To understand an external phenomenon we first need to recognize it, and then "measure" it.

1.3.1. The Measurement

The phenomenon or object to be measured, for example blood pressure, is called "variable". Actually, this is the terminology used by statisticians, whereas physicians, biologists and other life scientists are generally erroneously inclined to use the term "parameter" (see below).

A **variable** is any kind of observation that can assume different values for different subjects, times, places, etc. For example, height is a variable, as it can assume a different value for each individual observed. The opposite of the variable is the **mathematical constant**, a quantity that always assumes the same value. "Greek p" (π), which expresses the ratio between the circumference and the diameter of a circle, is an example of a constant, as it is always equal to 3.1415926. A **parameter** is a value that defines one mathematical curve within a specific family of curves. Usually, a change in the parameter determines changes in the shape, and/or width and/or position of a curve within a specific family of curves. For example (see Figure 1.1), if we consider the family of "normal" curves, the mean (μ) and the variance (σ^2) are its parameters, as their values fully determine a specific curve within the family: the mean determines its position, the variance its width. In practice, parameters are unknown quantities and the aim of the researcher is to estimate them. In this book we will use the terms parameter and variable according to the definitions given above.

A **measurement** can be defined as the assignment of numbers or symbols to the phenomenon or object being measured (the variable), according to a set of predefined rules. Each set of rules describes a **measurement scale** [30]. There are various types of measurement scales, as summarized in Table 1.1. These can be classified hierarchically based on the amount of information they convey. At the bottom of the hierarchy is the scale that coveys the least amount of information, the **nominal categorical scale**, generally referred to as the **nominal scale**. This scale classifies the observations in non-orderable categories which are mutually exclusive (that is, if an observation belongs to category A, it cannot also belong to category B) and exhaustive (that is, all observations must belong

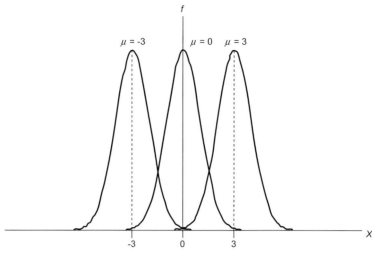

Normal curves with fixed σ and different μ values

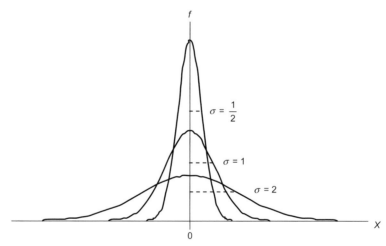

Normal curves with fixed μ and different σ values

Figure 1.1. Normal curves, defined by parameters μ (mean) and σ (standard deviation)

to one of the possible categories). A variable measured on this scale is called a **nominal variable** and is of the qualitative type. Examples of this kind of variable are race, marital status (married/not married/divorced), employment status (employed/unemployed/retired), and the codes derived from the coding dictionaries of medical terms, such as COSTART or MedDRA.

Table 1.1. Measurement scales

Scale	Type of variable	Definition	Example
Nominal	Nominal or qualitative	Nominal or qualitative.	Employed/ unemployed/retired
Ordinal	Ordinal or semi-quantitative (includes dichotomous variables)	Mutually exclusive and exhaustive categories for which it is possible to set an order, but it is not possible to determine the magnitude of differences among the categories.	Improved/stationary/worsened Dichotomous scale: positive/ negative
Interval	Quantitative	Characterized by the presence of a unit of measurement and the absence of a true zero point (defined as the absence of the quantity being measured). Because of the absence of a true zero point, the magnitude of differences between pairs of measurements does not change with the measurement scale, whereas the magnitude of ratios between pairs of measurements does change with the measurement scale.	Temperature in Celsius or Fahrenheit degrees
Ratio	Quantitative	Characterized by the presence of both a unit of measurement and a true zero point. Thus any value can be seen as a multiple of the unit of measurement (i.e. equal to x times the unit of measurement). Because of the presence of a true zero point, both the magnitude of differences and the magnitude of ratios between pairs of measurements do not change with the measurement scale.	Blood pressure in millimeters of mercury (mmHg), weight in kilograms or pounds

When the observations are classifiable in mutually exclusive and exhaustive categories, and the categories can be ordered using pre-defined criteria, it is said that the observations are measurable on an **ordinal categorical scale** or, simply, an **ordinal scale**. A variable that can be measured on this scale is called an **ordinal variable**. Examples are improved/stationary/worsened, below average/on average/above average, very negative/negative/normal/positive/very positive. In this kind of scale, all members of a given category are considered equal to one another, but different (better or worse) compared to members of other categories. However, it is not possible to quantify the magnitude of the difference between one category and another. For example, the difference between stationary and improved is probably not the same as that between worsened and stationary. Even though it is common to represent such ordinate categories with consecutive numbers, for example, worsened = -1, stationary = 0, improved = 1, these are not properly quantitative variables: in fact, because of the lack of a unit of measurement, the numbers assigned to each category do not represent quantities but only positions in a sequence. Since we cannot state that the distance between the categories 1 and 0 (which numerically is 1) is the same as the one between 0 and –1 (which numerically is also 1), indicators of central tendency such as the mean have no arithmetic meaning for these variables. Sometimes these variables are defined as semi-quantitative. Questionnaires, including those of quality of life, generally generate ordinal variables. A special case of ordinal variable is the **dichotomous** one, a variable that can only take one of two values, for example yes/no, successful/unsuccessful.

In the **interval scale**, it is not only possible to order the observations according to pre-defined criteria but also to establish the magnitude of the differences between any pair of measurements. The use of this scale implies the use of a unit distance, called **unit of measurement**, and of a zero point, both of which are arbitrary. The zero point is not a true zero, since it does not really indicate the absence of the measured quantity. Because of the lack of a true zero point, it is possible to quantify, independently of the measurement scale, the differences, but not the ratios between pairs of measurements (see example below). Typical examples of interval scales are the Celsius and Fahrenheit scales for measuring temperature. In these scales the unit of measurement is the Celsius or Fahrenheit degree and the zero point is arbitrary, since it does not indicate absence of heat.

Finally, at the top of the hierarchy is the **ratio scale**. In addition to the unit of measurement, the defining feature of this scale is the existence of a **true zero point**, which indicates the absence of the measured quantity. This scale is characterized by the fact that both differences and ratios between pairs of measurements are quantifiable independently of the measurement scale, i.e. it is possible to establish whether two differences or two ratios between pairs of measurements are different or not in a way which is independent of the scale of measurement. A typical ratio scale is the one for measuring weight. The statement that a person weighs 71 kg means that this person weighs 71 times the unit of measurement accepted by convention, in this case the kilogram. Furthermore a weight equal to zero means absence of weight.

To better understand the difference between an interval scale and a ratio scale, let us consider the Celsius (°C) and Fahrenheit (°F) scales for measuring temperature as examples of interval scales, and the scales for measuring weight in kilograms (kg) and pounds (lb) as examples of ratio scales. Equality of differences between pairs of values is independent of the measurement scale for both weight and temperature. For example, let us consider the statement "the difference between 30°C and 20°C is equal to the difference between 45°C and 35°C". This is still valid if the values are converted into °F: the first pair of values becomes 86°F-68°F and the second pair becomes 113°F-95°F and both differences equal 18°F. Conversely, whereas equality of ratios between pairs of values does not depend on the measurement scale for weight, it does for temperature.

For example, the equality between the ratios 40 kg/20 kg and 60 kg/30 kg is still true even after converting the weights into pounds: the first ratio becomes 88.18 lb/44.09 lb, the second becomes 132.27 lb/66.135 lb and they both still equal 2. On the contrary, whereas the ratio between 20°C and 10°C is the same as the ratio between 30°C and 15°C (ratio =2), the ratios between these pairs of temperatures expressed in °F are different: the first pair of values becomes 68°F and 50°F (ratio =1.36); the second pair becomes 86°F and 59°F (ratio =1.46). Therefore, while it is correct to state that a person of 80 kg weighs twice as much as a person of 40 kg, it is not correct to state that 20°C is twice as warm as 10°C. This is because there is a true zero point for weight but not for temperature.

Interval scales and ratio scales are **quantitative**: what makes a **scale** quantitative is the presence of a unit of measurement. Measurements made by instruments use interval scales or ratio scales and produce **quantitative variables**. A quantitative variable can be discrete or continuous. A **discrete variable** is characterized by interruptions in the values it can assume. Typical discrete variables result from counting and therefore assume values that are integer numbers. Examples of discrete variables are the number of heart beats in a given time interval, the number of cells in a given surface area and the number of events of a disease in a given population at a given time. A **variable** is **continuous** if its values are represented by a continuum limited only by the level of accuracy of the measuring instrument. Blood pressure, cholesterol level, weight are examples of continuous variables.

It should be noted that, strictly speaking, the variable age can be both continuous and discrete. The exact age at a precise moment is a continuous variable; for a given individual it could be 42 years, 137 days 7 hours 3 minutes 22 seconds. The age at the last birthday or the age rounded to the closest integer number are discrete variables. The same concept is valid for weight (exact weight vs. weight rounded to the nearest kg) and for all continuous variables.

The different types of scales generate different types of variables, which in turn require the use of different methods of statistical analysis. The methods used for the analysis of variables measured on interval scales or ratio scales are the same, but differ from those used for the other types of variables (nominal and ordinal). Furthermore, often the methods for the analysis of discrete variables differ from those for the analysis of continuous variables, mainly because their probability distributions have different shapes. An in-depth discussion of these topics is beyond the scope of this book.

1.3.2. Measurement Errors

Errors occurring in the process of measuring, though not part of the intrinsic variability of phenomena, contribute to the variability of phenomena as we know them.

First of all, it is crucial to understand the difference between random errors and systematic errors. These concepts will be useful throughout the book.

The **true** or **real value** of the phenomenon to be measured is the value we would obtain if the measuring instrument were perfect.

An error is defined as random if, in the course of repeated measurements, it produces departures from the true value that do not have a reproducible trend [27]. Rounding off decimals from two to one digit is a typical example of a **random error**: we underestimate the true value when the second decimal digit is a number between 0 and 4 and we leave the first digit unchanged; we overestimate it when the second decimal digit is a number between 5 and 9 and we increase the first digit by 1. It is impossible to predict which of the two options will apply to the next measurement.

An error is defined as systematic if, in the course of repeated measurements, it tends to produce results differing from the true value always in the same direction. The **systematic error** is also called **distortion** or **bias**. In this book we will generally adopt the term "bias" for systematic errors. If we measure weight with a scale that is not correctly calibrated, we make a typical systematic error because we always tend to underestimate or overestimate the true weight.

Both random and systematic errors have an impact on results; however, their effect is different. Increasing the number of measurements tends to decrease the impact of random errors on the indicators of central tendency, such as the mean or the median, because errors in opposite directions tend to compensate each other. Vice versa, systematic errors have the same direction on every measurement; thus, increasing the number of measurements does not attenuate their effect on the indicators of central tendency. This does not mean that random errors do not influence the result of measurements: they do increase the variability, i.e. the dispersion of the measurements around the true value. Random and systematic errors can have different importance, depending on the kind of measurement scale we use.

The smaller the measurement error, the greater the validity (i.e. the overall quality) of the measurement. The validity of a measurement can be described by two concepts: accuracy and precision. It is important to note that there is considerable confusion in terminology in the biomedical literature: the terms validity, precision, accuracy, reproducibility, etc. are frequently used with different meanings in different contexts. To add to the confusion, the same terms are also used with different meanings in the field of psychological and quality of life measurements. Here we offer two simple "technical" definitions, originally introduced by Cox [27] and Cochran and Cox [24], with no ambition of completeness or semantic correctness.

The **accuracy** of a measurement is the distance between the measured value and the true value (this implies knowledge of the true value or the assumption of such a value). The closer the measured value is to the true value, the more accurate the measurement is and vice versa. Let us assume we know that a given road section is 100 meters long (for example, on the basis of measurements conducted by a construction company working in the area) and that we accept this information as "true". Let us then imagine that we ask a student to measure that road section with two different measurement instruments, first with a stick, and then with a tape, both two meters long and both subdivided in centimeters. The student accepts our request and performs the two measurements, with the following results:

- stick   100.9 m;
- tape   102.8 m.

The measurement made with the stick turned out to be closer to the true value (100 meters) than the one made with the tape. Therefore, the first measurement was more accurate than the second one. Accuracy is a concept that can be applied to measurements performed with any kind of scale. With a quantitative scale, when numerous measurements are made under the same conditions, accuracy can be "estimated"(see chapter 5) by using an indicator of the central tendency of these measurements, such as the mean: accuracy is estimated by the difference between the value of this indicator and the true value.

Precision concerns the reproducibility of a measurement, i.e. the ability to obtain similar values when a measurement is repeated under the same conditions. Like accuracy, precision is a concept that applies to any kind of scale. With a quantitative scale, given a long series of measurements performed under the same conditions, precision indicates the dispersion of measurements around their mean. Variance and standard deviation around the mean (see section 5.4) are the measurements of dispersion most commonly used in the biomedical field. Precision is the opposite of dispersion. Let us imagine that we ask four students to measure the same road section with the stick and with the tape (four measurements do not really qualify as a long series, but keep the math simple, which helps in explaining concepts). The students accept and come back with the following results:

- stick   99.0 m, 99.5, 101.4 m, 100.5 m.
  mean: 100.1 m;
- tape   104.0 m, 102.5 m, 103.5 m, 100.0 m.
  mean: 102.5 m.

As stated above, the mean values can be used to estimate accuracy: they confirm that the stick is more accurate than the tape (100.1 m is closer to the true value than 102.5 m). Furthermore, the four values obtained with the stick are closer to each other compared to the four values obtained with the tape, i.e. the former have less variability around their mean than the latter. In other words, the stick achieved greater precision compared to the tape. In our case, the standard deviation of the measurements is 1.07 m with the stick, and 1.78 m with the tape. In conclusion, under the conditions of the test (that is, with those students, that environmental situation, those measurement instruments, etc.), the stick achieves measurements both more accurate and more precise (i.e. less variable, more reproducible) compared to the tape.

Accuracy and precision are not independent concepts. The relationship between these two concepts is complex. For example, if an instrument has poor accuracy, but good precision (that is, all measurements are systematically far from their true value, but with little dispersion), further increase in precision will not improve accuracy. On the contrary, if the instrument has good accuracy, increasing precision will result in increased accuracy under the same conditions. Finally, if there is no bias, i.e. accuracy is very high, precision and accuracy coincide. We will return to these concepts later, when we discuss strategies for increasing the accuracy and precision of an experiment (see chapters 8, 9 and 10).

A detailed discussion of the factors that influence precision and accuracy of a measurement is beyond the aim of this book. Briefly, they include the technical characteristics of the instrument, how well it works, the operator's ability to use it, the characteristics of the object (or subject) to be measured, and the environmental context (for example, wind, rain, light, etc.). Generally speaking, we can say that measurements on an ordinal or nominal scale are less accurate and less precise than measurements on a quantitative scale because they are influenced more by subjective factors.

1.4. Variability of Diagnostic Tests

The final step in "understanding" a phenomenon is generally that of evaluating, i.e. "judging" the measurement. In the medical field this often corresponds to making a diagnosis.

The evaluation of a measurement consists of comparing it to a reference entity, which is seen as "normal". When we state that our friend Barbara died young at the age of 40, we are evaluating Barbara's life span, measured in years, by comparing it to the life span that we consider normal and have chosen as the reference or term of comparison (say, 80 years). In this process the subjective factor can be very relevant. Often, the comparison with the reference occurs at a subconscious level and translates into a subjective evaluation. Subjectivity in the choice of the term of comparison is a huge source of variability. In the example above, if our social and cultural context were different and characterized by a shorter life expectancy (say, 35 years), our reference in the evaluation of Barbara's life span would also have been different and we would have concluded that Barbara died at an advanced age. The world of science is full of generic quantitative statements that refer to unspecified terms of comparison.

A procedure similar to the one described above, although somewhat less subjective, is used in the biomedical field when the quantitative result of a diagnostic test is transformed into a dichotomous result (for example, positive/negative, see above) for the purpose of making a diagnosis on a specific condition. This transformation occurs by means of a more or less arbitrary selection of a threshold value: if the measurement provides a result above the threshold value, the test is defined as positive, indicating the presence of the condition; if, instead, the result is below the threshold value, the test is defined as negative, indicating the absence of the condition. For example, if we choose a fasting blood glucose threshold value of 120 mg/ml for the diagnosis of hyperglycemia, a value of 119 mg/ml translates into a negative result, indicating absence of hyperglycemia, while a value of 121 mg/ml will translate into a positive result, indicating the presence of hyperglycemia. The transformation is typically carried out automatically by the measuring instrument itself.

A diagnostic test with a dichotomous result (positive/negative) can lead to two types of wrong conclusion:

- The result of the test is negative, but the subject actually does have the disease (**false-negative**).
- The outcome of the test is positive, but the subject actually does not have the disease (**false-positive**).

Table 1.2. Sensitivity and specificity of a diagnostic test in the population

Test	Disease	
	Yes	**No**
Positive	A (true-positive)	B (false-positive)
Negative	C (false-negative)	D (true-negative)
Total	A+C (subjects with the disease) (subjects without the disease)	B+D

Sensitivity, [A/(A+C)] x 100 = [true-positive subjects / all subjects with disease] x 100; Specificity, [D/(B+D)] x 100 = [true-negative subjects / all subjects without the disease] x 100

The probabilities of a test yielding false-negative and false-positive results are generally expressed in terms of sensitivity and specificity, respectively. Let us assume we perform the test of interest on all subjects of the population. We can summarize the results as in Table 1.2. The **sensitivity** of the test is the percentage of subjects with a positive test result among those affected by the disease, i.e. the probability of testing positive when suffering from the disease. The **specificity** of the test is the percentage of subjects with a negative test result among those not suffering from the disease, i.e. the probability of testing negative when not suffering from the disease. Taken together, sensitivity and specificity express the diagnostic accuracy of a test, that is, how closely the test predicts the actual frequency of the disease it is meant to diagnose.

Let us assume we use blood urea nitrogen (BUN) to make a diagnosis of renal failure and adopt the recommendation of a well known text of internal medicine, Harrison's Principles of Internal Medicine (Appendix: Laboratory Values of Clinical Importance), according to which the "normal" values of BUN are between 3.6 and 7.1 mmol/L. Let us also assume we adopt a threshold value of 8.5 mmol/L to make a diagnosis of renal failure. The diagnostic validity of the test with the above set threshold value can be "estimated" (see chapter 5) by measuring the BUN in two groups (samples) of subjects, one with and one without proven renal failure ("proof" based on a different diagnostic method). The outcome of the test is shown in Table 1.3 (fictitious data). The table shows few false-positives and therefore a high specificity, which means that the test is good at identifying the subjects without renal failure (more than 90% of the subjects not affected by renal failure are identified as such by the test). However, there are many false-negatives and therefore sensitivity is low, i.e. the test is poor at identifying subjects with the disease (in fact, only 70% of the subjects with renal failure are identified as such by the test).

Specificity and sensitivity (diagnostic validity) of a test depend on two orders of factors:
- The accuracy and precision of the measurement (see above);
- The chosen threshold value.

Table 1.3. Estimate of the sensitivity and specificity of BUN with a threshold value of 8.5 mmol/L as diagnostic test for renal failure using two samples (subjects with and without renal failure, respectively)

BUN	Renal failure	
	Yes	No
≥8.5 mmol/L (positive test)	A=35	B=4
<8.5 mmol/L (negative test)	C=15	D=46
Total	A+C=50	B+D=50

Sensitivity, [35/50] x 100 = 70%; Specificity, [46/50] x 100 = 92%

The role of the threshold value in determining the diagnostic accuracy of a test is often ignored. It plays the role of the reference mentioned in the beginning of this section. Let us apply a threshold value of 7.2 mmol/L to the same data used to generate Table 1.3. The situation changes dramatically, as shown in Table 1.4. Using a threshold value close to the normal range, the test has a very high sensitivity (almost 95% of the subjects with renal failure are identified by a positive test) but a very low specificity (only slightly more than half of the subjects without renal failure have a negative test).

Generalizing, the closer the threshold value is to the normal range, the higher the sensitivity and the lower the specificity, i.e. there will be few false-negatives and many false-positives. Conversely, the farther the threshold value is from the normal range, the higher the specificity and the lower the sensitivity, i.e. there will be few false-positives and many false-negatives. The choice of the threshold value for a given test depends on the disease under assessment.

It is important to make a final consideration before we move on. Even the most accurate of diagnostic tests will give a certain number of false-positives and false-negatives. Researchers and laboratory technicians are satisfied with a percentage of 1-2% for these kinds of error, but if the test is performed on a large population, this will result in a high number of incorrect diagnoses. For this reason, a single test is rarely sufficient for the conclusive diagnosis of a disease. This reasoning also applies to biomedical studies. If we select the subjects for a study on the basis of a single diagnostic test, an undefined (possibly high) percentage of enrolled subjects will not have the disease being studied. This will increase the variability of results. Thus, in biomedical studies, the diagnosis of the condition being studied should be very accurate. This is typically achieved by using more than one diagnostic criterion in a rigorous and standardized way.

Table 1.4. Evaluation of the sensitivity and specificity of BUN with a threshold value of 7.2 mmol/L as a diagnostic test for renal failure, using the same samples of Table 1.3

BUN	Renal failure	
	Yes	**No**
≥7.2 mmol/L (positive test)	A=47	B=20
<7.2 mmol/L (negative test)	C=3	D=30
Total	A+C=50	B+D=50

Sensitivity, [47/50] x 100 = 94%; Specificity, [30/50] x 100 = 60%

Summary

All biological phenomena, as we perceive them, are affected by variability. Variability can be divided into three main components: phenotypic (i.e. due to differences between individuals), temporal (i.e. due to changes over time, which can be cyclical – biological rhythms – or unpredictable) and measurement-related (i.e. due to the use of measurement instruments). Errors made in the process of measuring can be of two types: random errors, which generate measurements that oscillate unpredictably about the true value, and systematic errors (bias), which generate measurements that differ from the true value always in one direction. Two concepts, accuracy and precision, are useful for the evaluation of measurements. Accuracy refers to the distance of the measured value from the true value. Precision refers to the dispersion about the true value of measurements repeated under the same conditions.

A large part of the theory behind the planning of biomedical studies is devoted to optimizing the accuracy and precision of results.

2
Distinctive Aspects of a Biomedical Study
Observational and Experimental Studies

The aims of this chapter are, firstly, to introduce aspects which are common to all biomedical studies, and, secondly, to discuss the features that distinguish observational from experimental studies, the two fundamental categories of biomedical studies.

In this book, we use the expressions observational study and epidemiological study interchangeably; likewise, we use the expressions experimental study and clinical study interchangeably. We should stress, however, that the convention we have adopted, although useful for didactic purposes, is a simplification which is not always valid. Observational studies will be discussed in the next chapter.

2.1. Distinctive Features of Biomedical Studies

The aim of the researcher is to detect, against the background of biological variability, the effect of an attribute or behavior, which we refer to collectively as "characteristic" (e.g. age, smoking), or of a treatment (e.g. drug, surgical procedure), on a disease (e.g. myocardial infarction) or on a condition predisposing to a disease (e.g. high blood cholesterol). Researchers perform medical studies, i.e. studies on human subjects, to determine if and to what extent a cause-effect relationship exists between the characteristic or treatment and the disease or condition.

Medical studies are part of the broader field of biomedical research which, in addition to studies on human subjects, includes studies performed on animals and plants, as well as studies conducted on isolated organs and cell systems. All such studies are characterized by the presence of biological variability. We will focus our attention on medical studies. However, it is important to note that many considerations which apply to human studies can be extended to all biomedical studies. Biomedical studies as a whole are very different from deterministic studies, in which there is insignificant or no variability (studies in physics, engineering etc.).

All biomedical studies have (or should have) some common distinctive "methodological pillars". These features are discussed below.

The first fundamental feature is that *conclusions are extended from the sample to the population.* To simplify, for now, let us call "sample" the group of subjects under study (we will give a more technical definition in chapter 6). The set of procedures through which the conclusions drawn on the sample can be extended to the population from which it was taken is called **inference**. The branch of statistics concerned with the conditions under which such "passage" from sample to population is valid is known as inferential or inductive statistics, as opposed to descriptive or deductive statistics, which is concerned with describing a given sample without drawing conclusions about the population. The definition of inference will be discussed in detail in chapter 5.

The second fundamental feature is that *the data, i.e. the measurements performed on the subjects, are interpreted in the context of a statistical-probabilistic model.* The need to interpret data with a probabilistic key is the immediate consequence of what was discussed in the previous chapter. If there were no variability, we could determine the effect of a treatment (or of a characteristic, such as cigarette smoking) by simply observing and documenting the outcome on a single subject undergoing the treatment (or having the characteristic) of interest. The outcome would be of the deterministic type. Thus, repeating the study with the same treatment (or characteristic) under the same conditions, would always yield the same result, which could be immediately extended from that single subject to the entire population. Because variability exists, it is not possible to interpret biomedical data in a deterministic way: as soon as we add a second subject to the study, we will inevitably find that the result is different from the one given by the first subject; furthermore, the results observed on one group of subjects today will differ from those observed in the same group tomorrow. To be able to interpret data in a context affected by variability, we need a statistical model, and not just any model, but one "tailored" exactly to the problem, i.e. one that is adequate to represent reality. This model should allow the linkage between the phenomenon under study (the questions we want to answer) and the statistical-mathematical scheme that serves as the basis for the statistical analysis.

From this consideration derives the third common feature of biomedical studies. *Studies must undergo detailed and documented planning before starting and must then be performed with strict adherence to that plan.* Planning a study means building the link between the phenomenon under study and the results of the statistical analysis before the study is actually performed. This means defining the complex system of rules and assumptions that will form the frame of reference for performing the study, conducting the statistical analysis and interpreting the results. The document in which the planning of the study is described in detail and carefully justified is called the study protocol. The next section is dedicated to this topic. To better clarify what was stated above, let us consider the state lottery. This game is based on an underlying probabilistic model providing a series of rules which, *a priori* (before the game starts) link the stake to the possible outcomes of the game, and which *a posteriori* (after the game is over), when the winning numbers are revealed, determine the amount of the prize if the outcome is favorable. In the context of a biomedical study, this model can be translated as follows: the number chosen by the better is the hypothesis, which is formulated before the start of the study; the amount of the stake placed corresponds to the investment in the study in terms of sample size, precision and accuracy of the measurements, control of the sources of variability, etc.; the possible outcomes of the lottery are the possible outcomes of the study (possible *a priori*); at the end of the study the amount won (or lost) represents the degree of certainty with which we can accept (or reject) the hypothesis being studied. In both contexts, *a priori* the hypotheses are linked to the possible outcomes by means of probabilistic laws; a *posteriori,* the fairness of the relationship between payment and prize, or between investment into the study and strength of the data supporting the hypothesis, is ensured by applying the pre-defined probabilistic set of rules. In any betting game, if the rules are changed after the stakes have been laid, for example by adding new numbers, the fairness of the relationship between payment and prize is lost; likewise, when conducting a study, if this is not performed according to the pre-established plan, the underlying probabilistic model is altered; consequently, it is no longer possible to interpret the results because it is no longer possible to establish to what extent the results support the hypotheses. Thus, it is essential for the study to be performed according to the pre-established plan. Nevertheless, sometimes changes are unavoidable during the course of the study. When this happens, it is extremely important for the statistician to evaluate the impact of the changes on the probabilistic model used for the study. Study designs exist which allow changes based on the data collected during the study, but then the allowed changes are themselves part of the study plan. In other words, the rules governing the choice of one of several possible scenarios are pre-defined, as are the consequences in terms of analysis and interpretation of the data. Sequential and flexible plans belong to this category of study design (see chapter 11).

The fourth defining feature common to all biomedical studies is that ***reasoning, methods and conclusions are based on comparisons between groups.*** The comparison is made between one group of subjects receiving a given treatment or having a given characteristic, and another group of subjects not receiving that treatment or not having that characteristic. Depending on the type of study, the first group is defined as the **treatment group, active group, case group** or **exposed group**. The second is the **control group**. When the object of the study is a treatment, the control group may not receive any treatment, or may receive a placebo, i.e. a treatment which is missing the active substance, but is otherwise indistinguishable from the one under evaluation, or an active control, i.e. an alternative treatment, for which efficacy and safety are established. Within the same study there can be more than one treatment group (for example, more than one dose of the same drug) and more than one control group (for example, placebo and active control).

The fifth defining feature is that *the groups being compared should be as homogeneous as possible during the entire course of the study*, from the enrolment phase throughout all phases of evaluation. Ideally, the groups would only differ with regard to the treatment or characteristic under study, but otherwise be identical with regard to the distribution of all other characteristics that are not under study such as age, sex, race, area of birth, socio-economic status, concomitant treatments, etc. This ideal cannot be achieved. Indeed, one of the main objectives of biomedical research is to ensure that, through appropriate techniques, the groups being compared are as similar as possible and that any residual differences are random and not systematic. The reason is that a random error can be "eliminated" by taking an average of multiple measurements, while this is not possible for a systematic error, as discussed in the previous chapter. The expression normally used is that comparisons must be "**bias-free**" (i.e. free from distortion). This concept will be explained in detail in the following chapters; in particular, chapter 9 is dedicated to the major sources of bias.

The sixth and last defining feature is that *data from a biomedical study must be analyzed by appropriate statistical methods, defined in the planning stage.* The basic question is, "How likely is it that the difference observed between the groups under study occurred by chance?" As we will see in chapter 5, the answer to this question is not always straightforward. Generalizing, we can say that the role of the statistical analysis is to quantify the level of uncertainty of the conclusions made on a treatment or characteristic. The way in which the uncertainty (or the evidence) is measured depends on the statistical approach adopted. The frequentist approach is the most common one in the medical field and is based on the famous "p-value". With this approach, the answer to the basic question is indirect. The p-value represents the probability that differences between groups greater than or equal to the ones observed in the study could be produced by chance. The reasoning is as follows: if it is very unlikely that differences greater than or equal to the ones observed can happen by chance (i.e. if the p-value is smaller than a pre-set threshold) and there are no systematic differences between groups, then we accept that the observed difference is due to the treatment or the characteristic under investigation. This statistical approach is not the only one possible: for example, an alternative is the Bayesian approach. Chapter 5 is dedicated to these concepts.

If everything happens as described, it is possible to extend the results obtained from the sample to the entire population with characteristics similar to the sample examined. It is obvious that the validity of such conclusions is probabilistic in nature, i.e., it assumes the acceptance of a certain level of uncertainty.

As soon as the researcher has decided to conduct a study, he/she is immediately faced with a fundamental methodological choice. Two different approaches are possible, the observational one and the experimental one (see Figure 2.1).

These two types of study will be introduced in section 2.3 and 2.4 respectively.

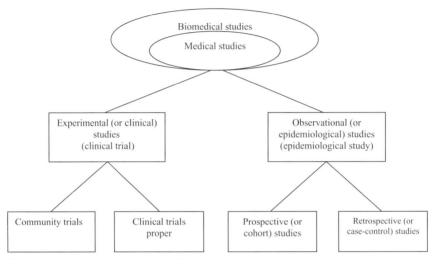

Figure 2.1. Classification of medical studies

2.2.   The Study Protocol

In the previous section we stressed the importance of planning biomedical studies and stated that all elements of the study plan are collected in a document known as the protocol. The **study protocol** has multiple functions. It is at the same time:

- A scientific document, because it describes all medical and statistical aspects of the study.
- An instruction manual, because it describes in detail how the study should be performed.
- A legal document, because it obliges the investigators to follow the procedures as described, which are to be officially approved by the authors (by signing the document) and by the competent independent authorities, i.e. the Ethics Committees, also known as Institutional Review Boards (IRB), and, at times, health authorities. In this sense, the protocol also serves the purpose

of protecting patients from procedures that are not properly evaluated and approved and therefore potentially dangerous.

Writing a protocol is a complex procedure that should not be underestimated. It is (or it should be) the result of long months of study and discussion among professionals with diverse expertise in the field of biomedical research, including the clinical personnel in direct contact with the study subjects, the pharmaceutical physician, the statistician, the data management expert, the drug supply manager, the operations personnel (responsible for selecting centers, controlling expenses, collecting data, and numerous other administrative and logistic functions), the legal and financial experts. Particularly important in building the protocol is the collaboration between the physician and the statistician. It would be diminishing and risky to assign the statistician to only the role of writing the section on statistical analysis because, as stated above, there is an unbreakable bond between objectives, design, end-points, probabilistic model, analysis and interpretation of results. Likewise, it would be diminishing and risky to preclude the physician from the possibility of commenting on the statistical analysis plan on the basis that he/she lacks the mathematical background: although this is generally true, there are many methodological aspects of the analysis plan that can benefit enormously from specialist medical knowledge.

Any study protocol must always cover the following fundamental areas:
- The rationale of the study.
- The objectives, i.e. the questions that it is expected to answer, asked in terms of medical-statistical hypothesis (chapters 4 and 5).
- The design, including the definition and justification of the sample size (chapter 6), the techniques to reduce systematic errors and to control variability (chapters 9, 10 and 11).
- The treatments under investigation and the concomitant treatments (chapter 7).
- The criteria for the selection (inclusion and exclusion) of subjects (chapter 6).
- The procedures for data management, quality control, and statistical analysis;
- Logistic, legal, and administrative aspects.

A good protocol is essential for the successful outcome of a study, be it clinical or epidemiological. Conceptually, the elements of a protocol can be classified into three groups:
- Medical and ethical aspects.
- Statistical aspects.
- Operational aspects.

With regard to the medical and ethical aspects, the fundamental task is to define the rationale and objectives, which must be relevant for advancing knowledge in the field, at the same time respecting every individual's right to receive the best possible therapy. Other key tasks include the definition of the target population (that is, the population to which we would like to extend the conclusions of the study) and the diagnostic tools for patient selection, the choice of the control treatment(s), the description of what constitutes a response to treatment, the context in which the study should take place. In clinical research, as in clinical practice, protecting the patient (or healthy volunteer) is of the utmost importance. And, just as occurs in clinical practice, there are many circumstances in which the ethical acceptability of a procedure is not universally acknowledged or a conflict exists between ethical and methodological needs. As an example, let us consider the chance assignment of patients to study treatments through randomization or the use of a placebo (see chapters 7 and 9). The ethics of clinical research, as well as the ethics of experiments performed on animals, is a complex matter that goes beyond the limits of this book, though some ethical issues will be discussed briefly. It is always appropriate for the researcher to read the protocol, putting him/herself in the patient's shoes (or in those of a parent or a son). Would the researcher hesitate to enter the study? Would he/she enroll a daughter or mother? If there is any hesitation or reluctance, it is necessary to dig deeper. Sometimes one can convince oneself (or be convinced by others) of the ethical acceptability of the procedures adopted in the study (the debate on the use of placebo is an interesting case in point). But other times it will be necessary to change them.

When looking at the statistical aspects, the fundamental task is to define the probabilistic model mentioned in the previous section. More specifically, this implies: translating the medical objectives into statistical hypotheses; adopting a set of probabilistic laws (each with an inevitable set of assumptions) based on the number and type of hypotheses and end-points; choosing a sample that is both qualitatively representative of the target population and quantitatively large enough to give the conclusions a sufficient degree of certainty; contributing to defining the design of the study so that it is appropriate to control bias and variability; defining the statistical analysis plan, such that it is pertinent both to the hypotheses and the design of the study.

The medical and statistical aspects of protocol development are closely interrelated. For example, consider how the "translation" of the medical objectives into statistical hypotheses requires very close interaction between these two areas of expertise.

Finally, the operational aspects of a study protocol should not be overlooked. These include the logistical aspects (procedures, drug supply management, case report forms collection, data management, etc.), the administrative aspects and legal ones. Close attention should always be given to the feasibility of the protocol. A balance between practical feasibility and methodological rigour is not easy to achieve and requires a great deal of experience. On the one hand, oversimplification of a study can make it difficult to answer the questions being posed. On the other hand, an excessively complex study is in our view the single most frequent cause of failure: the study looks perfect on paper, but is impossible for the patients and the staff to execute. If the study is too complex, sooner or later it will metaphorically implode. A growing number of things start going wrong at the same time. The study personnel experience an increasing amount of stress and frustration. The enrolled subjects do not receive the attention they deserve. The researchers start losing interest. At this point, keeping the study running requires a titanic effort and at times the only solution is to step back and decide to end the study prematurely. The discontinuation of a study before its completion for logistical reasons is probably the most frustrating experience in the career of a researcher, much more so than obtaining negative results. In fact, in the context of a well performed study, negative results are almost always of great scientific and practical relevance. A good researcher, no matter how enthusiastic he/she is about the hypothesis behind a study, should always be ready to accept negative results, or results that differ from those expected. It is in these circumstances that experience, scientific and moral rigour, and the ability to think laterally can yield an unexpected harvest: new research pathways and new hypotheses. On the contrary, prematurely ending an unfeasible study represents a total failure that has no value from any point of view, except perhaps that of teaching one not to make the same mistake again.

Once the protocol is written, it must be approved by an Ethics Committee which evaluates its ethical acceptability and scientific relevance. Changes to the protocol while a study is ongoing, formally known as protocol **amendments**, are necessary at times, but should be rare, motivated by strong reasons, and documented in detail. It is very important to evaluate the impact of such changes on the statistical model underlying the study. In fact, as we mentioned in the previous section, altering the probabilistic setting can threaten the possibility of reaching solid conclusions and, sometimes, may jeopardize the credibility of the results.

Many of the aspects described in this section may seem simple and obvious, but, in reality, are complex obstacles. We will return to each of these aspects later in the book, though not necessarily in the order defined above.

2.3. Observational Studies

In an **observational study**, also referred to as **epidemiological study**, the aim of the researcher is to study the relationship between a characteristic and an event without manipulating in any way the conditions under which the study is performed. The role of the researcher is limited to selecting the sample and thereafter "observing". The purpose of the observation is to determine the strength of the association between the characteristic and the event, and the circumstances under which the association is observed. In the presence of a strong association and plausible circumstances, a cause-effect relationship will be suspected. The stronger the association, the stronger the suspicion.

The **characteristic** under investigation can be a treatment (pharmacological or of a different nature), a demographic factor (e.g. age, sex, race), a behavioral characteristic (e.g. the number of cigarettes smoked per day or the number of calories taken daily in the diet), an environmental factor (e.g. exposure to pollen or to a specific industrial pollutant), a laboratory measurement (e.g. cholesterol levels in the blood), a genetic marker, and so on. The **event** can be the onset (or the diagnosis) of the disease under study, its recurrence or recrudesce, or death.

A characteristic capable of influencing the onset or progression of a disease in a predictable and reproducible way is called a **prognostic factor**. Strictly speaking, prognosis refers to disease progression and not to disease onset, but the term "prognostic" is often used in a more general sense embracing both onset and progression. Here we adopt the wider meaning. A prognostic factor can have either a negative or a positive influence on the disease. In the former case it is called **risk factor**. Cigarette smoking, for example, is a risk factor for lung cancer, because it is predictably and reproducibly associated with lung cancer. In fact, both the incidence and the prevalence (see section 3.1.1.) of lung cancer are always higher in smokers than in non-smokers and the probability of developing such a disease increases with increasing number of cigarettes smoked per day, as well as with the length of the smoking history of the subject. This has been repeatedly verified in many different populations. A prognostic factor capable of modifying favorably the onset or the progression of a disease in a predictable and reproducible way is called a **protective factor.** Examples of protective factors are the blood level of very low density lipoproteins (VLDL) and the level of physical activity in the natural history of hypertension.

Once again, what defines a prognostic factor (whether it is a risk or protective factor) is its ability to influence a disease in a predictable and reproducible way within a population. There are many other factors associated with the outcome of a disease but in a manner that is not predictable and reproducible. These are not prognostic factors. An example of such a factor is the study center in a multi-center observational study. Similar concepts also apply to experimental studies, even though the terminology is somewhat different (see section 2.4).

Generally, the level of certainty of the cause-effect link between the characteristic and the event is lower in an observational study compared to an experimental study with the same objectives (see chapter 9). As we will see, however, it is not always possible to use the experimental approach.

In summary, an observational study is characterized by the fact that the researcher does not intervene to influence or control the conditions of the study. Research of the factors that can modify the onset or progression of diseases by means of observational methods is at the heart of the discipline called **epidemiology**. Here we report the definition by Lilienfeld and Lilienfeld [67]: "Epidemiology is concerned with the patterns of disease occurrence in human populations and of the factors that influence these patterns. The epidemiologist is primarily interested in the occurrence of diseases by time, place, and persons. He tries to determine whether there has been an increase or decrease of the disease over the years; whether one geographical area has a higher frequency of the disease than another; and whether the characteristics of persons with a particular disease or condition distinguish them from those without it."

Pharmaco-epidemiology is the branch of epidemiology that studies the association between drugs (or other prophylactic or therapeutic procedures) and events (positive or negative) in the population by means of the observational methodology. Whereas in an experimental study the clinical researcher controls the administration of the treatment to the subject (deciding how, how much and when, see below), in an observational study the pharmaco-epidemiologist identifies and observes the subjects who are undergoing the treatment in question without exerting any such control.

Observational methods are only marginally discussed in this book. In chapter 3 we will discuss the classification of observational studies into prospective and retrospective studies, and look at the main characteristics of each.

2.4. Experimental Studies

The main feature of an **experimental study** is that the researcher controls the conditions under which the study is performed. Compared to the observational approach, the experimental approach generally allows a higher level of certainty in the evaluation of the cause-effect relationship between a characteristic and an event.

The characteristic under study, which in the context of an experimental study is often referred to as the **experimental factor**, is not simply "observed" in the population, as in the case of an observational study, but it is actually "assigned" by the researcher to the subjects. The range of interventions will obviously be restricted to those that are thought to influence favorably the course of the condition under study, generically referred to as "treatments" in the context of experimental studies (corresponding to the "protective factors" of observational studies). Going back to the example of cigarette smoking, it would not be acceptable if the researcher were to intentionally force some subjects to smoke and others not to. Therefore, the range of possible objectives of experimental studies in humans is more restricted than that of observational studies.

The assignment of treatments can be done by groups of study subjects or individually, subject by subject. An experimental study in which the treatments are assigned to groups of subjects is called a community study, while a study in which the treatments are assigned on a subject by subject basis is called a clinical study. In the language of experimental clinical studies, the term **trial** is often used interchangeably with the term study.

One of the first examples of a **community study** or **community trial,** reported in Lilienfeld and Lilienfeld's textbook [67], concerned the addition of fluorine to drinking water with the aim of reducing the onset of dental cavities [5]. Two cities of the state of New York, Newburgh and Kingston, were used as samples. Sodium fluorine was added to the drinking water of Newburgh starting May 1945, while the drinking water of Kingston was not treated. For 10 years (up to 1955) data were collected on the onset of dental cavities in a sample of children. Analysis of the results demonstrated a dramatic reduction in the incidence of dental cavities in Newburgh (exposed to fluorine in drinking water) compared to Kingston (not exposed), with a difference oscillating between 48% and 58%, depending on the age of the children. Children belonging to the first

age range, who were between 6 and 9 years old at the last follow-up visit, were
not born when the study began in 1945 and therefore were exposed to fluorine
from birth. Results demonstrated that this was the age range that showed the
most dramatic difference between the two cities, with approximately 60% less
dental cavities in Newburgh than in Kingston. This "internal consistency" gave
more strength to the conclusions of the study.

The second kind of experimental study, the **clinical study** or **clinical trial**,
is the main topic of this book. This type of study is also referred to as **clinical
experiment**.

In a clinical study the researcher achieves the maximum degree of control
over the experimental conditions.

The most rigorous control is exercised on the experimental factor, which, in
this context, corresponds to the treatments being compared in the study [80].
Typically, one clinical trial has one experimental factor, with the treatments
under comparison being the so-called "levels" of this experimental factor. There
are, however, study designs in which there is more than one experimental factor, each with its own set of levels, represented by treatments under comparison. In such study designs, the experimental factors are studied both individually and in combination (see chapter 10). A short diversion on terminology is
needed at this point. Strictly speaking, all of the treatments being compared in
a study, that is both the treatment(s) we are truly interested in and the control
treatment(s), active or inactive, should be defined experimental because they
are the levels of the experimental factor(s). This "purist" definition is very useful to distinguish between experimental and sub-experimental factors (see below). In practice, however, the term "experimental" is commonly used in referring to the novel treatment under study (rarely more than one in the same
study), for which efficacy and safety are still to be demonstrated, and which is
the reason for conducting the trial. Control treatments have already been "experimented" on (which is why they are chosen as controls) and we include
them in the study only in order to "experiment" on the new treatment(s). In the
rest of the book, we will use the expression experimental treatment(s) to indicate the new treatment(s), not yet tested or partially tested, while we will use
the expression study treatments to indicate all treatments being compared,
both the new treatment(s) and the control(s).

In a clinical trial, study treatments are controlled at two levels, the first being
the most important.

• First, subjects are assigned individually to the study treatments, with each
  subject receiving a single treatment or a single sequence of treatments (it
  should be kept in mind that a single treatment may be a combination of drugs
  and/or other therapeutic interventions). In the terminology of experimental
  studies, the expression **experimental unit** is used to indicate each subject
  undergoing a given study treatment (or sequence of treatments) [24, 27]. The
  entire set of experimental units represents the sample of the clinical study.
  Generally, the researcher assigns subjects to study treatments by means of a
  method of chance assignment called randomization. The methodological rea-

sons justifying this approach will be clarified in chapter 9. Randomization is often associated with "blinding" (also referred to as "masking"), which consists of making the study treatments indistinguishable from one another to both researchers and patients ("double-blind" study) or to patients only ("single-blind" study). Randomization and blinding, to which most of chapter 9 is devoted, have crucial importance in the methodology of clinical research.

- The second level of control consists of the set of rules, to be described in detail in the protocol, that defines how the study treatments are to be administered. At a minimum, the protocol must describe precisely the route of administration, the schedule including the days of the week (or month) and the time of the day at which the treatments should be given (and the degree of flexibility allowed), the relationship to meals and to liquid intake, the order in which the different components of the study treatment are to be taken (for example, different colored pills for different medications), and, finally, the duration of the treatment. In the case of more complex treatments, the protocol should give more details on the mode of administration.

In addition to the study treatments (the experimental factor), there are many other factors that are not directly under study, but that can influence the results (i.e. influence the effects of the experimental factor on the subjects). We will call such factors **sub-experimental factors,** following the terminology introduced by Pompilj [80]. We should warn the reader that this definition is not universally accepted. We do believe, however, that it is useful to understand some key methodological concepts. Examples of sub-experimental factors are:

- Demographic and anamnestic characteristics of the subjects included in the sample (age, sex, race, socio-economical status, clinical history, etc.).
- Previous and concomitant treatments, the latter being therapeutic interventions allowed by the study protocol, but not in themselves objects of the experiment.
- The institution (center) where visits and measurements take place (in a multi-center study).
- The type and stage of the disease under study (for example the stage of a cancer).

Sub-experimental factors that can influence the course of a disease in a predictable and reproducible way are defined **prognostic factors**, as already mentioned when discussing epidemiological studies. For example, age is a prognostic factor for many diseases, both acute and chronic, because it can influence the course of the disease in a predictable and reproducible way (in many diseases, the prognosis is worse with increasing age; for some cancers the opposite may be true). Vice versa, the center is definitely a sub-experimental factor as it may influence, at times heavily, the outcome of the treatment, but it cannot be defined a prognostic factor because its influence is neither predictable nor reproducible, either qualitatively (sometimes it is there, some time it is not), or quantitatively (a given center may sometimes favor and other times hinder the effect of the treatment).

The control that the researcher has on the sub-experimental factors is only indirect because study subjects are not directly assigned to these factors by the researcher. However, an indirect control on sub-experimental factors can be exercised in three ways.

- Through the set of rules and procedures predefined in the protocol. For example, the inclusion and exclusion criteria used to select the subjects for the study will determine the presence or absence in all subjects of a certain sub-experimental factor, considered very important for the study. Other sections of the protocol also regulate, often very precisely, the acceptability of some sub-experimental factors.
- Through randomization, which, as we will see in chapter 9, has the effect of balancing the groups under comparison with respect to both known and unknown sub-experimental and prognostic factors.
- Through a series of techniques, defined as "grouping" of the experimental units. Among these techniques are stratification, assignment in blocks, and pairing. We will come back to these concepts in chapters 9 and 10, dedicated to randomization and to experimental designs, respectively.

As Pompilj and Dall'Aglio remind us [80], "once we have identified the experimental factors and some of the most important sub-experimental ones, including some prognostic factors, we cannot conclude that we know all of the factors that can influence our experiment, because we should not forget that in the universe where the experiment takes place (where every phenomenon influences and is influenced by every other phenomenon), all other phenomena also influence the results of the experiment". Very often, these phenomena "totally escape our control; for this reason we tend to combine them into a single factor (assumed not interacting with others) to which we give the comfortable name of 'chance'." The effect of chance is called random error (see section 1.3.2), which is an error that does not systematically favor any of the treatments under comparison, because it is indeed the outcome of a combination of unknown factors (or factors which are known but not explicitly controlled). However, to be entitled to refer legitimately to chance and random error, the researcher must assign experimental units to treatments in a truly random fashion through the randomization process. In fact, as already discussed briefly, randomization not only allows a balanced distribution of patients among study treatments, but also ensures that any sub-experimental factor not explicitly controlled by the protocol, or even totally unknown, be distributed homogeneously among the groups under comparison.

There are two main advantages to controlling the experimental conditions:

- Reduction of bias, i.e. systematic distortion, which, as we said, is an error that systematically favors or hinders only one or some of the treatments being compared.
- Reduction of the "background noise", i.e. of the overall variability (real and measurement-related) and consequent increase of the probability of detecting a true signal (see chapter 4) when it exists, and of excluding it, when it does not exist.

These advantages render experimental studies generally more suitable than observational ones for establishing a causal link between a factor (characteristic or treatment) and an event.

Summary

Medical studies are part of the broader category of biomedical studies, characterized by the presence of biological and accidental variability. Medical studies can be grouped into two types: observational and experimental. In the former, the researcher simply observes the phenomenon under study; in the latter, the researcher directly controls the factor under study (the treatments).

These two types of study have, or should have, some common elements that are distinctive characteristics of all biomedical studies:

- Conclusions are extended from the sample to the population.
- Data are interpreted in the frame of a statistical-probabilistic model.
- The study is planned in advance and all the procedures are documented and justified in writing in the protocol before the start of the study; the protocol is to be followed rigorously throughout the course of the study and analysis of the results.
- The reasoning, the methods and the conclusions are based on comparisons between groups.
- The groups being compared are formed in a manner that prevents interference by systematic errors (i.e. are bias-free).
- The statistical analyses, decided upon during the planning stage, serve the purpose of measuring the degree of uncertainty of the conclusions.

Observational and experimental studies differ in many ways, due to the different degree of control that the researcher has over the conditions under which the study is performed. The consequences of such differences will be clarified later in the book.

3

Observational Studies

In this chapter we give a brief overview of observational studies, also referred to as epidemiological studies (as mentioned above, we use these terms interchangeably). The rest of the book is dedicated to clinical trials, which belong to the category of experimental studies (see chapter 2). We decided to devote some space to observational studies for three reasons: first, data from epidemiological studies are often required to plan and interpret clinical trials; second, to better understand the basic principles of experimental studies it is useful to understand those of observational studies; third, some of the methods of data analysis are common to both types of study. We will present a comparison between observational and experimental studies later in the book, once we have discussed experimental studies in detail (chapter 9). The reader who has a specific interest in epidemiology will find only general concepts in this chapter. For more on this topic we recommend the textbooks by Hennekens and Buring [57], Lilienfeld and Lilienfeld [67] and Miettinen [71] among many others.

In writing this chapter, we have two debts to acknowledge: one to Hennekens and Buring [57] from whose textbook we took numerous ideas and examples, and the other to Dr. Paolo Bruzzi, of the National Institute of Cancer Research, Genoa, Italy, who compensated for our lack of competence in the field by patiently reviewing our drafts and giving us valuable suggestions.

3.1. Basic Designs of Observational Studies

Based on the sampling method employed, observational studies can be of two types: prospective and retrospective. In **prospective studies** subjects are selected based on the presence or absence of a characteristic, whereas in **retrospective studies** subjects are selected based on the presence or absence of an event. Each type of study can be divided into different sub-types on the basis of the temporal relationship between the characteristic and the event: prospective studies can be classified into concurrent, non-concurrent and cross-sectional; retrospective studies into true retrospective, i.e. retrospective in the strict sense, and cross-sectional. This classification is presented in Figure 3.1.

The definitions "prospective cross-sectional" and "retrospective cross-sectional" may seem a contradiction in terms. In fact, considering the chronology of the studies, these can be prospective (the researcher observes the characteristic at the present time and waits for the event to occur later in time), retrospective (the researcher observes the event at the present time and goes back in time to look for the characteristic), or cross-sectional (the researcher observes both the characteristic and the event at the present time). Therefore, according to this classification, it would be correct to define the two types of cross-sectional studies as "cross-sectional with sampling based on exposure (exposed and non-exposed)" and "cross-sectional with sampling based on event (subjects with and without the event, called cases and non-cases)". However, the terms prospective and retrospective are commonly used not only with a chronological meaning but also with a logical one, i.e. the selection criterion of the subjects (selection of exposed/non-exposed in the former case, of cases/non-cases in the latter). The definitions in Figure 3.1 allow for this dual meaning and are used for the sake of brevity and also to stress that the prospective or retrospective logic applies also to cross-sectional designs.

Allowing for two types of cross-sectional studies is somewhat controversial: for example, in Lilienfeld and Lilienfeld's book [67] cross-sectional studies are described as a special category of retrospective studies, while in Miettinen's book [71] they are associated with prospective studies. Here we classify them in one category or the other depending on whether the starting point is the characteristic (risk or protective factor) or the event/disease. For example, let us suppose that we are interested in studying the relationship between obesity (potential risk factor) and depression (disease), and that we select the sample among patients who are being discharged from a given hospital. If we select patients based on the presence/absence of obesity (e.g. the exposed subjects come from the metabolic disease department, the non-exposed ones come from another department) and thereafter we evaluate the presence of depression, the study will be prospective cross-sectional. Vice versa, if we select patients on the basis of the presence or absence of depression (e.g. the cases come from the psychiatric department, the non-cases come from another department) and we then weigh each patient to determine the presence of obesity, the study is retrospective cross-sectional.

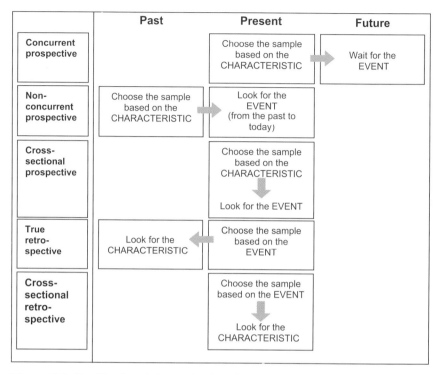

Figure 3.1. Classification of observational studies

In some cases it is difficult or irrelevant to classify a cross-sectional study as prospective or retrospective. For example, if we extract the whole sample from one population at exactly the same time and evaluate each individual for the presence of both the characteristic and the event at that point in time, it is both difficult and useless to classify the study in one or the other category.

3.1.1. Prospective or Cohort Studies

Concurrent prospective study. In a **concurrent prospective study,** the researcher first selects two groups of subjects, one with and one without the characteristic under study (for example cigarette smoking), but otherwise as homogenous as possible in every other respect, then observes them for a given period of time and documents if, when and how the event (for example lung cancer) develops. The aim is to determine whether the characteristic under study is a risk or protective factor for the event. Subjects who have the characteristic are often referred to as **exposed,** while those who do not have it are referred to as **non-exposed**.

Concurrent prospective studies are also referred to by many other names, for example, **cohort studies, incidence studies, longitudinal studies, follow-**

up studies, of which cohort study is the most commonly used. The word "cohort" was used in the ancient Roman army to indicate a subdivision of the legion. Just as the soldiers of the military cohort marched together, the members of a study cohort (the exposed and the non-exposed) live and age "together" (from a chronological point of view) and are therefore exposed to the same environmental factors, which are capable of influencing the onset and/or the progression of the disease under study. Some of these factors are known or at least suspected (pollution, working environment, etc.), but most are unknown.

A typical concurrent prospective, or cohort, study is shown in Figure 3.2. To conduct a concurrent prospective study the researcher proceeds as follows.

Ideally, two populations are identified, one comprising subjects exposed to a certain characteristic, the other, similar to the first, but comprising subjects not exposed to the characteristic. Both these populations may be obtained from the same database, for example the demographic registry of the Canadian state of Saskatchewan, which includes demographic and health data of most of the residents, or can come from different databases.

One cohort of exposed subjects and one of non-exposed subjects are selected at random from these populations, ensuring that each sample is representative of the underlying population. If the two populations belong to the same database, subjects to be included in the sample are extracted first, and later it is verified whether they belong to the exposed or non-exposed group. If each population has its own database, the extraction of exposed and non-exposed is direct.

In practice, it is not always possible to extract samples in a truly random fashion (e.g. it is rare to have a complete list of subjects exposed and non-exposed to the characteristic of interest); thus, the selection of cohorts of exposed and non-exposed subjects is often based on subject availability. For example, it is common for an epidemiological study to be performed within a certain hospital or in a restricted geographical area. In this case, the issue of the representa-

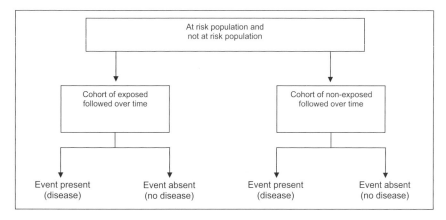

Figure 3.2. Concurrent prospective study

tiveness of the sample becomes problematic: what population should the sample represent? When representativeness of the underlying populations is in doubt, the risk of biased comparison is increased. In such cases, the emphasis is shifted from the principle of random sampling to the principle of comparability between groups, the aim being to make the cohorts under comparison as similar as possible to one another, by selecting them through procedures that do not introduce bias to the comparison (see below). In any case, it should be clear that by forgoing a truly random selection of subjects, the risk of bias is not trivial and there are problems in generalizing the results (see sections 3.2, 3.2.1 and 9.5).

Once the cohorts have been selected, they are followed for a sufficiently long period of time, during which all events of interest are recorded.

Finally, the incidences of the events of interest in the two cohorts are compared (see below).

Table 3.1. Data collected in a prospective study with characteristic and event of a binary nature and the same duration of follow-up for all subjects

		Subjects selected based on exposure		
		Exposure present (exposed)	Exposure absent (non-exposed)	Total
Subjects followed	**Event present**	a	b	(a+b)
to detect	**Event absent**	c	d	(c+d)
the event	**Total**	(a+c)	(b+d)	(a+b+c+d)

Let us give an example. We are interested in determining the link between cigarette smoking and lung cancer. The samples are selected on the basis of the characteristic under study, cigarette smoking: one cohort of smokers (exposed) and one of non-smokers (non-exposed). The two groups could be obtained by randomly sampling (if possible) the residents of a given town and recording, at the time of enrolment, whether each subject is a smoker or a non-smoker (see section 3.2.1). The researcher then follows the two groups for a period of time that is long enough for the event, the diagnosis of lung cancer, to occur (an appropriate time in this case could be ten years).

The concurrent prospective study is similar to the experimental clinical trial, the main difference between the two studies being that in the former the exposure to the characteristic is not assigned by randomization. This is a disadvantage from a methodological point of view, but it is an advantage from the practical one because it allows the effects of potentially damaging agents (the risk factors), to which subjects cannot be 'assigned', to be studied (this issue will be more extensively discussed later).

Let us start from the simplest situation, the one in which both exposure and event can be evaluated in terms of presence/absence, the duration of the follow-up is similar (theoretically identical) for all subjects and the risk of the event occurring is constant over the entire observation time. When the event of interest can occur multiple times in the same subject (for example, angina attacks, asthma episodes, etc), only the first occurrence will be considered. In this situation, the data from the prospective study can be illustrated in a two-way contingency table, as in Table 3.1.

Our goal is to verify whether the **incidence** of the event in the exposed, estimated by the ratio a/(a+c), is statistically and clinically different from the incidence in the non-exposed, estimated by the ratio b/(b+d). We remind the reader that incidence is the ratio between the number of new cases of the event (disease) occurring in a given population in a given time period and the number of individuals exposed to the risk of developing the event (disease) during that time period. It is clear that, given the assumptions just made, the denominators correspond to the total group of the exposed subjects (a+c) and the total group of the non-exposed ones (b+d). This type of incidence is properly called the incidence rate. Sometimes it is referred to as the cumulative incidence rate to stress that it depends on the observation period considered: for example, if the event of interest is death, it is easy to see that, if we wait long enough, the mortality rate will eventually reach 100%. In presenting the incidence rate, it is essential to report the time period to which it refers. Generally, incidence is expressed as number of cases per 1,000 individuals per year (or 10,000 or 100,000 depending on how frequent or rare the event is in the population). It is an estimate of the risk of developing the event in the time window considered. Incidences are often compared by calculating their ratio, called incidence ratio or **relative risk,** indicated with the abbreviation RR. Since RR is the ratio between the incidence of the exposed and the incidence of the non-exposed, RR=1 indicates that the two incidences are equal; RR>1 indicates that the exposed subjects have a higher incidence than the non-exposed ones; RR<1 indicates the opposite. Given the assumptions described above, the relative risk is estimated by $RR_{estimate}=[a/(a+c)]/[b/(b+d)]$: if the result is "significantly" different from 1 (see chapter 5), we can conclude that there is an association between the characteristic under study and the event of interest.

In real life, most studies have non-binary characteristics and events, have variable follow-up periods from subject to subject and the risk of the event occurring is variable over the observation time. In the example of smoking and lung cancer, the characteristic could be classified into multiple categories, based on the number of cigarettes smoked; the event could also be subdivided into multiple classes, based on the histological type of the tumor. Almost certainly the duration of follow-up would differ from subject to subject: some will abandon the study before its end, others will die before developing lung cancer; in some studies subjects are permitted to enter the study while it is already in progress. Also, the risk of developing cancer might change over time, for example it might increase. Under these conditions, the statistical analysis is clearly more complex.

With variable durations of follow-up it does not make sense to use the total number of subjects as the denominator to calculate the incidence, since this number varies over time. Therefore, the measure of incidence should be "adjusted" to account for the different exposure time of each subject.

Three methods are often used to calculate incidence in these cases.

The first method consists of calculating the total observation time for the cohort as a whole by adding up the observation times of all its subjects. The observation time of each subject is the time interval from the moment the subject enters the study to the moment one of the following occurs: the event happens, the subject leaves the study, the study comes to an end. The observation time is expressed in the appropriate time unit: person-years, person-months, person-days, etc. One hundred person-years could correspond to a hundred persons followed for one year, fifty followed for two years, ten followed for ten years and so on. The incidence is then calculated as the ratio between the number of new cases of the event (disease) that occur during the course of the study and the total observation time of the cohort, expressed in the chosen time unit. Again, for subjects showing more than one event, only the first one is considered. For example, expressing time as person-years and having observed 50 new cases in 370 person-years, the incidence rate of the event is 50/370 = 0.135, expressed as 13.5 events per 100 person-years of observation. This method gives an estimate of the mean incidence during the entire period covered by the study, and therefore makes sense only when it is reasonable to assume that the risk of an event occurring per unit of time is constant for the entire observation period.

The second method for calculating incidence, called actuarial, is based on the so-called survival tables. Briefly, one divides the observation time into intervals and assumes that the subjects who are in the study at the midpoint of each interval are exposed for the entire interval. Therefore, for each interval we are back to the simpler condition described above: a fixed number of subjects, all monitored for the same time period. Consequently, the incidence can be calculated as illustrated above. In reality, the situation is more complex. First, to apply this method, the entire cohort of subjects must enter the study at the same time; if this is not the case, for each subject, the calendar time must be replaced by a time scale in which the study start coincides with the time the patient entered the study. Second, it should be kept in mind that some of the subjects who are lost to follow-up before developing the event could have later developed it. It is not possible to discuss such complex aspects in this brief overview: we refer the reader to Colton's textbook [26] for an introduction to survival tables and to the book by Marubini and Valsecchi [69] for an exhaustive coverage of the topic. The actuarial method assumes that the risk is constant within each interval and that the interval risks are independent of calendar time.

The third method does not require the assumption that the events of interest occur at a constant rate in the different time intervals. This method consists of calculating the "incidence density", which can be seen as an extreme case of the actuarial method. The observation time is divided into intervals of an infinitesimal length (a situation similar to the one we will find in section 5.1.2 when discussing the probability density function). The incidence density can be calculated in several ways, for example by applying the Kaplan-Meier method, also known as the product-limit technique. For more details on this topic we refer to the above-mentioned book by Marubini and Valsecchi [69]. Both the actuarial and the product-limit methods require large samples: for this reason they can rarely be used for sub-groups of subjects selected based on sex, age, etc.

The considerations on incidence introduced in this section are also useful for the analysis of events in clinical trials, often adverse events.

Non-concurrent prospective study. The second kind of prospective study is the non-concurrent one. Figure 3.3 helps to clarify the difference between concurrent and non-concurrent studies.

In concurrent prospective studies, exposed and non-exposed subjects are selected at the present time, i.e. at the start of the study (in 2005 in the figure) and are followed in the future until the end of the study (2015 in the figure). In **non-concurrent prospective studies,** the researcher goes back in time (to 1995 in the figure), selects the exposed and non-exposed subjects and then tries to find all the relevant information on these subjects, up to the present time.

The methodological characteristics of the two types of study are identical. However, in practice, there are two major differences:

- Non-concurrent studies have much shorter execution times and much lower costs.
- In non-concurrent studies, it can be more difficult to retrieve information, especially that about exposure, but also information related to the occurrence of the event. Often, such information can only be obtained if well-designed and complete databases are available because the memory of interviewed subjects is an unreliable source, especially if the study goes far back in time.

Cross-sectional prospective study. The third type of prospective study is the **cross-sectional prospective** or **transversal prospective study**. As for all prospective studies, subjects are selected on the basis of the presence/absence of the characteristic of interest. What is specific to the cross-sectional type is that the event is searched at the present time. For example, one could select two groups of subjects, one obese and one non-obese and evaluate on the same day the frequency of exertion angina by submitting all subjects to a standardized stress test (e.g. treadmill or cycling).

The differentiation between cross-sectional prospective studies on the one side and concurrent and non-concurrent prospective studies on the other is based on the duration of the process connecting the event to the potential risk/protective factor. An example from Miettinen [71] is enlightening. Let us consider a study in which over a 24 hour period both the diet and a potential effect are monitored: if the effect of interest (event) is high level of blood glucose at the end of the 24 hours, the study is concurrent (or non-concurrent) prospective; if instead the effect of interest is obesity, then the study is cross-sectional prospective.

Compared to the concurrent and non-concurrent prospective studies, the cross-sectional prospective study has the one major disadvantage that the researcher does not know for certain if the characteristic (for example obesity) was acquired before or after the event (for example exertion angina).

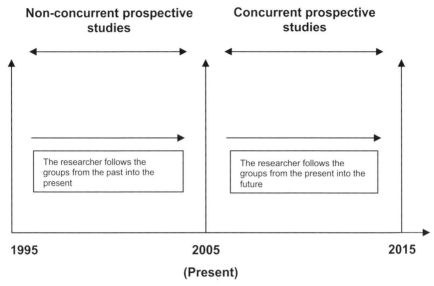

Figure 3.3. Concurrent and non-concurrent prospective studies

Cross-sectional prospective studies are also called **prevalence studies** because they allow calculation of prevalence rates (also referred to simply as **prevalence**) of the event of interest among the exposed and the non-exposed. We remind the reader that the prevalence is the ratio between the total number of subjects with the event (disease) in a given population at a given moment in time and the total number of subjects constituting that population at that same time. These studies are not suitable for calculating incidence because incidence refers to a time interval, while prevalence refers to a single point in time.

3.1.2. Retrospective Studies or Control Cases

True retrospective study. In the **true retrospective studies** (which, from now on, we will simply call retrospective), the researcher selects two groups of subjects, respectively with and without the event of interest at the time the selection is made ("today") and searches the past of each subject for a given length of time for information on the exposure to the characteristic under study. The subjects affected by the event are called **cases**; those not affected by the event are the **controls** (the "non-cases"). Whereas in the prospective study the sample selection is based on the characteristic of interest, in the retrospective study it is based on the event of interest. However, the aim is the same, namely to verify whether exposure to the characteristic under study has an impact on the event, that is, whether it is a risk or protective factor.

Because in retrospective studies the comparison is made between subjects with the disease (affected by the event) and subjects without the disease (not affected by the event) and because the subjects with the disease are called cases and those without are called controls, retrospective studies are also known as **case-control studies.**

A typical retrospective or case-control study is presented in Figure 3.4.

To conduct a retrospective study one proceeds as follows.

Ideally, a population of subjects with the disease of interest (cases) and one of similar subjects but without the disease (controls) are identified. These populations may come from the same database or from different databases. Thereafter, two representative samples are randomly extracted from these populations. As with prospective studies, this is often not possible; therefore, one forgoes representativeness and concentrates on building groups of cases and controls that are as similar as possible to each other (see below).

The selected groups of cases and controls are then studied retrospectively to verify whether or not, from a given time in the past up to the present, there has been exposure to the characteristic under study.

Finally, the measures of association between exposure and event obtained in the two groups are compared (this phase presents some complications, which will be illustrated later).

In the example on the association between cigarette smoking and lung cancer, the cases are subjects with diagnosis of lung cancer, while controls are lung cancer-free subjects. The sample of cases could be obtained by selecting a group of hospitals and enrolling all lung cancer patients (or a random selection thereof) from the oncology departments, while the sample of controls could include all patients (or a random selection thereof) from non-oncological departments of the same hospitals. Once comparable (unbiased) groups are obtained, the researcher documents for each subject whether the characteristic under study is or has been present, i.e. whether the subject is or has been a smoker. It is often useful to also collect quantitative data on the characteristic, for example, how many cigarettes the subject smokes or smoked per day.

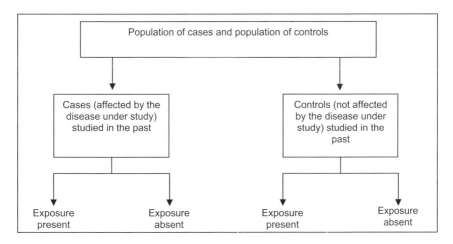

Figure 3.4. Retrospective or case-control study

Adopting the same simplification used for prospective designs, data from a retrospective study, in which both the event and the exposure are classified as present/absent and the observation times are similar (theoretically identical) for all subjects, can be illustrated in a two-way contingency table, similar to table 3.2.

Again, the final objective is that of verifying whether the incidence of the event among the exposed is statistically and clinically different from that among the non-exposed. However, in retrospective studies, a/(a+c) and b/(b+d) do not estimate these incidences because the denominators (a+c) and (b+d) do not really represent the total number of exposed and non-exposed subjects who experienced a events and b events respectively. In other words, in retrospective studies the cumulative incidence rates cannot be calculated. Consequently the relative risk of exposed versus non-exposed cannot be estimated. Nevertheless, in retrospective studies a measure of the association between exposure and event, i.e. an indirect estimate of the relative risk, can be obtained by calculating the **odds-ratio** (OR).

The **odds** of an event are defined as the ratio between the probability of the event occurring and that of it not occurring. This term was originally used in horserace betting, where it indicated the reciprocal of the bet value set by the odds maker: a horse given 2 to 1 winning (odds = $1/2$) means that for this horse the probability of the event "victory" is half that of the event "defeat" (consequently, by betting 1 dollar on victory, one would win 2 dollars if the horse wins). Under the assumptions of binary event and characteristic, fixed duration of follow-up and constant risk, in a retrospective study the odds of the event occurring among the cases can be estimated with the formula [a/(a+b)]/[b/(a+b)], while the odds of the event occurring among the controls can be estimated with the formula [c/(c+d)]/[d/(c+d)]. Then, the ratio between these odds can be calculated as equal to ad/bc, as can be demonstrated by simple algebraic passages. Under the same assumptions, in a prospective study (see Table 3.1), the odds of the event occurring among the exposed can be estimated with the formula [a/(a+c)]/[c/(a+c)], while the odds of the event occurring among the non-exposed with the formula [b/(b+d)]/[d/(b+d)]. The ratio between these quantities is again equal to ad/bc. In conclusion, for both the prospective and the retrospective studies, an estimate of the OR is given by the ratio between the cross-products of the frequencies in the two-way table.

Table 3.2. Data collected in a retrospective study with binary characteristic, binary event and same duration of follow-up for all subjects

		Subjects selected based on exposure		
		Exposure present	Exposure absent	Total
Subjects selected based on event	Event present (cases)	a	b	(a+b)
	Event absent (controls)	c	d	(c+d)
	Total	(a+c)*	(b+d)*	(a+b+c+d)

* these totals do not represent the totals of exposed and non-exposed in whom a events and b events respectively occurred

The meaning of OR is similar to that of relative risk: if OR=1, we can conclude that the exposure is not associated with the event; if OR>1, the exposure is positively associated with the event (it is a risk factor); if OR<1, the exposure is negatively associated with the event (it is a protective factor) (see [57] or [67]).

It should be noted that, under the hypothesized conditions, OR estimates RR only if the event/disease of interest is rare (as can be demonstrated by simple algebraic passages). However such limitation to rare events can be circumvented in many cases, in particular when:

- The population under study is dynamic, so that, if the incidences could be directly calculated, person-time instead of number of subjects would be used as denominator.
- A special form of case-control study, proposed by Miettinen, is used, in which the cases, instead of being compared to the non-cases, are compared to a sample of subjects extracted from the general population (consisting of cases and non-cases).

We refer the reader to Miettinen's book [71] for a more comprehensive discussion of these topics.

In retrospective studies, as in prospective studies, characteristics and events are often not binary and subjects are often lost to follow-up, so that it is not possible to establish whether they were exposed or not to the characteristic of interest in the past. Under these conditions statistical analysis becomes more complex.

Cross-sectional retrospective studies. While in true retrospective studies the exposure to the characteristic is sought in the past, which can also extend to the present, in **cross-sectional retrospective** or **transversal retrospective studies** the exposure to the characteristic is sought only in the present, for example subjects smoking at the time of occurrence of the event (see Figure 3.1).

The distinction between cross-sectional retrospective and true retrospective studies is made based on the duration of the process connecting the event to the potential risk/protection factor. For example, let us consider a study performed over a 24 hour period on patients with hyperglycemia (the event): if the risk factor of interest is the diet during the 24 hours before testing blood glucose levels, we have a true retrospective study; if instead the risk factor of interest is obesity, we have a cross-sectional retrospective study.

In the cross-sectional retrospective study the researcher does not know for certain whether the characteristic (for example heroin use) is acquired before or after the occurrence of the event (for example depression). Therefore, the cause-effect relationship is more difficult to establish. In all other methodological aspects cross-sectional retrospective studies are identical to true retrospective studies.

3.1.3 Sample Size

In the previous sections we stated that the objective of an observational study is to show that the groups under comparison have incidences of the event which are different in clinical and statistical terms, i.e. that there is a clinically and statistically meaningful association between exposure and event. This requires that the magnitude of the difference considered clinically meaningful be pre-established and that the size of the sample be such that we may be 'reasonably' sure to achieve a statistically significant result if that clinically meaningful difference (or one even greater) really exists. To meet this objective in observational studies, concepts similar to those introduced in chapters 5 and 6 for clinical trials apply, although the specific techniques are different. These techniques are not presented in this book.

3.2. Bias and Confounding

We have already stated that an epidemiological study, unlike an experimental study, does not have the advantage of the chance assignment (through randomization, see chapter 9) of subjects to exposure or non-exposure to the risk factor of interest, nor has the advantage of the control over the experimental conditions.

For these reasons it is less easy to obtain homogeneous groups in observational studies than in experimental studies. At the end of the study, any difference between the groups being compared could of course be due to chance, but could also be due to bias. Furthermore, differences between groups can also contribute to generating a phenomenon known as confounding. Therefore, the researcher confronted with a result indicating an association between the exposure to a characteristic and a disease should always ask him/herself:

1. Could the result be due to chance?
2. Could it be due to bias?
3. Could it be due to confounding?

Question 1: chance and statistical analysis. The statistical analysis allows the first question to be answered. As was mentioned in the previous chapter, and will be discussed in detail in chapter 5, the purpose of the statistical test is to quantify the probability that a result is due to chance. If this probability is small enough, one accepts that there is a real difference between the groups.

Question 2: bias or distortion. **Bias**, also referred to as **distortion**, is any systematic error (see section 1.3), which in epidemiology causes an incorrect estimate of the association between exposure and event. Bias is caused primarily by the researcher and/or by the subjects under study and can occur at any phase, from the selection of subjects (selection bias) to their evaluation (observation bias, often determined by the subjects' poor recollection of past events). Bias cannot be evaluated through the statistical analysis (see below). A **selec-**

tion bias occurs when the systematic error is introduced during the selection of subjects to be included in the study. This may concern the mechanism used for the selection of subjects (different from group to group), or the mechanism by which a subject is assigned to one group or another. An example of the first type of selection bias is when cases are selected from a hospital in one region and controls from a hospital in another region, the two regions having different socio-economic and cultural backgrounds. The second type of selection bias, also called classification bias, may occur when in a case-control study the knowledge of the exposure influences the assignment of uncertain cases to the diseased or non-diseased groups. Let us suppose that the hypothesis under study is the existence of a link between cigarette smoking and cancer. The researcher confronted with opaque spots on the chest x-ray of a heavy smoker could assign him hastily into the diseased group, without requesting the further investigation required for a definitive diagnosis. A cohort study can also be affected by classification bias when knowledge of the presence or absence of the event influences the assignment of subjects to the exposed or not exposed group.

The **observation bias** includes the forms described below.

- Recollection bias: the ability to remember is different between subjects with and without the disease, which may influence the assessment of exposure.
- Interviewer bias: occurs when questions are asked in a different manner, depending on the group to which the subject belongs, possibly influencing the answers.
- Bias caused by subjects who are lost to follow-up: occurs when subjects who are lost to follow-up differ systematically from the ones remaining in the study.
- Response bias: occurs when the subjects who answer to the questions differ systematically from those who do not.

In case-control studies, the most dangerous forms of bias are selection and recollection bias, while in cohort studies, one should be most concerned with the bias caused by subjects who are lost to follow-up, although selection bias is also dangerous.

In section 3.2.1 we will discuss the most important methods for controlling bias in observational studies.

Question 3: the phenomenon of confounding. The term **confounding** takes several different meanings in the biomedical field. Without going into definitions that are too technical (see Armitage and Colton's encyclopaedia [4]), we will discuss here the two most common forms of confounding, namely the biological and experimental ones. The common root of all manifestations of confounding is that "the effects of some factors are mixed". In the epidemiological field, confounding refers to the contamination of the effect of interest, i.e. the effect of the characteristic/exposure on the event, by factors external to it. In the experimental field, confounding refers to the inseparability of certain effects (see chapter 10) in a given design. Whereas in the former case confounding is considered a "problem" which leads to a wrong conclusion (biased estimates), in the latter it is an intentional characteristic of the design, that is, the information on some effects is intentionally "sacrificed" (i.e. one accepts less precise estimates of these effects) with the purpose of estimating other effects with greater precision. In this section we will discuss confounding in epidemiology, while we refer the reader to section 10.9 of this book for an example of a clinical trial design with confounding, and to Cox [27], Cochran and Cox [24] and Fleiss [39] for a deeper discussion of this concept in the experimental field.

Even within the epidemiological field there is little agreement among researchers on confounding. Among the various definitions found in the literature, we have chosen the one given by Hennekens and Buring [57] because, in our opinion, it is rigorous and at the same time operationally useful, in the sense that it can help the researcher to address the problem (see section 3.2.2).

There is confounding when the magnitude and, sometimes, even the direction of the estimate of an association between a characteristic/exposure and an event/disease is modified by the presence of a third factor with specific features (the confounding factor, see below). Confounding, as well as bias, lead to the over- or under-estimation of the true association between exposure and disease and can even change the direction of the observed effect.

For a factor to be confounding, the following three conditions enter into play:
• It must be associated with the characteristic/exposure.
• It must be a risk or protective factor for the disease under study, independently of the characteristic/exposure;
• It must be distributed in an unbalanced manner between the groups under comparison.

Fulfilment of the first two conditions qualifies a **factor** as **potentially confounding**. To better clarify the meaning of such a factor, let us refer to figure 3.5. In case A the "third factor" is potentially confounding because it is associated with the exposure and, independent of this, it affects the event/disease. If, however, as illustrated in case B, the exposure expresses its effect on the event by affecting the "third factor", which in turn modifies the risk of the event, then this third factor is not a potentially confounding factor but rather an intermediate step in the causal chain between exposure and event.

We provide four examples to illustrate Figure 3.5. The first two illustrate case A (a potentially confounding factor). Let us suppose that a study reached the

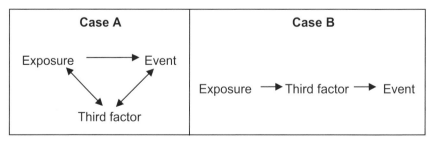

Figure 3.5. Potentially confounding factor (case A) and not potentially confounding factor (case B). (Reprinted from: Epidemiology, Hennekens CH and Buring JE, 1987. Copyright Little Brown and Co, Boston-Toronto. Reproduced with permission)

conclusion that an association exists between increase in physical exercise and reduction of the risk of myocardial infarction. A potentially confounding factor is age, as young people tend to exercise more and, independent of exercise, they tend to have a lower risk of myocardial infarction. Let us then suppose we are interested in studying the association between smoking and pancreatic cancer. A potential confounding factor in this case is alcohol: the propensity to smoke is more frequent in drinkers than in non-drinkers; furthermore alcohol, independent of smoking, is a risk factor for pancreatic cancer.

The next two examples illustrate case B (not a potentially confounding factor). In the case of the association between physical exercise and myocardial infarction, daily fluid intake is not a potentially confounding factor: even though it is associated with physical exercise (the more one exercises the more one drinks), there is no known independent association between fluid intake and risk of myocardial infarction in people who do not exercise. Let us then suppose that a study has demonstrated a negative association between moderate alcohol consumption and the risk of infarction (moderate consumption reduces risk). A factor that could be erroneously considered potentially confounding is the level of high density lipoproteins (HDL) in the blood. In fact, some studies have shown that alcohol increases the level of HDL and that high levels of this class of lipoproteins are associated with a reduction in the risk of myocardial infarction. However, it has also been demonstrated that the effect of alcohol on myocardial infarction is due, at least in part, to the fact that it increases the level of HDL. Therefore, the level of HDL cannot be considered a potentially confounding factor because one of the mechanisms of action of alcohol on the risk of myocardial infarction is indeed an increase of HDL.

So far, we have always talked of potentially confounding factors. For a potentially confounding factor to actually confound a study, that is to really behave as a **confounding factor**, it must be distributed unequally between the groups. The association existing between a potentially confounding factor and a risk factor makes the occurrence of this imbalance probable. However, if for whatever reason such imbalance does not materialize, the potentially confounding factor remains "innocuous". Let us return to the example on smoking, alcohol consumption and pancreatic cancer. It is likely that in a study comparing smokers and non-smokers, the percentage of drinkers will differ between the groups (because of the association between the propensity to smoke and the propensity to consume alcohol). However, if in the actual study the imbalance with regard to alcohol consumption between the two groups under comparison does not occur, this factor does not cause confounding, i.e. it cannot lead to overestimation of the risk of pancreatic cancer induced by smoking.

The effect of confounding can be positive or negative: in the first case, the confounding factor increases the magnitude of the observed association relative to the true one; in the second, it reduces it. Therefore, the terms "positive" and "negative" in this context refer to the effect of the confounding factor on the magnitude of the estimate of the effect of the exposure on the event, compared to the real one.

Sometimes the terms confounding and bias are used interchangeably. This is incorrect. We have a bias when the systematic imbalance between the groups under comparison is introduced by the design or the procedures of the study, whereas we have a confounding when the systematic imbalance is intrinsic to the problem being studied, because of the association between the potentially confounding factor and the exposure. As we will see, confounding can be controlled at least in part through the statistical analysis, whilst bias cannot. Furthermore, in a given study, confounding can occur without bias, and vice versa. For example, in a study in which a selection bias for a prognostic factor has occurred, there will be no confounding if this factor is part of the causal chain between the characteristic under study and the event (see figure 3.5, case B).

In experimental randomized studies (see chapter 9), the random assignment of the subjects to the treatments is such that the concept of potentially confounding factors does not apply, whereas the possibility of bias, to which a large part of this book is dedicated, remains.

Finally, the reader should keep in mind that, at times, the term confounding is used interchangeably with the term **spurious association.** Like many other terms in our field, this one is also used with multiple meanings: sometimes, mostly by physicians, it is used to indicate "false association", and at other times, mostly by statisticians, to indicate an association observed between two factors which is actually caused by a third factor. In both cases, the definition of spurious association is more generic than that of confounding.

In section 3.2.2 we will cover the most important methods for controlling the phenomenon of confounding in observational studies.

3.2.1. Control of Bias in Epidemiology

Bias cannot be evaluated quantitatively *a posteriori* by means of the statistical test for the between-group comparisons. Statistical techniques that can somewhat "purify" the results from the influence of bias do exist, but are exploratory in nature (see section 9.1). In fact, bias can be prevented or reduced only through careful planning of the design and correct implementation of the study. Special attention must be paid to the following aspects:
• Choice of the population.
• Method of data collection.
• Sources of information on exposure and disease.

Choice of the population. There are many ways to reduce bias through the choice of the population. The random selection of subjects from the population they are intended to represent dramatically reduces bias but, as stated previously, this is rarely possible in epidemiology in the way it is possible in clinical trials. However, to obtain unbiased estimates of the association between exposure and event, a comparable distribution of baseline characteristics (e.g. demographics, socio-economic factors, etc) between the samples of cases and controls or of exposed and not exposed is more important than the samples representativeness of the underlying populations. Fortunately, only the latter requires chance extraction of the sample from the population. Therefore, it is crucial that the process by which subjects are selected be the same for all groups, so that selection bias, if any, will occur to a similar degree in all groups.

In retrospective or case-control studies, these considerations are very important for the selection of the group(s) of controls. For diseases requiring hospitalization, hospital controls are often used. On the one hand, in a case-control study the selection of hospital controls (i.e. controls selected from the same hospital(s) from which the cases are selected) can increase the comparability between cases and controls in terms of desire to participate, factors influencing the choice of a particular hospital, and ability to recollect information related to the event and the exposure. In this way, the probability of three types of bias, i.e. non-response, selection, and selective memory, is reduced. On the other hand, when cases and controls are selected from a hospital population, one could easily run into one of the following two problems:

- The hospital controls do not have the same degree of exposure to the risk factor under study as the general population of controls, i.e. they do not accurately reflect the population that is free from the disease of interest.
- The hospitalization rates are different between cases and controls.

As an example of the first problem, let us assume that we are interested in studying the association between cigarette smoking and lung cancer and want to select the cases and the controls for this study from the same hospital. The population of cases could be that of the patients hospitalized for lung cancer (the sample of cases for the study is randomly chosen from this population), while that of the controls could be patients of similar sex and age who are hospitalized in another department, say the neurology department (the sample of controls for the study is randomly chosen from this population). If the propensity to smoke in the population of patients in the neurology department differs from that of the general population of subjects without lung cancer (e.g. it is higher, given the correlation between smoking and some neurological diseases) and we, unaware of this difference, perform the analyses as if the sample were representative of the general population for smoking habits, the association between cigarette smoking and lung cancer would be estimated in a distorted way (underestimated, in this example).

Concerning the second problem, let us refer to the example given in Table 3.3., which illustrates (lower section) data from a hypothetical case-control study which investigates the association between transient ischemic attack (TIA) and congestive heart failure (CHF), by using patients with colon cancer as controls. The idea for this example was taken from lecture notes by Bruce S Shoemberg (National Institute of Health, Bethesda, USA). In the example, CHF is the potential risk factor, while TIA is the event of interest. In the upper left section of the table, a hypothetical population of 1000 patients with TIA and one of 1000 patients without TIA are presented, while in the upper right section, the hypothetical hospitalization rates for TIA, colon cancer and CHF are presented (note for cardiologists and oncologists: the numbers are invented!). By applying these hospitalization rates to the above-mentioned populations, we obtain the corresponding populations of hospitalized patients, as illustrated in the central section of the table. Finally, let us hypothesize that we are performing a case-control study with the objective described above. To this end, we randomly select 100 cases and 100 controls from the hospitalized populations. The data for the two samples are reported in the lower section of the table. While in the population there is no association between TIA and CHF (OR=1), in the case-control study CHF appears to be associated with TIA; more precisely, CHF appears to be a risk factor for TIA (estimated OR=3.45, which means that the occurrence of TIA is about three and a half times more frequent in patients with CHF than in controls). This happens exclusively as a consequence of the different hospitalization rates between patients with TIA and patients with colon cancer.

Because of such problems, more than one control group is often used in retrospective studies.

In prospective (cohort) studies the choice of control groups must take into account one of the most dangerous forms of bias for these studies, namely the loss of subjects to follow-up, which may cause a difference between the groups under comparison in the ability to obtain information on all the subjects of the sample. To reduce the risk of such a bias, epidemiologists often restrict the population to the members of a particular institution, for example to subjects using the same health care provider or insurance company, etc. This approach makes the loss of subjects to follow-up less likely; furthermore, sometimes it also allows access to centralized databases specific to that institution. Another method for limiting such bias is to choose a population with an above-average risk of developing the event: subjects belonging to high risk populations are often more motivated to participate in studies compared to subjects with average or low risk.

Method of data collection. The main objective is to guarantee that data collection is similar in all groups under comparison. Two elements can contribute to reducing bias: the construction of a specific instrument for data collection (e.g. questionnaire, interview, physical examination) and the appropriate use of this instrument by the study personnel.

Closed questions must be used, i.e. answers must be chosen from a pre-determined list. Furthermore, questions must be very specific; for example, any reference to time must be precise. Measurements must be conducted by properly trained personnel and follow a standardized protocol. When different treatments are compared, their masking (i.e. blinding, see chapter 9) is to be maintained to the maximum level possible, which implies that the personnel involved in data collection should, as far as possible, not be aware of which group each study subject belongs to. It is also useful to ensure that the study subjects are unaware of the hypothesis being tested. For example, in a case-control study on the relationship between alcohol consumption and myocardial infarction, the study could be presented to the subjects as a survey on the dietary habits of patients. For this purpose, instead of focusing only on alcohol consumption, the

Table 3.3. Retrospective study investigating the association between Transient Ischemic Attack (TIA) and Congestive Heart Failure (CHF) *

Population	TIA		Hospitalization rates	
	Present	**Absent** (Patients with colon cancer)	**Disease**	**%**
CHF				
Present	100	100	TIA	10%
Absent	900	900	Colon cancer	50%
Total	1000	1000	CHF	40%
OR	(100 x 900) / (100 x 900) = 1.00			

Hospitalized Population	TIA	
	Present	**Absent** (Patients with colon cancer)
CHF		
Present	46 (#)	70 (##)
Absent	90 (###)	450 (####)
Total	136	520

Case-control Study	TIA		**Method of patient selection**
	Present (Cases)	**Absent** (Controls with colon cancer)	
CHF			
Present	34	13	100 cases and 100
Absent	66	87	controls are randomly
Total	100	100	selected from the
			hospitalized (presence/
OR Estimate	(34 x 87) / (13 x 66) = 3.45		absence of CHF is
			proportional to that
			of the corresponding
			populations)

* Fictitious data have been chosen to illustrate the problem caused by different hospitalization rates between cases and controls. (#) = sum of patients hospitalized for TIA ($\rightarrow$ 100 x 0.1 =10) and patients hospitalized for CHF ($\rightarrow$ 90 x 0.4 = 36, where 90 results from 100-10); (##) = sum of patients hospitalized for colon cancer (100 x 0.5 = 50) and patients hospitalized for CHF (50 x 0.4 = 20, where 50 results from 100-50); (###) = 900 x 0.1; (####) = 900 x 0.5
CHF = Congestive Heart Failure, TIA = Transient Ischemic Attack, OR = Odds Ratio

questionnaire should take into account a variety of other factors.

It is clear that one cannot always pursue the blinding of observers with respect to the group to which the subjects belong and the blinding of subjects with respect to the study objectives. However, "dummy" questions can be included in the data collection instruments to serve as an alarm system for the epidemiologist, with the aim of getting a general sense of the likelihood of bias having occurred during the evaluation phase. For example, in a case-control study investigating the regular use of aspirin as a protective factor for myocardial infarction, questions concerning the use of other drugs not associated with the risk of myocardial infarction can be added to the questionnaire. If the groups do not differ with respect to the frequency of the use of these drugs, the epidemiologist is reassured that observation bias was unlikely to have occurred; vice versa, if such differences do occur, the presence of various forms of bias, such as recollection bias, may be suspected. In addition, questions concerning factors for which association with myocardial infarction is well known could be added. If this association is confirmed, the hypothesis that no bias has occurred is substantiated; the opposite outcome will give way to the opposite suspicion.

Another method is to build a questionnaire that contains multiple questions aimed at obtaining the same information in different ways: consistency in the answers to these questions is checked. To control the bias that may be introduced by the examiner, information on the duration of the interview or exam can be collected. Finally, one could ask the examiner to judge the reliability of the answers obtained from each subject examined: data analysis could be conducted both including and excluding results from subjects considered unreliable.

Sources of information on exposure and disease. Pre-existing databases or archives are the sources least likely to be affected by bias, since the information is collected before the occurrence of the event of interest. However, this type of information may be incomplete and the frequency of missing data may vary from group to group.

It is useful, although not always feasible, to use multiple sources that allow cross-checks. For example, in archive-based studies one could use both the hospital records and the records of the physicians caring for the study subjects outside the hospital; in studies based on questionnaires, confirmation of selected data could be sought by examining the physicians' archives; data from death certificates could be compared with those from hospital records, and so on.

Exposure and event of interest must be meticulously defined and the definitions must be based as much as possible on standard criteria (e.g. diagnostic criteria established by international guidelines) in order to limit liberal interpretation by the study personnel.

3.2.2. Control of the Phenomenon of Confounding

In the planning phase of a study, the best method for controlling the phenomenon of confounding would be the random assignment of the study subjects to the exposure. However, this cannot be done in epidemiological studies. Therefore, in such studies, confounding is controlled through the following techniques:

- Restriction (used only in the planning phase).
- Stratification and matching (used both in the planning and analysis phases).
- Adjustment (used only in the analysis phase).

Restriction. The phenomenon of confounding occurs only if the potentially confounding factor is unbalanced, i.e. it appears with different frequency in different groups being compared. One way to prevent this is to apply the method of restriction: the inclusion/exclusion criteria in the study are restricted in such a way that only specific categories of the potentially confounding factor can be included. In some instances, through restriction, the risk of confounding for a given factor can be completely eliminated: for example, if the confounding factor is sex, one can enroll only males or only females. In other instances, it can be minimized: for example, if the potentially confounding factor is age, one can enroll only subjects within a very restricted age range.

Restriction is easy to use but has some inconveniences:
1. It is not always applicable, because often the potentially confounding factor is unknown.
2. It reduces the number of subjects who can participate in the study.
3. It does not always eliminate the problem, because confounding may still occur within the restricted category.
4. It does not allow assessment of whether the association between exposure and disease is different at different levels of the potentially confounding factor.
5. It reduces the ability to generalize results.

Stratification and matching. To reduce imbalance with respect to potentially confounding factors, stratification and matching techniques can be applied. **Stratification** is achieved by dividing cases and controls or exposed and non-exposed into subgroups (strata), based on the level of the factor of interest or, in case of multiple factors, on the combination of levels. For example, if we want to stratify by sex and presence of diabetes, we have to consider four subgroups (combination of the two levels of each factor) and then make sure that the proportion of subjects belonging to each stratum is similar in cases and controls or exposed and non-exposed. **Matching** is achieved by pairing each case with a similar control (or multiple controls) with respect to one or more pre-established factors of interest. For example two subjects are matched if they are of the same sex, race, age range, socio-economic level, etc.

These two techniques force the distribution of potential confounding factors to be similar in the groups under comparison.

With reference to applicability of these methods, stratification does not present major inconveniences, except that it makes the study design more complicated, increasing the probability of making mistakes. Matching, on the other hand, is used frequently in epidemiological studies, but presents many limitations.

- It is difficult to apply and requires much time. For example, in a study with two groups, if we divide age in five categories, sex in two and race in three categories, there are 30 (5x2x3) possible combinations to be considered in matching the subjects. Because of its complexity, matching is not used frequently in large cohort studies, but it is often used in case-control studies, which tend to be smaller.

- It is not possible to evaluate the effect of the potentially confounding factor on the result observed in the study because the distribution of this factor has been forced by design to be similar in cases and controls.

- It may be more difficult to control other potentially confounding factors that were not used for matching (for example, when matching is applied to one factor, the stratified analysis of other factors may be more complex).

In spite of these limitations, a "parsimonious" application of matching is often useful.

To be effective, the two techniques described above must be considered both in the planning and analysis phases. More precisely, when matching has been used in the design, it should be explicitly taken into account by the statistical analysis, that is, forced similarities between subjects of the same block must be taken into account (pairs, triplets and so on, depending on the number of groups under comparison). This is achieved by using specific statistical methods. If matching is not accounted for in the analysis, the true association between exposure and event/disease of interest is underestimated (see for example [57]).

If stratification is used in the design, the analysis must evaluate the association between exposure and event/disease within each stratum of the potentially confounding factor. If, for example, sex is a potentially confounding factor, the association between exposure and disease should be calculated separately for males and females. If, in addition to sex, race is also a potentially confounding factor (e.g. with three categories: whites, blacks, other), the association should be calculated separately for the following six strata: white females, black females, females of other races, white males, black males, males of other races. The **estimates** within a stratum are called **stratum-specific**. By design, stratum-specific estimates are not influenced by the potentially confounding factor used to build the strata since there is no variability with respect to this factor within a stratum.

Sometimes a study is not designed with stratification, but the analysis is performed in a stratified manner, i.e. the strata are defined in the analysis phase. In these cases, we speak of **a posteriori stratification** to distinguish it from the one defined in the planning phase, known as **prospective stratification**. The latter is to be preferred because the former can be influenced by knowledge of the results. In addition, with an a posteriori stratification, one must face data-related issues such as incomplete or inadequate data concerning the potentially confounding factors, or strata very unbalanced in size (because not planned). Such issues, by design, are avoided by a prospective stratification.

Adjustment. Once the stratum-specific estimates of the association of interest between exposure and disease are obtained, it can be useful to calculate an overall estimate of the association, based on the stratum-specific estimates. Generally these **estimates** are referred to as **adjusted** with respect to the factor (or factors) considered, while those calculated without considering stratification are known as **non-adjusted** or **crude**. Different methods exist to combine stratum-specific estimates into a single adjusted estimate. These methods are based on the calculation of weighted means of the stratum-specific estimates. Methods vary depending on the type of weighting that is used in calculating the weighted means (see for example [57]).

A method for verifying if a potentially confounding factor is really confounding, i.e. if confounding did occur, is that of comparing the raw estimate of the exposure-disease association with the estimate adjusted for the factor under examination. If the two estimates differ, the potentially confounding factor is really confounding. We should point out that this method is only valid if the measurement of the effect of the risk factor is made in terms of difference between risks or ratio of risks (relative risk), while it is not valid if it is measured in terms of odds ratio, unless the conditions are met under which the odds ratio can be interpreted as relative risk (see section 3.1.2). In the Encyclopaedia of Biostatistics edited by Armitage and Colton [4], under "confounding", an example is reported in which, when the odds ratio is used to measure the association, the crude and the adjusted estimates are not the same, despite confounding not being present.

Finally, it is important to point out that the adjustment for a factor that falls under case B of Figure 3.5, i.e. an intermediate step in the causal chain linking the exposure to the event, is to be avoided, since it causes an underestimation of the association between exposure and event of interest.

How to choose the potentially confounding factors. The choice of candidate factors to be considered as potentially confounding factors is difficult. In the previous section we saw that these can be truly identified only at the time of the statistical analysis. But selection of the potentially confounding factors must be done in the planning phase if we are to properly collect the data necessary to assess whether the suspected factors are truly confounding or not.

It is obvious that it is not possible to collect data on all factors for which a confounding role cannot be excluded a priori. A selection must be made based on the knowledge of the disease and on information collected in other studies. Lacking any indication on potential confounding factors, as a minimum, information must be collected on factors such as sex, age, race, that do have the role of risk or protective factors for many diseases. It is important for the data to be collected in a complete way. For example, smoking can be a risk factor for many diseases, but often it is not sufficient to collect such data as smoker/former smoker/never smoked because some diseases are linked to how much the subjects smoke (or have smoked).

When the potentially confounding factors are many, the stratification and adjustment methods presented above cannot be used to study the effect of all these factors simultaneously. For example, let us suppose that in the study of the association between myocardial infarction and physical activity there are four potential confounding factors: sex, age (strata: <50; 50-59; 60-69; ≥70), cigarette smoking (strata: never smoked, former smoker, smoker) and body mass index, defined as the ratio between weight and height (strata: <0.4; 0.4 - <0.6; 0.6 - <0.8; ≥0.8). These variables would require a total of 2×4×3×4=96 strata to cover all the possible combinations of sex, age, smoking and body mass index levels. Even if the sample were large, it is likely that many strata would be empty or scarcely populated.

Bias, confounding and biological plausibility. In an observational study there are two considerations that may at times clarify doubts on whether or not an observed association represents a true cause-effect relationship: the biological plausibility of the outcome, and the confirmation of the result under different circumstances. If an observed association between a characteristic and an event has a solid biological basis, it is less likely to be caused by bias and/or confounding than one that lacks such a basis. In the case of lung cancer and smoking, many cell biology studies have proven the carcinogenicity (i.e. the ability to modify cells in a cancer-causing way) of tobacco combustion products, and many animal studies have linked chronic exposure to cigarette smoke with the onset of various cancers, among which is lung cancer. Vice versa, if an epidemiological study concluded in favour of a strong association between drivers wearing red clothing and deaths in automobile accidents, the lack of a solid biological plausibility would raise the suspicion of bias and/or confounding. The second consideration, that of replicating a result under different circumstances, probably has even more value in excluding bias and confounding.

Two comments should be added on biological plausibility. The first one is that biological plausibility used to justify a result should itself be evaluated in a critical manner: physicians and biologists are capable of "creating" a biological plausibility even for the most absurd association, in order to justify the results of a study (generally due to excessive "closeness" to the study, occasionally for authentic dishonesty). The second comment goes in the opposite direction: the fact that an association is unexpected and lacks a solid biological basis does not necessarily mean that it is untrue. The history of epidemiology is rich in results initially considered implausible for not meeting the expectations of the researchers or the prevailing opinion of the scientific community, but which later were found to be true through other epidemiological, clinical and/or pre-clinical studies. We will mention three examples to emphasize the point: the association between fluoride treatment and increased incidence of bone fractures (fluorine increases bone density, therefore a reduction in fractures was expected) [84]; the association between treatment with fenoterol and increased lethal asthma attacks (fenoterol is a powerful bronchodilator, therefore a reduction in serious asthma attacks was expected) [28]; the association between the reduction of the incidence of some infections, including tuberculosis, and the increase of the incidence of asthma (the opposite was expected) [94].

Finally, investigation of the possible causes of bias and confounding is in itself a powerful generator of hypotheses to be verified in subsequent studies. Returning to the apparently absurd relationship between the colour of the drivers' clothing and death from car crashes, this observation could actually be due to the fact that subjects who prefer the colour red tend to have certain personality traits such as aggressiveness, which could predispose them to car accidents. The hypothesis that aggressiveness predisposes one to car accidents can itself be made the objective of a later study.

3.3. Advantages and Disadvantages of the Different Types of Observational Studies

As always, each type of study presents advantages and disadvantages and the advantages of one type of study are often the disadvantages of another.

This section focuses mainly on the comparison between concurrent prospective studies and true retrospective studies. Many of the conclusions, however, can be extended also to non-concurrent prospective studies and cross-sectional prospective studies on one side, and to cross-sectional retrospective studies on the other. In the final part of this section, some specific considerations on these types of studies are provided.

From a methodological point of view, concurrent prospective studies are better overall than retrospective studies for two main reasons:

- They generate data susceptible to forms of bias that are more easily controlled (for example, the loss of subjects to follow-up can be limited by trying to motivate the subjects participating in the study) and therefore allow more reliable comparisons between groups.
- They allow the incidence rates of the exposed and non-exposed to be estimated.

On the down side, however, these studies are more complex, expensive and lengthy. If the disease under study is rare, the sample size required to conduct a prospective study and the time required for the disease or event to appear could be prohibitive, to the point that the study is totally unfeasible.

The great advantage of retrospective studies is that they are much faster and less expensive. The event has already occurred and the characteristic of interest can be searched for in the personal and clinical history of each study subject relatively rapidly and economically. Instead, in concurrent prospective studies, one must wait for the event to occur, often for many years: the duration of the study may outlast the duration of the career of the researcher.

The biggest disadvantage of retrospective studies is the lower reliability of the information, and consequently of the conclusions, compared to prospective studies. As stated previously, in retrospective studies, the documentation on the characteristic of interest is obtained by enquiring into the clinical records and the memory of the subjects under study (and/or of relatives or health care providers). Unfortunately, both sources are generally incomplete and inaccurate. Let us suppose that the risk factor under study is cigarette smoking. Subjects, in recalling their smoking history, may consciously or subconsciously reduce the number of cigarettes smoked per day (or, in some circumstances, increase that number), they may not remember having been smokers, or have preconceived ideas about what constitutes smoking ("smoking less than 10 cigarettes per day is not really smoking"), etc. Unfortunately, such errors in detection of the characteristic of interest tend not to occur with the same frequency in cases and controls, because the presence or absence of the event tends to influence the degree of accuracy in detecting the characteristic. Going back to our example, it is likely that cases in whom lung cancer has been diagnosed tend to minimize their smoking history more than controls without a diagnosis of lung cancer. In this way bias is introduced, inevitably distorting the conclusions of the study. In concurrent prospective studies, major errors in the detection of the characteristic of interest are less likely because often it can be directly observed. Furthermore, since the characteristic is documented before the onset of the event, the tendency for errors to systematically go in the same direction is less likely. It is for this reason that generally the reliability of the evidence generated in prospective studies is greater than that generated in retrospective studies. The other major disadvantage of retrospective studies is that they do not allow an estimate of the incidence of the event in the groups with and without the characteristic under study and therefore do not allow a direct estimate of the relative risk. However, we have shown that often an indirect estimate of the relative risk of exposed to non-exposed can be obtained using the odds ratio (see section 3.1.2).

Tables 3.4 and 3.5 list the advantages and disadvantages of concurrent prospective and true retrospective designs.

A final remark on the comparison between concurrent prospective and retrospective studies is that the former are advantageous for studying the relationship between rare characteristics/exposures and relatively frequent events, whereas the latter are advantageous for studying the relationship between rare diseases and frequent characteristics/exposures. The advantage is represented mainly by a smaller sample size compared to the alternative design. In addition, the former are generally well suited for studying multiple effects of a given exposure, while the latter are indicated for studying multiple risk factors for a given disease.

A few brief considerations on non-concurrent and cross-sectional prospective designs and cross-sectional retrospective designs will conclude this section. As discussed previously, in general the advantages and disadvantages of these designs are the same as those of concurrent prospective designs and true retrospective designs, respectively. Two specific considerations apply however.

Non-concurrent prospective studies, like retrospective ones, do not require that the researcher wait for the event to occur (often a very long time). In addition, from a methodological point of view, they have the same advantages as concurrent prospective designs. Therefore, they would appear to be the ideal choice. Unfortunately, from a practical point of view, conducting non-concurrent prospective studies is often limited by difficulties in finding the needed information. Retrospective searching for data on the exposure is more difficult than on the event for several reasons, especially because many databases are set

Table 3.4. Concurrent prospective studies

Advantages	Disadvantages
• The natural temporal sequence is followed, by starting from the exposure and going on to assess the event. This allows for less bias in collecting the information	• The costs are high (e.g. it is necessary to monitor subjects periodically over time)
• The estimate of the incidence of the event is possible and the estimate of the relative risk is direct	• The study duration is long (especially if the disease under study is rare and/or the latency time between exposure and disease/event is long)
• Classification errors are relatively infrequent	• The occurrence of events may be influenced by the study itself
• It is possible to obtain information on subjects who no longer have the characteristic under study	• A selective loss of subjects to follow-up (i.e. more in one group than in the other) may occur
• The latency between the start of exposure and the event, and that between the end of exposure and the reduction of its effect can both be measured	• A limited number of hypotheses may be studied
• The risk of other diseases related to the characteristic/exposure under study can be studied	• Hypotheses generated after the start of the study cannot be added to its objectives
• Indispensable for rare exposures	

Table 3.5. Retrospective studies

Advantages	Disadvantages
• The costs are relatively low	• The reverse temporal sequence is followed, by starting from the event and going back to assess the exposure. This increases the likelihood of some forms of bias, such as recollection and evaluation bias (if one knows that the subject is a case, the search for the exposure could be more careful, and findings more frequent, than if one knows that the subject is a control)
• The study duration is relatively short	
• Multiple risk/protection factors can be examined	
• Indispensable for rare diseases	• Only approximated relative risks can be calculated through odds ratios
	• The accuracy and completeness of information can be unsatisfactory

up to be searched for event, not for exposure and because subjects generally re-member better the onset of a given disease/event than exposure to a given risk factor. In addition, it can be difficult to reconstruct the incidence of the event of interest, since it is difficult to find information on subjects who have moved to other areas or died. For these reasons, non-concurrent prospective designs are used where databases (paper-based or electronic) exist, which allow a compre-hensive follow-up of cohorts over time in a relatively easy and complete way. A field in which non-concurrent prospective studies have yielded very important results is that of investigation of adverse effects, mainly carcinogenic, of occu-pational exposures, such as the association between exposure to asbestos and the onset of mesothelioma of the lung. Where a suspicion of this kind is raised, it is not acceptable for the worker to continue to be exposed to a potential haz-ard while waiting for the result of a concurrent prospective study. On the other hand, in these cases it is almost always possible to reconstruct a cohort of work-ers exposed in the past to the suspected risk factor and to evaluate the risk of disease or death after the exposure. This is typically accomplished through local registry offices, which are often very reliable sources for diseases such as can-cers.

In cross-sectional studies, characteristics and events are searched for only in the present, therefore the possibility of bias is lower compared to other types of prospective or retrospective studies, even though not eliminated (for example, in a retrospective cross-sectional study cases may tend to "lie" consciously or subconsciously about their current smoking status more frequently than con-trols).

Cross-sectional studies, both prospective and retrospective, have the disad-vantage that the researcher does not know if the characteristic (for example, being a smoker) was acquired before or after the onset of the event. In the lat-ter case, smoking cannot be considered a potential risk factor for cancer devel-opment. Therefore, the cause-effect relationship is more difficult to establish in cross-sectional studies than in other types of prospective and retrospective studies.

Summary

Observational studies can be of two types:
- Prospective (also known as follow-up, longitudinal or cohort studies).
- Retrospective (also known as case-control studies).

In prospective studies, the researcher selects two groups of subjects, referred to as the exposed, i.e. those with the characteristic under study, and the non-exposed, i.e. those without that characteristic (for example smokers and non-smokers), but otherwise as homogenous as possible. The researcher then "ob-serves" each subject for a given period of time and documents if, when, and how the event of interest (for example lung cancer) occurs. In retrospective studies, the researcher selects two groups of subjects, referred to as cases and controls, with and without the event of interest respectively and for every subject searches for information on exposure to the characteristic under study.

Prospective studies can be classified in three types, based on the chronological relationship between the study, the event and the characteristic: concurrent (the exposed and non-exposed subjects are selected at the beginning of the study and are followed prospectively into the future, up to the end of the study); non-concurrent (the researcher goes back in time, selects exposed and non-exposed subjects and then tries to trace the information relative to the event of interest, up to the present); cross-sectional (the subjects are chosen based on the presence/absence of the characteristic of interest in the present, and the event is also searched for in the present).

Retrospective studies can be classified in two types based on when information on the exposure is sought: if the research goes back in time, the study is truly retrospective, while if it is limited to the present, the study is cross-sectional.

Since in epidemiological studies one cannot use randomization to assign subjects to exposure or non-exposure to the characteristic of interest, it is more difficult to obtain unbiased groups (that is, groups that are homogenous for multiple factors and differ only by chance), compared to experimental studies. The non-randomized assignment of subjects increases the likelihood of a systematic error, referred to as bias or distortion, as well as that of a phenomenon known as confounding, where an association is established between a characteristic of interest and an event, which in fact is determined by a third factor. The confounding factor has three features: 1) it is associated with the characteristic of interest; 2) it has an effect on the event independent of the effect of the characteristic of interest; 3) it is unevenly distributed between the groups under comparison.

Both prospective studies (concurrent, non-concurrent and cross-sectional) and retrospective studies (true and cross-sectional) are susceptible to different forms of bias and to confounding. However, the prospective are generally more accurate than the retrospective, but are more complex and expensive.

4

Defining the Treatment Effect

4.1. From the Single Measurement to the Signal

In this book we will use the term "signal" to define the summary variable which, at a group level and in comparative terms, is used to formulate the hypothesis to be tested, in order to evaluate the effect of the experimental treatment under study. It should be noted that in clinical research the term signal is often used with a different meaning, to indicate an increased frequency of a given adverse event in the experimental treatment group over the control group, to the extent that the adverse event is suspected to be causally related to the experimental treatment. In this book we will use this term in the literal sense of "a sign to convey a command, direction, or warning" (Webster's New World Dictionary, [103]).

Generally, multiple signals are defined and evaluated in one study. The definition of each signal requires a detailed description of the expected effect of the experimental treatment in qualitative, quantitative and comparative terms. To this end, the researcher must proceed through a logical sequence of steps, some at the level of the individual patient, others at the level of the treatment groups under comparison.

In this section we will provide a brief outline of such steps, which we have grouped in four stages (Figure 4.1).

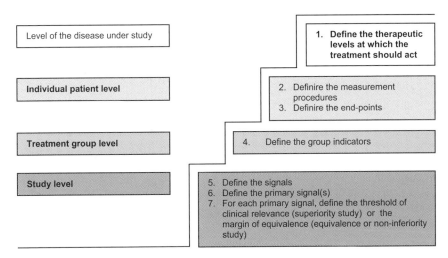

Figure 4.1. Logical sequence of steps to define and quantify the signal

Stage one. Disease level

1ˢᵗ step: define the main therapeutic level. First of all, we must define the "therapeutic levels" and, for each therapeutic level, the aspects of the disease on which our treatment is supposed to act. We call "**therapeutic level**" the level of therapeutic benefit, from transient improvement of some symptoms to complete cure, that we expect to achieve with the experimental treatment. Frequently, multiple therapeutic levels must be studied to assess adequately the effect of a treatment on a disease, and, for each therapeutic level, multiple aspects must be examined. However, it is crucial to define the main therapeutic level and aspect to which we want to link the primary end-point/signal (see below).

Stage two. Individual patient level

2ⁿᵈ step: define the measurement procedures. At an individual patient level, it must be decided how to best measure each therapeutic level and aspect selected for the study. From a statistical point of view, this corresponds to identifying the variables. The decisions concern the type of measurement (scale and instrument), the measurement technique (instructions on how to perform the measurement), the number of measurements (one or more can be envisaged for each patient) and their chronology (i.e. the timing and sequence of the measurements).

3ʳᵈ step: define the end-points. Each set of measurements, as defined in step 2, must be combined into a single "summary" variable for the individual patient. These are the **outcome variables** commonly referred to as **end-points**. Obviously, if only one measurement is chosen for a given aspect of the disease, it will coincide with the end-point.

We will illustrate the steps we have described so far with a brief example (a more detailed example is provided in section 4.6). Hypertension is the disease of interest. We want to study the effect of a treatment on arterial blood pressure (the therapeutic level). To this end, we choose two variables, the systolic blood pressure (SBP) and the diastolic blood pressure (DBP), which detect two different aspects of the selected therapeutic level. SBP and DBP are measured with an instrument called sphygmomanometer. We decide to perform the measurements always on the patient's right arm, with the patient in a seated position, in the morning, just before beginning the treatment (the so-called "**baseline**" time-point) and at the end of the treatment, say, after 8 weeks. We chose the instrument and train the users. Furthermore, we decide that the differences between values at baseline and week-8 for SBP and DBP, respectively, are the end-points of the study. Thus, the end-points are the changes in SBP and DBP from baseline to the end of the 8th week of treatment. Clearly, we could have taken alternative approaches: for example, we could have decided to measure SBP and DBP at the end of each week of treatment until the end of the study and to use as end-points the mean of all SBP and the mean of all DBP measurements. In this case, the end-points are the mean SBP and DBP levels during treatment. The choice of the end-point should take into account statistical considerations (see section 4.4), but must be ultimately guided by a clinical rationale: in the first scenario our main interest is the final effect of the treatment (after 8 weeks), while in the second our main interest is the ability to control blood pressure in a stable manner over time.

Stage three. Treatment group level

4th step: define the group indicators. Next, we must decide how to "synthesize" each end-point at a treatment group level. This means that, for each end-point, the values obtained from all patients constituting a treatment group must be summarized into a single indicator of the effect of the treatment on a given aspect of the disease of interest (for example, the arithmetic mean, the geometric mean, the median, the proportion, the count, etc.). The choice of this indicator, which we will call **group indicator**, depends on both the type of end-point and its distribution (see chapter 5). Unlike the previous step, here the choice is mainly statistical (see section 4.4).

Stage four. Study level

5th step: define the signals. For each group indicator we must define the way in which the treatment groups are mathematically compared. If the indicator is a mean, we might compare the groups by using the difference of means; if the indicator is a proportion we might use the ratio of proportions. We have finally defined the indicator of the overall effect of the treatment in comparative terms. This is the **signal**.

*6th **step: classify hierarchically the end-points and signals into primary and secondary.*** The process is not over yet, because almost inevitably we will have selected numerous end-points and corresponding signals. If this is the case, a hierarchical ordering must be established by identifying the primary ones (possibly just one, see below). The others will be secondary.

*7th **step: define the threshold of clinical relevance/non-relevance.*** At this point, the approach changes depending on whether we have decided to perform a study aimed at showing superiority, equivalence or non-inferiority. **Superiority studies** have the objective of demonstrating that the experimental treatment is superior to the control; equivalence studies, that of demonstrating that the treatments under comparison are equal; non-inferiority studies, that of demonstrating that the experimental treatment is not inferior to the control. For superiority studies, for each primary signal, we must decide by how much the effect of the experimental treatment must be superior to that of the control treatment in order to declare the difference clinically (or biologically) relevant. Frequently, this process is referred to as the definition of the threshold of clinical relevance or clinical significance of the signal. We will use the expression **threshold of clinical relevance**, since we prefer to reserve the term "significance" for statistical differences. This threshold must not be defined at the level of the single patient, but at the level of the signal. The threshold of clinical relevance is essential for defining the hypothesis system to be subjected to statistical verification (see chapter 5) and for defining the sample size of the study (see chapter 6). For equivalence or non-inferiority studies, for each primary signal, we must define the "delta of clinical non-relevance" or **margin of equivalence**. This is the maximum tolerable difference between the treatment groups that is still consistent with the statement that they are similar (in the case of equivalence studies) or that the experimental group is not inferior to the control (in the case of non-inferiority studies). Again, the definition of this threshold is essential for setting up the system of statistical hypotheses and for deciding the sample size of the study. Finally, when we have multiple primary end-points/signals, it is necessary to decide the type of approach to adopt for the complex question of multiple comparisons (see below).

We now return to the example of the hypertension study in which two treatments are compared to illustrate the final four steps. We now choose the dichotomous variable response/non-response for SBP as the only primary end-point. Response refers to a single patient ("**responder**"): let us assume that a patient is a responder when the mean of his/her SBP measurements performed in the final four weeks of treatment (which we call "final mean SBP") is less than 90 mmHg, while a patient is a non-responder when his/her final mean SBP is equal to or greater than 90 mmHg. Next, we move from the single patient to the treatment group and choose, as the group indicator, the proportion of responders in the treatment group (given by the ratio between the number of responders and the total number of subjects in that group). We then move to the signal, i.e. to defining the overall effect in comparative terms between treatment groups: we choose as the signal the ratio between the proportion of responders in the two treatment groups. Finally, let us assume that we want to perform a superiority study. As a final step, we must establish the threshold of clinical relevance for the primary signal. We decide that this threshold is 50%, i.e. we consider the difference between groups relevant from a clinical point of view when the experimental treatment group has a number of responders equal to one and a half times that of the control group, or more. Any smaller difference is not clinically meaningful.

From this overview it should be clear that the definition of the treatment effect we want to study is a conceptually complex process that starts with defining the aspects of interest of the disease under exam and progresses from the individual patient to the treatment group and from the individual treatment group to differences between groups.

We should point out that there is considerable confusion in the terminology in this field and the term "end-point" is used to indicate any one of the above mentioned steps, both in lay terms and in the scientific literature.

It is also important to note that in the study protocol the individual components contributing to the definition of the signal do not appear one after another in the logical order described above. For example, the end-points are described in different sections, including the ones on measurement methods and on statistical methods; the signals are usually defined in the section on objectives and then covered in depth in the statistical methods section; the group indicators are generally mentioned only in the statistical section. Nevertheless, the logical process linking the measurement performed on the single patient to the objective of the study follows the sequence described above.

Table 4.1 illustrates schematically the use of these elements in the planning of a superiority clinical trial.

The ultimate objective is to decide whether, in statistical terms, the estimated value of the signal stands above the background noise of variability (biological and measurement-related), i.e. whether or not it is the expression of a real effect of the experimental treatment. If we do conclude that the effect is real, we must still ask ourselves if it is also clinically relevant. To this end, we use the pre-defined threshold of clinical relevance as a term of reference.

For an equivalence or non-inferiority study, Table 4.1 must be modified. For these types of study, the sample size is determined based on the threshold of clinical non-relevance through techniques that differ from those used for superiority studies. The statistical methods are also different (generally, based on confidence intervals). In this book we concentrate on superiority studies, unless specifically indicated otherwise. A brief introduction to the problem of equivalence studies is presented in section 11.1.

The concepts of the internal validity and external relevance of the trial should be considered in defining the end-points and signals and in quantifying the signals. By **internal validity**, we mean the ability to draw valid comparative conclusions, and to derive from these valid conclusions on the causal relationship

Table 4.1. Use of the primary end-point, signal and threshold of clinical relevance in a superiority clinical trial

Planning phase		
End-point - 1 -	**Signal** - 2 -	**Threshold of clinical relevance** - 3 -
The statistical analysis is planned on the basis of the end-point. The plan requires defining the group indicator, the method by which groups are compared (the signal) and the tests for verifying its statistical significance.	The signal expresses the effect of the treatment in comparative terms. It is typically defined as the comparison between group indicators and is treated as an unknown entity to be estimated.	The threshold of clinical relevance is necessary for the construction of the system of statistical hypotheses as one of the key components for the determination of the size of the study (other crucial elements are the design of the study and the estimate of the variability of the end-point). Furthermore, it serves as point of reference for judging the clinical relevance of the result.
Analysis phase		
The statistical analysis is carried out on the data obtained from the sample, as described in -1-. Then the estimate of the signal as defined in -2- is obtained. • If the estimate of the signal stands above the variability in statistical terms, we conclude that there is a real effect of the treatment (assuming absence of bias). • If this estimate is equal to or above the threshold defined in -3-, we conclude that the effect is clinically relevant.		

between the treatment and the effect. By **external relevance**, we mean the ability to achieve the practical goals that the researchers set for themselves, such as using the study to achieve regulatory approval of a new treatment, or to differentiate the profile of the new treatment from that of existing treatments, to demonstrate health economic value of the new treatment justifying a target market price, etc.

In section 4.2, we will discuss in greater depth the steps at the level of the single patient, which have the goal of defining the end-point. In section 4.3 we will do the same for the steps at the treatment group level, which have the goal of defining the signal. Sections 4.4 and 4.5 will be dedicated to statistical considerations (which have a key role in determining the internal validity of the study) and to marketing and regulatory considerations (which have an important role in determining the external relevance of the study), respectively. In section 4.6 we will provide another example, more detailed than the one reported above, which will be useful to illustrate in practical terms some of the concepts introduced at a theoretical level in Section 4.1. In sections 4.7 to 4.9 we will address some important problems related to the definition of end-points and signals. The statistical analysis of the end-points and the determination of the sample size (see Table 4.1) will be discussed further in chapters 5 and 6, respectively.

4.2. Identification and Quantification of the End-Points (Individual Subject Level)

We will use the terms end-point and outcome variable interchangeably. In the previous section, we learned that a detailed definition and description of the measurements to be used for evaluating one or more aspects of the disease of interest are necessary steps, but not sufficient to define the end-point. This concept will be illustrated by an example in section 4.6.

4.2.1. Methodological Characteristics of the End-Point

To be methodologically valid, the end-points of a study should be:
- Appropriate to answer the questions set out in the objectives of the study.
- Precisely defined and measurable.
- Hierarchically classified into primary and secondary.
- Statistically analyzable.
- Selected and defined a priori.
  Each of these methodological characteristics requires some comment.

1. First of all, total clarity on the objectives of the study is crucial. ***The end-points must "serve" the objectives.*** The lack of a logical relationship between objectives and end-points is among the most frequent methodological weaknesses in research protocols. This can be due to the fact that the design of protocols involves months of discussion, divergent opinions of experts (real or supposed), and multiple small changes. As a consequence, both objectives and end-points can undergo a slow process of transformation, which can make them very different from what was initially intended.

2. ***The end-points must be defined with meticulous precision.*** An example of what this implies is illustrated in section 4.6. They should also be measurable by means of a pre-specified measurement scale. As discussed in section 1.3.1, depending on the type of scale used, different variables are obtained, ranging from the nominal categorical (lowest level) to the properly quantitative (highest level). Any measurement instrument, whether a psychological questionnaire or a psycho-social or quality of life one, an electronic instrument or a mechanical one, must be properly validated before it is used in a clinical study (see section 4.8).

3. ***It is essential to hierarchically classify the end-points into primary (few, possibly only one) and secondary.*** The selection of the **primary end-points** is a methodological imperative. The conclusions from a study should be drawn from the results of the primary end-points. The results of the **secondary end-points** can strengthen or weaken the conclusions and generate new hypotheses, but never reverse the conclusions. The reasons for

such categorical statements will be illustrated later in this chapter (section 4.7). Very briefly, the problem is that with increasing numbers of end-points and statistical comparisons in the same study, the risk of obtaining false-positive results increases. In other words, there is an increasing risk of obtaining results that are statistically significant purely by chance. The selection of a restricted number of primary end-points (ideally only one) and the use of appropriate statistical techniques, reduces such risk to "acceptable levels" (according to convention). Having seen the results of the study, under no circumstance should one give in to the temptation of transforming secondary objectives and related end-points into primary (and vice versa). Unfortunately, in our experience, such "exchanges" are not rare, especially in the academic and pre-clinical environments. This happens not because clinical researchers in the pharmaceutical industry are more skilled or more honest than their academic and pre-clinical colleagues, but because clinical research sponsored by industry is controlled more rigorously by regulatory authorities. The ethical and practical implications of such "exchanges" (if made consciously) are identical to those of the fabrication of data. The a priori definition of the study objectives and of the hierarchy of the end-points in the study protocols reduces the magnitude of this problem.

4. ***The evaluation of the effect of the treatment on the end-point must be carried out by means of the statistical analysis.*** The physician/biologist and the statistician must work together to obtain from the literature and from previous studies information concerning the distribution (see chapter 5) of all end-points. This information is necessary in order to design a correct and complete analysis plan for each of the study end-points. Most importantly, the statistician must have information on the characteristics and variability of the distribution of the primary end-point (or end-points if more than one has been pre-selected as primary) in order to define the sample size, i.e. how many subjects are required to obtain statistically significant conclusions, when the experimental treatment is efficacious in the circumstances and under the assumptions defined by the protocol (see chapters 5 and 6). The more unreliable and fragmentary this information, the more incomplete the analysis plan and uncertain the conclusion of the study. A variable with unknown distribution in a population which is at least similar to the study population should not be used as a primary end-point of a study. This is crucial if the study is pivotal (see section 4.2.2).

5. ***All the end-point related aspects described above must be defined a priori*** (i.e. before starting the study) and justified and described in the protocol. A study in which this occurs a posteriori, i.e. after generating the results, loses its legitimacy, especially if results are "positive". Clearly, the reason for this is that the researchers must not adjust the end-points to fit the results. This does not mean that it is wrong to perform unplanned analyses on data collected in a study. Quite to the contrary, in our opinion, unplanned

analyses (called *post-hoc*) are legitimate, as long as they have a purely exploratory purpose, i.e. the purpose of generating hypotheses, not to confirm them, and as long as the post-hoc nature of the analysis is clearly declared at the time of presenting and publishing the results.

4.2.2   Discriminating between Primary and Secondary End-Points and between Efficacy and Safety/Tolerability End-Points

Must all end-points of all studies have all of the characteristics described above?

Before answering this question let us clarify further the meaning of the terms "primary" and "secondary" and introduce the terms "confirmatory" and "exploratory", often used to qualify the end-points and the objectives of clinical studies.

We refer to **objectives** as **primary** or **confirmatory** when their aim is to answer conclusively one or more questions. The **end-points** (possibly only one) built to verify these objectives are themselves primary or **confirmatory**. **Objectives** are **secondary** or **exploratory** when their goal is either to help to interpret the primary objectives or to generate new hypotheses. The **end-points** linked to these objectives are themselves secondary or **exploratory**. In some circles, the objectives/end-points supporting the primary ones are called secondary, and those linked to other hypotheses are called exploratory. We will use the terms secondary and exploratory interchangeably, to indicate all of the non-primary objectives and end-points.

Often, the terms confirmatory and exploratory are also used to qualify different types of study. With reference to the phases of clinical research (mentioned in passing in chapter 1 and properly discussed in chapter 12), phase III studies are often referred to as confirmatory, whereas phase II studies are referred to as exploratory. This does not mean that all end-points in phase II are exploratory and all in phase III are confirmatory. Here the terms confirmatory and exploratory are used with a different meaning, i.e. to indicate the role of the study in the clinical development process. In fact, the two phases have different aims, each with confirmatory and exploratory objectives and end-points (see chapter 12).

The aim of phase II studies is to establish the biological activity of the new treatment and, if pertinent to the treatment, the dose (or doses) to be studied in phase III, while the aim of phase III studies is to establish the clinical efficacy and safety. Therefore, the former are generally confirmatory with respect to end-points derived from laboratory, imaging or instrumental measurements, while the latter are generally confirmatory with respect to clinical end-points. In phase II studies, examples of end-points with a confirmatory objective are: the reduction of tumor volume between the first and last day of treatment (or other pre-defined evaluation time points) in cancer patients; the mean viral load in the last month of treatment in HIV patients; diastolic pressure at the final measurement in patients with hypertension; change in the concentration of high-density lipoproteins (HDL) between the baseline measurement and the mean of the last two measurements in patients with heart failure, and so on. In phase III studies, on the other hand, the confirmatory end-points must reflect a tangible clinical benefit to the patient, such as survival time and quality of life (see also section 12.2.4). These kinds of end-points are generally missing or exploratory in phase II studies. It should be noted that, for some diseases, the end-points of phase III studies can be the same as those of phase II studies (see also section 4.9). For example, in the development program of a bronchodilator, a valid end-point both for phase II and phase III studies can be a measurement of the respiratory function such as the area under the time-response curve for forced expiratory volume in 1 second (FEV1) obtained in the last day of treatment and "adjusted" (by difference or analysis of co-variance) for the value of the same curve obtained at baseline. This is possible when the end-point in question is a validated surrogate (see section 4.9) of a clinically meaningful outcome. Generally, in these cases, the phase II primary end-point is evaluated over a shorter duration of time as compared to the same end-point in phase III. For example, in phase II clinical trials in asthma, FEV1 is evaluated after up to two weeks of treatment, whereas in phase III trials, it is evaluated at the end of a three to six month treatment period. Only **pilot studies** are generally completely exploratory: they are performed in the early stages of the clinical development process, when there is not yet enough information to plan a study that leads to valid conclusions.

To avoid confusion, we will not refer to a phase III study as confirmatory, but will use the term **pivotal** to indicate a **study** with the purpose of conclusively answering one or more questions regarding clinical efficacy. The terms confirmatory and exploratory will be reserved for end-points (as opposed to entire studies) to indicate the goal of conclusively answering a question and that of generating hypotheses (i.e. new questions), respectively. Both phase II and phase III studies can have confirmatory and exploratory end-points.

Let us now return to the question asked at the beginning of the section: must all end-points of all studies have all of the characteristics described in section 4.2.1? In theory, the answer should be yes. Indeed, all of the end-points must be appropriate to address at least one of the objectives of the study, all must be hierarchically classified as either primary or secondary; all must be meticulously defined a priori and analyzable. The only concession made to secondary end-points (including those of safety and tolerability, see below) concerns the sample size. Typically, the calculation of the number of subjects to include in a study (i.e. the sample size) is based only on the primary end-points. It is the very fact that the sample size is based on the primary end-points that makes them confirmatory. Because the sample size calculation is not based on the secondary end-points, the amount of information on their distribution, variability, etc., to be obtained in the planning phase, can generally be less than that required for primary end-points.

Nevertheless, one should resist the temptation of defining the end-points in an approximate way, and of introducing an excessive number of end-points, even when they are exploratory. It is true that with exploratory end-points the consequences of wrong conclusions (i.e. false-positives and false-negatives) are less serious than for confirmatory ones, since any hypothesis generated by a positive result must be confirmed by further studies in which the end-point in question is elevated to primary. But it is also true that no researcher would want to embark on studies to verify hypotheses that have no foundation (false-positive), or to discard hypotheses that could be true (false-negative). In addition, the proliferation of end-points increases the operational complexity of the study and the likelihood of overall failure (see below).

The other important distinction to make is that between an **efficacy end-point**, and a **safety** or **tolerability end-point**. The distinction between the terms "safety" and "tolerability" is not always straightforward. Broadly speaking, safety refers to outcomes that may be a true danger for the patient's health, whereas tolerability refers to outcomes that are bothersome, but not dangerous. For example, itching is generally considered a tolerability end-point because, although potentially extremely bothersome for the patient, in itself it is not life threatening, nor puts the patient at risk of permanent disability. Clearly, there is a considerable element of subjectivity in this disctintion. Furthermore, in many situations safety and tolerability are used interchangeably. In every clinical study the safety and tolerability of the treatments under comparison must be carefully assessed. Therefore, a number of safety and tolerability end-points are added to the efficacy ones.

Safety and tolerability end-points do not tend to be classified as exploratory or secondary, but in practice are treated as if they were: they generally satisfy all of the characteristics defined in section 4.2.1, with the exception of the one illustrated in point 4 (i.e. it is not required to know all of the statistical characteristics necessary for the sample size calculation, since the sample size is not based on these end-points). Safety/tolerability end-points (few, ideally only one) are considered primary end-points only if the primary objective of the study concerns the safety or tolerability of the experimental treatment.

In our opinion there are three reasons that legitimize treating the safety/tolerability end-points as secondary, even if from a clinical point of view they are not.

1. The first is a practical one: it would be impossible to size the study to account for all of the safety and tolerability end-points.

   The other two reasons are statistical in nature: they are the basis of an approach to safety and tolerability end-points which is more conservative for the experimental treatment than for the comparator(s), i.e. tends to favor the latter. Generally, such is the preferred approach for safety and tolerability end-points.

2. Whereas for efficacy end-points, false-positives (made more likely by multiple comparisons) tend to favor the experimental treatment, for safety/tolerability end-points, these same false-positive results tend to damage it.

3. For safety/tolerability end-points, the overall goal is generally to demonstrate that the treatments being compared have similar effects, not that one treatment is superior to the others. This reminds us of the above-mentioned equiv-

alence and non-inferiority studies. For such studies, the common statistical analyses are not appropriate, for reasons that can only be clarified later in the book. Therefore, since the standard statistical test does not apply, the multiple comparison issue does not apply either. An introduction to equivalence studies, which includes a few specific points on safety/tolerability end-points, will be presented in chapter 11.

4.3. Identification and Quantification of the Signals (Group Level)

We saw in section 4.1 how the final goal of the process is the definition of the signal for each end-point of the study. In addition, for each end-point selected as confirmatory or primary (ideally only one, see section 4.7), the difference in effect between the experimental and control treatment groups that must be observed to declare the result clinically relevant (in a superiority study) or compatible with equivalence (in an equivalence study) must be expressed in quantitative terms.

When the measurement scale is quantitative, defining the group indicator and then the signal can be relatively easy: typically, the so-called measures of central tendency, such as the mean, mode, and median are used. For example, if the measurement is diastolic blood pressure (DPB) expressed in millimeters of mercury (mm Hg) and the end-point is the difference between DPB measured at the end of the study and that measured on the same subject at baseline, the group indicator can be the mean or the median of the DPB differences between baseline and end-of-study for all subjects in the group, and the signal can be the difference between the mean or the median of the two groups under comparison. Note that with more treatment groups, the transition from group indicator to signal can become complicated. For instance, if we have more than one experimental treatment (typically, different doses or formulations of the same active principle) and more than one control, we may want to compare a "mathematical elaboration" (for example, the mean) of the means of all experimental treatments versus the same elaboration of all control groups.

When the measurement scale is qualitative (nominal scale) or semi-quantitative (ordinal scale), the definition of the signal can be more complex. For example, let us assume that the measurement scale is "worsened/unchanged/improved" and that the end-point is "responder/non-responder", having defined as "responder" a patient that scored "improved" or "unchanged" in each of the last three visits of the study. The group indicator could be the proportion of responders and the signal could be the difference between the proportions of responders in one treatment group and that in the other treatment group. However, under some circumstances, it is not appropriate or convenient to convert a categorical variable into a dichotomous one, as we have just done. As an alternative, we could keep the original 3-category measurement scale of the end-point (worsened/unchanged/ improved) and change the group indicator to a table of frequencies (or percentages), also called **contingency table**, in which the percentage of patients in each category within each treatment is reported (with 100% representing all patients assigned to that treatment). The signal could then be the difference between the percentages of the groups under comparison, category by category.

As stated previously, the signal must be predefined for all the end-points of the study.

Let us first consider superiority studies. The final step is that of quantifying the threshold of clinical relevance for each primary signal. Typically, this is done in terms of the difference between indicators of central tendency (mean, median, mode). Therefore, variability is not explicitly included in this definition. Nevertheless, in order to be able to discriminate relevant from irrelevant differences, the researcher must have knowledge of the variability of the end-point. Let us suppose that the signal is defined as the difference between the mean walking distances (on a treadmill) at the end of treatment of the two groups under comparison. A 50 meter difference will have a completely different meaning if the variability of the end-point, expressed for example in terms of standard deviation, is of the order of 100 meters or 1000 meters! Intuitively, the threshold of clinical relevance for an end-point with high variability must be higher than for one with low variability. A frequently used pragmatic approach is to define the threshold of clinical relevance in terms of multiples or submultiples of the standard deviation. For example, a difference between groups of the order of one half of the standard deviation is usually accepted as relevant from a clinical point of view. However, this can vary enormously from disease to disease.

When the signal is expressed as a difference between frequencies or percentages in a contingency table, the threshold of clinical relevance could be expressed as a fixed difference, equal in all categories, or as a difference changing from category to category, always pre-specified in the planning stage.

Equivalence and non-inferiority studies are planned starting from a difference judged a priori as clinically not relevant. The researcher must therefore establish this margin of equivalence. The approach is similar to that taken in defining the threshold of clinical relevance in superiority studies, even though, for reasons that will be clarified later, the definition of the margin of clinical equivalence for equivalence and non-inferiority studies is more convoluted and complex than that of the threshold of clinical relevance for superiority studies (see section 11.1).

4.4. Statistical Considerations

Statistical considerations do not fall into one specific step in the definition of end-points and signals: they should accompany biological and medical considerations throughout the entire process, as they are crucial to the internal validity of the trial.

Statistical considerations should not take the highest priority, whilst forgetting that the problems addressed are of biological and/or medical nature. For example, if we choose an end-point only so that we can use a new statistical method, recently published in a prestigious journal, the choice will probably be wrong.

However, the opposite attitude is much more frequent and just as wrong. Often, a primary end-point is chosen of which little or nothing is known in terms of distribution and variability. When this happens, it would be best to reconsider the choice made, because many aspects of the design and analysis of the study will be complicated, difficult to plan and justify correctly. As a consequence, results will be unreliable. If the chosen variable cannot be changed (for example, because the alternatives are no better), it will be necessary to make assumptions and to establish the threshold of clinical relevance based on the number of patients that it is reasonable to enroll in the study (see chapter 6). However, no matter how complicated and frustrating, we must seriously ask ourselves whether it would not be better to start the process of selecting the signal all over again, approaching it from a different angle.

The right approach is that of seeing statistics as an indispensable tool for answering the researcher's questions. The questions are biological and medical in nature. The statistician helps the physician/biologist to formulate them in a way that is statistically "manageable", since the answers are not interpretable without the correct statistical approach.

With regard to the choice of primary end-point(s), the contribution of the statistician is two fold: to assess their accuracy and precision (see 1.3.2) and to define the most appropriate methods of analysis. For example, when the measurement scale is quantitative and the pre-treatment measurements are highly correlated with the post-treatment ones, an end-point based on the difference between pre- and post-treatment measurements is more precise, i.e. less variable, than an end-point based on a single measurement taken post-treatment. Let's assume that in a study on an antihypertensive agent we measure DBP before and after the treatment: we must choose whether to base the primary comparison on the absolute values of the post-treatment measurements (end-point: "DBP level after X days of treatment") or on the difference between pre- and post-treatment measurements (end-point: "change in DBP after X days of treatment"). Not only medical considerations, but also statistical ones, should guide the choice between these two end-points. If from previous studies we could estimate the correlation between the pre- and post-treatment measurements in a population similar to that of our study, we would use this information to choose our end-point: if the correlation is low (for example, less than or equal to 0.5), we would be inclined to use "DBP level after X days of treatment"; vice versa, if the correlation is high (for example, greater than 0.5), we would prefer "change in DBP after X days of treatment" (see for example [39]). This choice is justified because in the first case the variability of "DBP level after X days of treatment" is less than that of "change in DBP after X days of treatment", while the opposite is true in the second case. The inspection of a simple scatter plot of post- vs. pre-treatment measurements can reveal the degree of correlation between the two measurements and, therefore, can help to choose the right end-point. When the measurement scale is categorical, the response can have a non-linear relationship with the baseline value and, in such cases, the analysis of the changes from baseline can be problematic.

Another choice, not always easy, is that between change and percentage change from baseline. As before, from a statistical point of view, one should choose the end-point that shows less dependency from pre-treatment measurements. Inspection of scatter plots of change and of percentage changes vs. pre-treatment values is often sufficient to make this choice. The use of the wrong end-point may have a negative impact on both accuracy and precision.

A frequently encountered situation in which the statistician has a crucial role is when the end-point is related to events. How do we transform the "raw" count of events into the end-point? Should we use the event rate, calculated as the total number of events divided by the total number of person-years of observation (e.g. a patient observed for two years is equal to two patient-years)? Or would it be better to use the total number of events occurring in a given period of time, grouped in pre-specified classes? Or would the responder status be best, the patient qualifying as responder if experiencing at least one event? Or would it be preferable to focus on the time interval from the start of treatment to the first occurrence of the event? Assuming that in the circumstances of the experiment all of these potential end-points are clinically meaningful, statistical considerations will help in making the choice. These will be influenced by whether it is best to hypothesize a constant or variable rate for the observation period, whether the event of interest is rare or frequent, whether or not the events occur in an independent and random fashion, and so on. This information is crucial to allow the statistician to recommend the most appropriate end-point, be it dichotomous or categorical, a numerical count or related to survival.

If we decide to change from a continuous end-point to a dichotomous one, for instance from the continuous variable "reduction of LDL (low density lipoprotein) cholesterol" to the dichotomous variable "LDL reduction above or below a given threshold", we must realize that the power of the statistical test to be used in the latter case may be reduced (see chapters 5 and 6).

The statistician guides the definition of the group indicator because it depends to a large extent on the type and shape of the distribution of the endpoint (see chapter 5). However, in this case, too, the collaboration between statistician and physician/biologist is precious, since the latter must always check that the statistical approach is intelligible. If the choice of the group indicator is perfect from the point of view of statistical properties, but is not understood by the majority of non-statisticians, what good is it?

Finally, the statistician must help the physician/biologist to define the signal. Generally, the contribution of the statistician is that of recommending the definition that maximizes the power and precision of the study, i.e. its ability to distinguish the signal from the background noise. Sometimes the statistical model behind the "best" signal may be very complex. In this case, the statistician must make sure that the signal (and the estimate that will be obtained for it) is easy to interpret by the health professional who is not statistically inclined. Obviously, in all of this, the statistician must constantly pay attention to the numerical aspects of the study. For example, in studies with dichotomous end-points (such as success/failure), the statistician must remind the physician/biologist that the relative risk, i.e. the ratio between the absolute risks, is preferable to the difference between absolute risks when the true proportions of successes in the groups under comparison are very small. On the contrary, the odds ratio (see section 3.1.2), which is often appealing to the statistician for its mathematical features, suffers sometimes in interpretability on the side of the physician/biologist.

4.5. Practical, Regulatory, Marketing and Pharmaco-Economic Considerations

As stated above, statistical considerations are fundamental to choosing end-points and signals because they guarantee the internal validity of a clinical study. However, ***practical considerations*** are also very important and should never be forgotten. A sure recipe for failure is over-complicating the protocol of a study. This can happen in many ways, for example by including too many end-points, imposing complex and invasive measurements which require an excessive effort on the part of the patients and staff, defining abstruse signals not easily interpretable by those who will assess the final results, and so on. In our search for the optimal design, we must always strive for the greatest possible level of simplification.

It is evident that the external relevance of the study should be kept in mind when choosing end-points and signals. In this context, external relevance means that the conclusions of our study must be relevant to the "external world". For example, they must be useful for achieving the approval of the product by regulatory authorities, a reasonable price and/or reimbursement by payers, a good positioning versus competitors, etc. In real life, regulatory, marketing and pharmaco-economic considerations receive great attention, especially if the study is sponsored by a pharmaceutical company. What is the benefit of performing a methodologically "perfect" study with a primary end-point that is not accepted by the regulatory authorities, and therefore does not contribute to the registration of the treatment? What is the point of performing a study that contributes to the registration of an unmarketable drug? Obviously, these considerations play a role not only in the choice of end-points and signals, but in all aspects of the trial that contribute to defining the target product profile

We will start with the ***regulatory aspects.*** General methodological guidelines exist, many released by the International Conference of Harmonization (ICH). In addition, several regulatory authorities, especially the US Food and Drug Administration (FDA) and the European Medicines Agency (EMEA) have released a number of therapeutic area-specific guidelines. The interested reader can consult the web-sites www.fda.gov and www.emea.eu.int. Let us suppose, for example, that we are planning a pivotal phase III study in patients with mild Alzheimer's disease and that we select symptomatic improvement as the therapeutic level of our experimental treatment (i.e. we have no ambition of curing or modifying the natural course of the disease). A guideline released in July 1997 by the Efficacy Working Party of the EMEA [35] provides the minimum regulatory requirements for a symptomatic treatment to be considered efficacious in Alzheimer's disease: each of two independent studies must show a statistically significant difference for two pre-defined primary end-points, one measuring the cognitive ability of the patient and the other reflecting the clinical relevance of the cognitive improvement, in terms of ability to function (activities of daily life), or overall status (overall clinical evaluation). The requirement of statistical significance for both end-points eliminates the problem of statistical multiplicity (see section 4.7). The guideline neither specifies how the signals should be defined, nor indicates the threshold of clinical relevance. If the "activities of daily life" end-point is chosen as co-primary, together with cognitive ability, the "overall clinical evaluation" end-point can be included among the secondary ones, together with individual symptoms, and vice-versa. However, the guideline warns that, in order to claim efficacy for any individual symptom, an additional pivotal study in which the chosen end-point is declared as primary must be performed. The guideline does not impose the use of specific measurement instruments, but does highlight some features that must be taken into account in choosing these instruments (validation, sensitivity, precision, relationship between complexity of administration and type of patients under study, etc.) and does mention some suitable assessment scales, such as the ADAS (Alzheimer's Disease Assessment Scale) for the cognitive domain and the CDR (Clinical Dementia Rating) scale for the overall clinical evaluation.

Generally the regulatory guidelines reflect the current level of knowledge of the scientific community (they are often developed following a "Consensus Conference"). Therefore, it is unlikely that the physician and statistician, having accurately studied the literature and addressed in depth the basic questions both medically and statistically, reach conclusions contrary to the content of these documents. In fact, it is often convenient to start the literature search from the references reported in the regulatory guidelines. If in doubt, it is good practice to discuss with the regulatory authority directly.

The importance of the **marketing aspects** for a pharmaceutical company is self-evident. Marketing decisions require not only an in-depth knowledge of the therapeutic state of the art, but also insight on future trends in the area and on activities of competitors. Let us suppose we are developing an antihypertensive drug to be administered daily. Two pivotal studies are ongoing with the aim of confirming a mean reduction of 10 mmHg at the end of 10 days of treatment. While the studies are underway, we discover that another company is developing a similar compound, also administered daily, for which the predicted effect is a mean reduction of 20 mmHg in 10 days. What do we do? Do we throw everything away? Pretend we do not know and continue as planned? It is intuitive that solutions to this kind of situation are not easy and that there is no cook-book formula to give to the reader. Situations like this require a 360-degree analysis of the problem, which is to involve experts in many fields and to include a reassessment of the therapeutic level that our compound could potentially tar-get. It could be that our treatment, in addition to reducing the mean blood pres-sure, could also reduce sudden pressure peaks and prevent the complications that arise from them. If data support this hypothesis, it could be appropriate to start a new study in which the primary end-point measures this aspect, for ex-ample the number of times (in a predefined number of measurements) DBP is below a certain threshold (clearly, measurements must be as frequent as possi-ble in order to detect transient events). Alternatively, it could be logical to di-rectly measure the most severe complications, such as those requiring hospital-ization: the primary end-points of the new study could be the number of hospi-talizations and their mean duration. A different approach could be to study the safety profiles of the two treatments, if we believe that the competitor's product has problems that our product does not have. If so, an additional study with a safety primary end-point could be a reasonable approach.

Pharmaco-economic end-points (see section 4.9) are often included in phase III pivotal studies, even though they are generally not primary. Their use has been increasingly frequent in recent years, as the requirements for pricing and reimbursement of pharmaceuticals have become more and more stringent. These days, most pricing and reimbursement authorities explicitly request pharmaco-economic data.

4.6. Selection and Characterization of the Primary End-Point and Signal: an Example

In this section we will illustrate the process of selection and characterization of the primary end-point and corresponding signal through an example taken from the field of respiratory medicine. We will follow the sequence of steps (grouped in stages) introduced in section 4.1.

We are responsible for the development of a new inhaled corticosteroid and wish to evaluate its efficacy in the treatment of asthma. To simplify matters, we shall ignore the evaluation of safety and tolerability.

4.6.1. Stage One: Define the Main Therapeutic Level

The *first and fundamental step* is that of choosing the main therapeutic lev-el that the treatment will target. Do we want to cure asthma, i.e. completely eliminate the disease, as is the case of antibiotics with some infections? Or do we want to reduce the frequency of severe asthma attacks, which are so dan-gerous for the patient and often require hospitalization? Or do we want to simply improve the symptoms of the patient? These three examples represent three different therapeutic levels at which the treatment could theoretically aim.

Therapeutic levels frequently used in clinical research include the following: prevention, cure, mortality, survival time, remission time, frequency and/or duration of exacerbations, frequency and/or duration of hospitalizations, clinical symptoms and signs (symptomatic treatment), quality of life, direct and/or indirect costs. The main therapeutic level for which we want to demonstrate efficacy is only occasionally obvious, as in the case of a generic copy of an existing drug. Instead, in most cases this fundamental choice is far from obvious and requires an in depth evaluation encompassing the pharmacological properties (if the treatment is a drug), the complexity of the treatment, the unmet therapeutic needs of the disease and the risk one is willing to take (in both scientific and financial terms). For pharmaceutical companies (who develop the vast majority of drugs), the expected financial return plays a very important role in the choice of the therapeutic area and of the main therapeutic level. Key determinants of the return on investments are: the prevalence of the disease (market size), the market price and level of reimbursement likely to be granted by payers (private insurance companies and public health care systems), the profit margin (which in turn is determined by many factors, including the cost of goods and the expenses for development and marketing). The fact that the drug development has one foot in science and the other in marketing is ethically challenging for many researchers, young and not so young (including the authors of this book).

Returning to our new corticosteroid, we know that the inhaled steroids available on the market (beclomethasone, budesonide, fluticasone, etc.) are effective in reducing asthma symptoms as well as the frequency of the exacerbations in the majority of patients. However, we also know that a small but meaningful percentage of asthma patients (5-10%) responds poorly to inhaled corticosteroids. These patients are prone to serious, sometimes lethal, attacks which are responsible for the majority of hospitalizations and direct and indirect costs caused by this disease. Let us suppose that the results of in vitro and in vivo experiments performed before starting clinical trials indicate that the action of our compound on airway inflammation is stronger than that of fluticasone, and that recently completed clinical studies show a trend towards reduction of severe exacerbations. We may have a drug that meets a real medical need (steroid-resistant asthma) with important socio-economic implications. The market interest for a drug that is effective in this population is high and the company is ready to invest in a study with the aim of confirming the potential of this new corticosteroid on severe exacerbations. These practical and scientific considerations compel us to choose the reduction of severe exacerbations as the primary therapeutic level of the study. Naturally, we will also be interested in exploring the potential of our drug at other therapeutic levels, both "higher" (for example, mortality) and "lower" (for example daily symptoms). However, it is absolutely essential to decide on one principal therapeutic level, from which the primary end-points and signals (ideally only one) will be derived. The primary therapeutic level will also influence in a decisive way the design of the study (patient selection, duration, control treatments, etc.). Furthermore, it is necessary to consider the problem of multiple comparisons (see section 4.7) from the very beginning of the planning process.

4.6.2. Stage Two: Define the Primary End-Point (Individual Patient Level)

The choice of the main therapeutic level represents a first and decisive step towards the definition of the overall response to be submitted to hypothesis testing, i.e. the signal. In our case, prevention of severe asthma attacks is the level at which we want to attack the disease. Next, we must define precisely the primary end-points, which must allow measurement of the efficacy of the treatment at the chosen therapeutic level in the individual patient. For reasons that will be discussed in section 4.7, it is imperative to minimize the number of primary end-points, typically to one or two at most. Let's assume we agree to have only one primary end-point.

Before continuing with this example, we would like to emphasize once more the importance of referring to guidelines which are accepted by the scientific and regulatory community, resisting the temptation of "doing it ourselves". In the case of asthma, the guideline of the Global INitiative for Asthma (GINA, www.ginasthma.com) is an obligatory reference.

First of all, the measurement procedures must be defined (*2ⁿᵈ step*). What constitutes a "severe attack"? How is it measured? We decide to use respiratory function to define the onset and severity of an asthma attack. Among the many possible measurements, we choose the Peak Expiratory Flow Rate (PEFR) for the following reasons:

1. PEFR is a frequently used variable in clinical practice and clinical research; therefore, data on its distribution and variability in asthma patients are available.
2. There is a clear correlation between the level of PEFR (generally expressed as a percentage of the "normal" value in healthy subjects of the same race, age and sex, or as a percentage of the "optimal" value for the patient) and the severity of clinical symptoms.
3. The instrument for measuring PEFR (peak flow meter) is portable and easy to use, so that the patient him/herself can measure PEFR one or more times a day at home or work, this being indispensable for detecting the onset of an attack.
4. The peak flow meter is inexpensive.

As illustrated in this example, clinical, statistical and practical considerations come into play in choosing the primary end-point. It is extremely important to consider each of these components. The practical ones are especially prone to be overlooked by researchers in the planning phase. Practical difficulties later can turn into a nightmare. Had we chosen for measuring respiratory function the spirometer, a more expensive and complex instrument than the peak flow meter, would we have been able to provide one to each patient? And would the patients have been able to use it?

Having chosen PEFR as the measurement, we must decide how it should be used to detect a severe attack. Based on the literature (especially the national and international guidelines) and on experience (in the absence of a standard criterion), we decide to define an asthma attack (exacerbation) as "severe" when PEFR measured in the morning by the patient decreases below 60% of the patient's optimal value for two or more consecutive days (the optimal value is to be established for each patient in the early phase of the study, before treatment begins). A new attack will have to be separated from the previous one by at least three days with morning PEFR values greater than or equal to 60% of optimal value; consequently episodes separated by less than three days will be considered part of the same attack. The example illustrates another important concept: when the phenomenon to be measured is an event, it is critical to establish the criteria defining its beginning and end, since both the number of events and their duration depend on these criteria. If during the course of one week a patient has a morning PEFR below 60% of optimal value on Monday, Tuesday, Thursday, and Friday, how many severe attacks should be assigned to that patient? Four? Two? One? Using our definition, the patient will have had only one severe asthma attack, since the two pairs of consecutive days with morning PEFR below 60% are separated by less than three days.

At this point we must move from the measurement to the end-point, which, as we have learned, is the single summary variable which expresses the response to the treatment for one patient (**3rd step**). We could express the end-point in terms of "responder"/ "non-responder" (patient with or without severe attacks for the entire course of the study, respectively), or as the mean number of attacks per patient per month or year (rate), or as the yearly rate of attacks adjusted by the number of days in which the patient is at risk, etcetera. In our example, the researcher chooses this last option. To clarify, let us suppose that a patient experiences three severe attacks during the 90-day course of the study and that the total number of days with severe attacks is 10. The end-point for this patient will be obtained by the ratio between 3 and 80, 80 being the difference between the duration of the study and the number of days in which the patient has severe attacks (i.e. 80 is the number of days in which the patient is at risk of developing an attack), the result multiplied by 365.6 (to annualize the rate). The value of the end-point for this patient will then be equal to 13.7 severe attacks per year at risk.

In summary, the primary end-point chosen for our study is the yearly rate of severe asthma attacks adjusted for the days in which the patient is at risk (for brevity, we will refer to our primary end-point as the "annualized rate of severe attacks"), where a severe attack is defined by morning PEFR values less than 60% of the patient's optimal value for two or more consecutive days. A new attack must be separated from the previous one by three or more days with morning PEFR values greater than or equal to 60% of the optimal value.

4.6.3. Stages Three and Four: Define the Group Indicator, the Signal, and the Threshold of Clinical Relevance (Treatment Group and Study Levels)

At this point we should move from the single patient to the treatment group and then from the single treatment group to the comparison between treatment groups. How will we "synthesize" the end-point in each of the treatment groups (group indicator, *4th step*)? How will we express this quantity in comparative terms between two treatment groups (the signal, *5th step*)? One approach could be to synthesize the end-point in each treatment group by calculating the mean of all individual values in the group and express the signal as the difference between the group means. Another approach could be to choose the median as the group indicator and express the signal as the difference between group medians. In our example, we decide to use the mean as group indicator and to express the signal as the ratio of group means (mean annualized rate of the group treated with the new corticosteroid divided by the mean annualized rate of the control group). A result equal to 1 would indicate that the treatments are equivalent; a result below 1 would indicate the superiority of the group receiving the experimental treatment; a result above 1 would indicate that the control group is superior.

The *6th step* is to order hierarchically the end-points and respective signals, identifying the primary one(s), which in our example we have already done (we are assuming that the study has several other end-points which we treat as secondary). Having decided to show superiority of our new steroid over fluticasone, the *7th and final step* is to decide the threshold of clinical relevance for the primary end-point, i.e. how large must the difference be between the response to the new treatment and that of the control treatment, to be considered clinically relevant. As pointed out in section 4.3, this threshold must be expressed in quantitative terms. Let us return to our example. If our new corticosteroid were to reduce the mean annualized rate of severe asthma attacks by 0.1% compared to the standard treatment (i.e. prevent 1 attack in 1000), would we be satisfied as researchers? If we were the health authority, would we approve the drug? If we were the reimbursement authority, would we be willing to recommend it for reimbursement? And if we were patients, would we be willing to buy it, paying a price higher than that of the drug that we are usually taking? The answer to all of these questions would probably be "no". What if the reduction was 1%? 5%? Clearly this choice is important and difficult. Knowledge of the variability of the end-point in the absence of treatment (and/or in the presence of the standard treatment) can be very useful in establishing the threshold of clinical relevance: if the literature suggests that fluctuations of 3-4% in the yearly rate of severe attacks are common, it would be reasonable to choose as our threshold of clinical relevance a difference between the treatments under comparison of at least 5%. However, other considerations must enter into play, most importantly the severity of the disease and the therapeutic level that the treatment aims to achieve. A much lower threshold of clinical relevance will be acceptable for a treatment aiming at curing AIDS compared to one aiming at treating symptoms of allergic rhinitis! Finally, as usual, practical considerations are of great importance.

As we will see in chapter 6, all other considerations being equal, the smaller the threshold of clinical relevance, the greater the sample size must be, i.e. the number of patients to be included in the study. Choosing a threshold of clinical relevance that is too small can be a disastrous error, resulting in a study of little clinical interest that is very complex and costly, and ultimately unethical!

For our new corticosteroid, after careful evaluation we decide that the threshold of clinical relevance is 10%, i.e., in order to declare the success, the new steroid group must reduce the annualized rate of severe asthma attacks by at least 10% compared to the control group. In other words, the signal must be less than or equal to 0.9.

Let us assume that the results of the study show that the mean annualized rate of severe attacks is 19.2 in the group treated with the new corticosteroid and 27.4 in the control group. Thus, the effect of the experimental treatment is 0.7, indicating a 30% reduction in the number of severe asthma attacks in the group treated with the new corticosteroid compared to the group treated with fluticasone (control treatment). This is below (i.e. better than) the predefined threshold of clinical relevance. In conclusion, our data lead us to believe that our new treatment is promising compared to the standard one (which we have used as control). Therefore, we decide to continue the development of the new compound.

Finally, if we decide to use more than one primary end-point in the same study (this does not apply to our example), the complex question of multiple comparisons, which will be presented in section 4.7, must be faced.

It should be noted that the same process must be followed for each of the secondary end-points and signals that we decide to include in the study, with the possible exception of the definition of the threshold of clinical relevance (but some would argue for predefined thresholds of clinical relevance for secondary end-points as well).

This example illustrates how much attention must be paid to defining the end-points of a study and the corresponding signals. Unfortunately, however, the study protocol often provides only a "shopping list" of measurements. No effort is made in the protocol to define how the measurements are transformed into end-points and the end-points into signals, or to identify one or more end-points as primary, or to define how to evaluate the treatment with respect to the chosen end-points.

4.7. More Than One Question in the Same Study: the Problem of Multiple Statistical Tests

The scientific and logistical complexity of clinical research, the very high costs, and the long duration are such that many clinical studies are unique events, unlikely to be repeated. It is therefore typical and completely understandable that

a long list of questions (each representing a potential objective) and end-points is put forward when the planning of a study begins and grows even longer as the planning continues. It is equally typical (and equally understandable) that the investigators do not want to limit themselves to comparing one experimental treatment with only one control, but would rather have more (for example, a placebo and an active control, or 3-4 different doses of the experimental drug). Returning to the example of the previous section, even if we consider only the comparison between the experimental treatment and one active control, and only the primary objective (severe asthma attacks), it would be very interesting to examine severe attacks, not only in terms of changes in lung function (PEFR in our case), but also in terms of hospitalizations. We would then have two primary endpoints:
1. Annualized rate of episodes, as defined by a predefined reduction of PEFR.
2. Annualized rate of episodes, as defined by an admission to hospital.

Furthermore, as mentioned at the beginning of section 4.6, we would probably also be interested in evaluating other dimensions of the effect of our new corticosteroid (different therapeutic levels and/or different aspects of the same therapeutic level), such as the effect on nocturnal symptoms, quality of life, tolerability, etc. Clearly, each of the selected dimensions can in turn be explored through multiple end-points. In addition, in a study of long duration, many variables are measured more than once.

As a consequence, it is very common for a single study to envisage dozens of questions (objectives) and end-points and hundreds of measurements for each patient.

The problem of **multiple end-points** and resulting **multiple** statistical **tests** is one of the most critical and complex in the field of clinical research methodology. In summary, multiple statistical tests can derive from the combination, in the same study, of three "multipliers":
1. Multiple objectives, from which multiple end-points and signals are derived.
2. Multiple measurements of the same variable analyzed individually (i.e. not combined into a single summary variable for each patient), resulting in multiple end-points for the same type of measurement.
3. More than two treatments, resulting in multiple signals for the same end-point.

An in-depth discussion of the problems underlying multiple comparisons is beyond the aims of this book. Therefore, we will provide only a brief overview.

The problem can be deconstructed into three main components: statistical methodology, clinical interpretation and practical feasibility.

Statistical methodology. The inclusion in a single study of multiple end-points (and corresponding signals) of equal importance carries a "price to pay" in order to reduce the danger of false-positives, i.e. of statistically significant results favoring the experimental treatment when in fact no true difference from the control exists (results due to chance). This problem occurs when the pre-defined decision rule allows success to be claimed when even only one (or some) of the multiple comparisons yields a significant result. Instead, if the decision rule requires that all of the comparisons must be significant to declare success, there is no additional price to pay: in this case, the probability of false-positives will not increase (in fact it decreases). These concepts will be better understood after reading chapter 5, in which the logic of the statistical testing is discussed. Here we provide a few rules, which for the moment the reader must accept "in faith".

- All other conditions being equal, the threshold of statistical significance of each test must decrease, as the number of primary comparisons (and therefore of statistical tests) increases, unless a statistically significant result is required for all of them (see above). The threshold of statistical significance is typically 0.05 (i.e. 5%). In order to claim that a treatment "wins" over another in statistical terms, the outcome of the statistical test must not exceed the threshold of statistical significance. Thus, reducing this threshold makes statistical "success" more difficult. This is the "price to pay" mentioned above, defined in statistical terms as **adjustment for multiplicity**. A reduction of the threshold of statistical significance for each test will either cause a decrease of the probability of success of the study, if the sample size is maintained unchanged, or an increase in the sample size, if the probability of success is to remain unchanged.

- As a consequence, assuming that the other conditions remain unchanged, the number of subjects to be included in the study must increase as the number of comparisons to be submitted to statistical testing increases (see chapter 6).

- The statistical methods needed to overcome these problems are often quite complex. This fact should not be underestimated, because the communication between statistical and biomedical disciplines becomes more difficult and often the quality of the final product (i.e. the correct interpretation of the results) suffers.

The above reasons explain why a hierarchical classification of end-points into primary and secondary is imperative in the planning of clinical trials.

It should be noted that in practice the problem of multiple comparisons is restricted to the primary end-points. Conceptually, secondary end-points cannot be used to confirm hypotheses and therefore lie outside the problem of multiple comparisons. Nevertheless, when results from many tests are interpreted, even if only for the purpose of generating hypotheses, it is always a good idea to keep the problem of multiplicity in mind.

The ideal situation from a methodological point of view is that of only one primary end-point, translated into one signal and one statistical comparison between treatments. In our experience this "methodological purity" is not always achieved (often for very good reasons, see above). The farther we are from the ideal situation, i.e. the more end-points and comparisons we use for confirmatory purposes, the more serious are the methodological issues that must be addressed.

Clinical interpretation. The greater the number of end-points, the harder the overall interpretation of the results will be, unless we obtain homogeneous results for all of the end-points (a rare event!). Returning to our example, let us suppose that we give in to the insistence of our colleagues and elevate the annual hospitalization rate to the status of primary end-point (we have two now), without defining a decision-making rule to establish the success of the study. The corresponding primary signal will be, for example, the ratio between the mean values of this rate in the two groups under comparison (of course we will need to define precisely the threshold of clinical relevance, as for the other primary end point). Let us suppose that, at the end of the study, we find that our new corticosteroid is superior to the control treatment based on one primary end-point (severe asthma attacks defined by PEFR) but not on the other (severe asthma attacks defined by hospitalization). What is our conclusion? Does the new drug work or not? It is clear that it is necessary to define in advance the decision-making rules, allowing for all possible combinations of results. In the example, we could decide that both end-points must be significant, or that at least one of them must be significant and the other not show a conflicting trend, etc. Each of these solutions leads to a different sample size of the study. As should be clear by now, things are difficult enough with two primary end-points; with more than two, predefining the criteria for success becomes extremely complex.

Practical feasibility. The quality of any experiment depends on the quality of the data collected. There is no defense against data of poor quality (missing data, transcription errors, systematic measurement errors, etc.). The operational, logistic, and data management issues of a clinical study are beyond the purpose of this book. However, we must remind the reader that these issues are complex, requiring sophisticated specialist competencies and experience, and that their importance is often underestimated, if not ignored completely, by physicians, biologists and clinical scientists in general. A study with dozens of end-points, many of which are measured repeatedly, requires burdensome case record forms and generates an enormous amount of data. All data must be entered into the database by manual typing or electronic transfer. Thereafter, the data must be "cleaned", a somewhat unsophisticated term, but one that describes the process very well: the data manager must find missing data, correct obvious errors, ask the investigator to correct mistakes and reconcile conflicting entries, etc. Each of these steps is prone to errors and there will always be a breaking point, beyond which the errors will be so numerous as to compromise the quality of the study. When this happens, the inclusion of numerous secondary end-points, which originally had the aim of widening our knowledge by making the best use of the study, ends up reducing (or destroying) the reliability of the results, including those of the primary end-points, with the final outcome of making the worst possible use of the study.

4.8. Validation of Measurement Scales

The term **validation** is often abused or used with an ill-defined meaning. In fact, this term has precise technical meanings which, however, may differ in different disciplines. When applied to processes (computerized or not), validation indicates "a documented program which provides a high degree of assurance that a specific process will consistently produce a product meeting its predetermined specification and quality attributes" [17]. When applied to analytical methods (for example, the assay measuring the concentration of a compound in biological fluids), validation must demonstrate that the procedure under evaluation is able to predict accurately and precisely the concentration of the compound. Therefore, validation indicates "a documented program which provides a high degree of assurance that the analytical method will consistently result in a recovery and precision within predetermined specifications and limits" [17]. The "documented program" is also standardized, as the main elements it must comprise are precisely defined.

When considering measurement scales, the definition of validation is less standardized. If the reader were to perform a literature search on validation of measurement scales, he/she would find a very heterogeneous series of papers, which recommend different types of information to support the validation of a measurement scale. As we cannot cover this topic in any reasonable detail, we will briefly touch upon the minimum requirements to validate a measurement scale.

Any measurement scale must be validated through dedicated studies, performed on a well-defined patient population, following a pre-specified protocol. These studies have three key objectives:
- Obtain information on the types of mistakes made with a given measurement scale.
- Obtain information on the behavior of the scale when repeated measurements are taken in the absence of any change in the subject's health status (precision and reproducibility).
- Evaluate the ability of the scale to detect clinically relevant changes of the subject's health status (**responsiveness**).

As for all other biomedical studies, a comparative logic is applied in validation studies. The new measurement scale is compared with the one considered the best, because of scientific merit or (more often) because it is the one most commonly used (the reference scale is sometimes referred to as the "gold standard").

The first objective is met through the following assessments:
- Sensitivity and specificity of the scale, if pertinent (see section 1.4).
- Internal consistency, when the scale is a questionnaire with multiple questions, for example, using an index known as Cronbach alpha coefficient [4].
- Distribution of the new scale in the population of interest (shape and basic parameters, see section 5).
- **Degree of agreement** between the new scale and the gold standard. On this

topic we refer to a paper by Bland and Altman [14], where the authors elegantly explain why the correlation coefficient should not be used to measure the degree of agreement between two measurements and present a more appropriate approach for obtaining this type of information.

Moving on to the second objective, the best way to obtain information on the reproducibility of a scale is to plan for multiple measurements on each subject, taken close enough in time that changes in health status are unlikely. Two types of information should generally be acquired: the **intra-observer reproducibility** (measurements repeated on the same subject by the same observer) and the **inter-observer reproducibility** (measurements repeated on the same subject by different observers). Clearly, a scale that allows high reproducibility (i.e. low variability) of repeated measurements is desirable.

The level of reproducibility of the scale also influences the degree of agreement between the new scale and the reference scale (the gold standard): if a scale has low reproducibility, i.e. if repeated measurements obtained with this scale have high variability, the degree of agreement between the two methods of measurement will also be low [14].

Finally, to meet the third objective, we must obtain a measure of the association between the changes over time of the scale being studied and the changes over time of other indicators of the subjects' health status (e.g. clinical tests, the gold standard scale). Therefore, the study must be planned so that the measurements of interest are repeated over a time frame sufficient to detect changes in the subjects' health status.

4.9. Special Types of End-Points

Before concluding this chapter, it is important to discuss briefly the following special types of end-points: surrogate, composite, quality of life, and pharmacoeconomic.

The so-called **surrogate end-points** are indicators of biological activity ("biomarkers") capable of replacing a clinical end-point.

We report the definition of biomarker, clinical end-point and surrogate end-point given by the "Biomarkers Definition Working Group" of the US National Institute of Health (NIH) [13], together with some examples.

1. A **biomarker** is defined as "a characteristic that is objectively measured and evaluated as an indicator of normal biological processes, pathogenic processes, or pharmacologic responses to a therapeutic intervention". For example, the plasma concentration of the enzymes angiotensin I, angiotensin II, renin, and the hormone aldosterone are biomarkers of one of the pathological processes leading to arterial hypertension. The blood levels (number/mL) of CD4+ lymphocytes and of the HIV virus (HIV viral load) are biomarkers of the progression of the HIV infection.

2. A **clinical end-point** is "a characteristic or variable that reflects how a patient feels, functions, or survives". In patients with hypertension, examples of

clinical end-points are mortality from myocardial infarction, from all cardio-vascular accidents and from all causes. In patients with HIV infection, clinical end-points are the length of time between conversion to HIV positive serum and diagnosis of full-blown AIDS or death, mortality from opportunistic infection and mortality from all causes.

3. A **surrogate marker** (or end-point) is "a biomarker that is intended to substitute for a clinical end-point. A surrogate end-point is expected to predict clinical benefit or harm (or lack of benefit or harm)". Arterial blood pressure is a surrogate end-point (partial, see below) of mortality from cardiovascular accidents, while blood levels of CD4+ lymphocytes is a surrogate end-point (again partial, see below) of the overall mortality in HIV/AIDS patients.

The interest in surrogate end-points in clinical research stems from the fact that sometimes they allow conclusions to be reached about the efficacy (or tolerability) of a treatment more rapidly than would be possible using the corresponding clinical end-point. This is especially important when a new treatment targets diseases with no cure and high mortality. Naturally, the validity of the conclusions based on a surrogate end-point depends on the validity of the surrogate. The "perfect" surrogate end-point has two fundamental characteristics [4, 83]:

1. It is highly correlated with the corresponding clinical end-point.
2. It is capable of capturing completely the "net effect" of a treatment on the corresponding clinical end-point, where "net effect" indicates the overall effect resulting from all mechanisms of action of the treatment.

While there are many biomarkers that can satisfy the first criterion, none can really satisfy the second one, i.e. so far no biomarker has proven capable of completely capturing the "net effect" of a treatment on a clinical end-point. Colburn, in a paper of 2003 [25], states that "as more than 100,000 proteins are in the human body and most, if not all, act on a variety of biological processes, why should a single protein biomarker provide that kind of insight?" Returning to the example of the blood levels of CD4+ lymphocytes in HIV/AIDS, this biomarker is a weak surrogate of survival time in HIV infection: in fact, it can explain no more than 30% of the net effect of the antiretroviral treatments on survival [25]. Strictly speaking, therefore, CD4+ lymphocyte blood level is not a surrogate end-point.

In some cases, the effect of the mechanism of action captured by a biomarker is so partial with respect to the multiplicity of mechanisms of action of the treatment that it points in a direction which is opposite to the net effect of the treatment on the clinical end-point. For example, sodium fluoride increases bone density (biomarker), but it also increases the risk of bone fractures (clinical end-point) in postmenopausal women with osteoporosis, instead of decreasing it as one might expect. This occurs because the mechanism of action captured by the biomarker (increase in bone density), which should increase the mechanical resistance of bone, is not only antagonized, but reversed by other mechanisms of action of the treatment which are not captured by this biomarker and act more powerfully in the opposite direction. In the example, it was demonstrated that fluoride not only increases bone density, but also modifies the bone architecture in a manner that reduces its resistance.

Acknowledging the impossibility of reaching the perfect surrogate, in clinical practice a less rigorous definition of surrogate end-point is accepted, in the sense that a biomarker that captures even partially the net effect of the treatment on the clinical end-point is elevated to the rank of surrogate end-point. The proportion of the net effect that must be captured by a biomarker to consider it a surrogate end-point is an arbitrary decision. For example, according to the FDA, the blood level of CD4+ lymphocytes cannot be considered a surrogate. Generally, it is only through clusters of partial surrogate end-points that the perfect surrogate is approached. These clusters are examples of composite end-points, which we will touch upon later in this section. The combination of blood levels of CD4+ lymphocytes and of viral load appears to capture approximately 70% of the net effect of antiviral drugs on the survival time. It is for this reason that the FDA accepted such a cluster of biomarkers as a surrogate end-point of survival time in pivotal studies in HIV infection/AIDS [25].

Composite end-points are variables built by combining different end-points with the purpose of obtaining a single summary end-point. It is obvious that this combination cannot be just a simple numerical exercise, but it must have a clinical meaning. This technique is frequently applied to evaluations of the quality of life (see below), and when the end-points are events. For example, in a cardiovascular study the individual end-points could be death, myocardial infarction and other cardiac events requiring hospitalization; in such a study the composite end-point could be the onset of any one of these events. The main advantage of using composite end-points is the increase in the statistical power of the study (see chapter 5), for two reasons. First, when each individual end-point has a low incidence, the composite end-point will have a higher incidence: in these circumstances, the treatment difference that can be considered of clinical relevance is bigger than in the case of low expected incidences. Second, the problem of multiple comparisons is reduced (or eliminated). The main disadvantage is the difficulty in interpreting the results of the composite end-point when the effect of the treatment is not homogeneous in all of the individual end-points that contribute to the composite one.

In the last 20 years, there has been a tendency in clinical research to pay more attention to the patient's perception of **quality of life**. Quality of life is by definition a multidimensional concept, which encompasses clinical symptoms, mood, level of physical, intellectual, social activity, etc. A typical instrument for evaluating quality of life, therefore, includes different sections, called domains or dimensions, each intended to measure a specific aspect through a series of questions. A scale is associated with each question, typically a score ranging between two extremes, where one extreme represents the worst condition (for example, disfiguring lesions and stigmatization, making social interaction almost impossible), while the other extreme represents the best condition (for example, no impact of the disease on social interaction). Generally, the scores of the individual questions constituting each domain are summed; domains are then combined (sometimes by simple sums, other times by using a weighing system) to obtain a global score, a typical example of a composite end-point. It is crucial to use validated quality of life questionnaires (see section 4.8). Quality of life questionnaires are generally classified as generic or specific for the disease under study. Frequently used questionnaires belonging to the first category are the SF-36 [102], the Sickness Impact Profile [10] and the Nottingham Health Profile [58]. These questionnaires are very useful when it is not known on what dimension the treatment under study acts and when comparisons across different diseases are to be made, as health policy makers often must do. However, because these instruments are relatively poor in capturing changes in the health status of the patient, disease-specific questionnaires are often used. A vast literature on quality of life in clinical trials exists: among the many excellent papers, we recommend the one by Fletcher et al [41].

Finally, we shall briefly touch upon the so-called **pharmaco-economic end-points**. These end-points allow the evaluation of direct and indirect costs (for example, linked to introduction of a new treatment on the market) and the assessment of efficacy vs. costs or more broadly of benefits vs. risks, taking into account not only clinical efficacy and safety, but also economic and organizational aspects. There is no consensus as to which are the most relevant pharmaco-economic end-points. Among the most commonly used are the following: frequency and duration of hospitalizations, frequency and duration of absence from work, gain in years of life adjusted for quality of life (Quality-Adjusted Life Years, QALY), time with neither symptoms from the disease nor toxicity from treatments, again adjusted for quality of life (Quality adjustment to Time Without Symptoms of disease and Toxicity, Q-TWIST). The last two indexes combine the concepts of quality of life with that of survival. On this topic we recommend the article by Powe and Griffiths [82].

Summary

The definition of the effect of a treatment is a conceptually complex process that starts with defining the aspects of interest of the disease and then proceeds in progressive steps to define, for each aspect of interest, the measurements to be performed on each patient, the variable that summarizes the measurements in the individual patient (the end-point), the group indicator and, finally, the overall effect expressed in comparative terms between two treatment groups (the signal).

The confirmatory (primary) end-points must have all of the characteristics defined in section 4.2.1. Primary end-points are generally related to efficacy. The exploratory (secondary) end-points must have the same characteristics, except the one concerning the sample size, as the size of a study is not based on secondary end-points. The more the end-points depart from these characteristics, the more cautious one must be in interpreting the results, even when they serve only to generate new hypotheses.

In practice, safety and tolerability end-points are treated as secondary, even though, from a clinical point of view, they are not. The reason why this is generally considered acceptable is because the potential error made by not ordering the safety/tolerability end-points hierarchically is of a conservative type, that is to say, it works against the experimental treatment.

The process of defining the end-points and signals has several leading actors: the physician/biologist, the statistician, regulatory, marketing and pharmaco-economic experts.

Measurement scales must be validated prior to be used in clinical studies. Validation requires that information be collected on the errors that can occur in a single measurement (for example through analysis of the sensitivity and specificity of the scale and the characterization of the distribution of results in the population of interest), as well as in repeated measurements on the same subject. In addition, the scale should be assessed for its ability to capture clinically relevant changes in the health status of the patient and for the degree of agreement with a previously validated reference scale (gold standard).

Surrogate end-points, used frequently in clinical practice, are instrumental or laboratory measurements used as substitutes for clinically relevant end-points, i.e. end-points that measure directly how the patient feels, functions, survives. The validity of surrogate end-points must be evaluated carefully before using them in clinical trials. Composite end-points and quality of life questionnaires are other frequently used types of end-points. Pharmaco-economic end-points are increasingly used in clinical trials; these end-points have the goal of assessing the relationship between costs and benefits of treatments and ultimately of evaluating the sustainability of a newly marketed treatment by a given health care system.

5

Probability, Inference and Decision Making

In writing this chapter we have three special debts of gratitude to acknowledge. One is to Professor Theodore Colton for the frequentist approach, outlined with simplicity and rigor in his textbook on clinical trials [26]. The second is to Professor Ludovico Piccinato, of the University of Rome, since our outline of the Bayesian approach is based on one of his books [76] and on a presentation he and one of the authors gave to a medical audience on the comparison between the Bayesian and frequentist approaches. The third is to Professor Adelchi Azzalini, of the University of Padua, for his precious suggestions and advice.

We will start this chapter with an example. The result of a clinical study on patients with intermittent claudication demonstrated that the mean walking distance on a treadmill was 472 meters for patients who received treatment A and 405 meters for patients who received treatment B. Having documented a mean difference of 67 meters in favor of treatment A, can we conclude that treatment A is superior to treatment B under the conditions of the study? Furthermore, if we do conclude that treatment A is better than treatment B, should every doctor prescribe treatment A to his/her next patient with intermittent claudication?

The first is a typical question of inference: what conclusions can we draw on the overall population from the results of our study?

The second question concerns decision making: what treatment should we choose for our next patient, based on the information obtained from the present study and from previous studies on the same topic?

The feature common to the two questions is that the answers are given with a degree of uncertainty. The level of uncertainty will be different in different circumstances, but very rarely will it be absent. If the level of uncertainty is low, the conclusions will be strong. Thus any decision based on such conclusions or "evidence" will be reliable. Vice versa, if the level of uncertainty is high, the conclusions will be weak, at times impossible to reach. Thus any decision based on such conclusions will be questionable, because it will not be based on evidence, but on experience, instinct, faith, or quite simply on chance.

From what was stated above, we can understand how important is it to measure the degree of uncertainty. The probability theory provides us with tools and methods to make these kinds of measurements. Any detailed discussion of this theory is beyond the boundaries of this book. In this chapter we will only introduce some key concepts on probability, inference and decision making. In summarizing numerous concepts in the relatively short span of this chapter, we will touch upon many of them in a superficial manner, with emphasis on the logical rather than the mathematical aspects. The reader interested in delving deeper into the topics covered in this chapter and in the practical aspects of conducting statistical analyses should refer to the above mentioned textbook by Colton and to that by Armitage and Berry [3] for the frequentist approach, to the book by Berry [12] and an article by Parmar et al [74] for the Bayesian approach. A comprehensive overview of Bayesian methods applied to clinical and epidemiological studies is offered by the recent book by Spiegelhalter, Abrams and Myles [97]. For Bayesian applications in oncology, we recommend Tan et al [98] and for applications to rare diseases Spiegelhalter et al [96].

This chapter ends with a section on the so-called "Evidence-Based Medicine", which gives special importance to the methodological aspects of decision making under conditions of uncertainty.

5.1. Probability

5.1.1. Definitions

What do we mean by probability? Although we all have an intuitive sense of what probability is, it is very difficult to define it properly. In giving a definition, we must ensure that it reflects our intuitive understanding of the concept, but also that it is operationally useful, i.e. it allows the necessary mathematical procedures.

Many definitions have been given, none of which are completely satisfactory. Here we will present two of them, the "frequentist" and the "subjective". We will build the definitions around a specific event, namely a complete recovery from a disease after treatment.

In the frequentist approach, the probability of an event is defined as the relative frequency at which the event occurs in an infinite (or very long) series of tests repeated under identical (or very similar) conditions. The relative frequency is the ratio between the number of tests where the event occurs and the total number of tests performed. This frequency approximates the probability as the number of tests performed under similar conditions increases. In our example, a single test consists of treating one patient and recording whether he/she recovers (the event happens) or not (the event does not happen). The relative frequency of recovery is the ratio between the number of patients who recover and the total number of patients studied. The probability is the relative frequency we would obtain if we could hypothetically evaluate the results from an infinite number of tests performed under identical conditions. Based on this definition, the probability can take numerical values between 0 and 1. Often it is expressed as a percentage, with values between 0 and 100%.

In the second **approach**, the "**subjective**" one, probability is defined as "the level of trust that a person has that an event will occur". This definition is much broader than the previous one (it also applies to events for which it is very difficult to perform repeated tests, even conceptually), but it has the shortcomings of being neither operational nor adaptable to real life. One way to remedy these shortcomings is to adapt the definition to the betting world. With this approach, the probability of an event is defined as "the sum of money one is willing to bet to receive 1 if the event happens and 0 if it does not. The probabilities of events should be assigned so that it is not possible, in a set of bets, to surely win or surely loose" [29]. If we apply this definition to our example, the probability of recovery is no longer seen as an objective documentation of a fact, but as a subjective evaluation of the value of the treatment, based on all available information. This evaluation is expressed in terms of the amount of risk one is willing to run in a hypothetical fair bet on whether or not the event "recovery" will occur.

Table 5.1. Laws (or axioms) of probability forming the basis of probability theory

- For each event, the probability of it happening is equal to or greater than 0.
- If the event is certain, the probability of it happening is 1.
- Given two non-compatible events (that is, they cannot happen at the same time), the probability that at least one of them will happen is represented by the sum of the probabilities of each event happening.

Assuming the laws described in Table 5.1, both definitions have an operational content that allows to construct the entire mathematical system underlying the probability theory.

To the non-expert reader it may seem incredible that the whole mathematical system behind the probability theory, which allows to address the most diverse and complex probabilistic situations, is based on the simple rules reported in Table 5.1! This is indeed the case, but we will make no attempt to elaborate further.

5.1.2. Probability Distribution and Probability Density Function

Let us return to variables affected by uncertainty. First, we shall try to link the concept of probability with these variables, by using clinical research terminology and examples.

Let us consider a generic end-point (outcome variable), which we will indicate as X. As a remainder, the concept of end-point is covered in detail in chapter 4: briefly, it is a precisely defined indicator of the health status of a single patient, affected by a specific disease and undergoing a specific treatment. For example, in hypertension, X could be the change from baseline to the end of the treatment of the patient's diastolic blood pressure, measured with a sphygmomanometer under preestablished conditions. In rheumatoid arthritis, X could be the mean of a predetermined number of pain scores, measured on a predetermined scale and obtained at predetermined intervals during the treatment. In peripheral arterial disease or intermittent claudication, X could be the walking distance, measured at the end of the study on a treadmill (of a specific model, with defined characteristics, etc.).

We mentioned in section 1.1.3 that, in the jargon of statistics, X is called a variable. More precisely it is defined as a **random variable**, where the term random indicates the uncertainty relatively to the specific value that the variable will take in a given patient, in a given experiment, at a given time, etc. Conventionally, the random variable is represented by a capital letter, while its specific values are represented by the same letter, but in low case. In this chapter the terms random variable, outcome variable and end-point will be used interchangeably, however we will try to use the first one when discussing methodology, and the other two when dealing with applications.

The random variable X will take different values x_1, x_2... in the different units of the population. A **population** is defined as the totality of subjects (units) who have a predefined set of characteristics. For example, the totality of patients in the world who have high blood pressure constitutes the "population of patients with hypertension"; all patients with diastolic blood pressure above 110 mmHg (the accepted limit for severe hypertension) make up the "population of patients with severe diastolic hypertension". Usually it is not possible to observe an entire population, which therefore is a theoretical concept. However, this does not mean that the concept of population is not useful. On the contrary, it serves the important purpose of providing the logical frame of reference in which we can place and give meaning to the individual measurements.

In order to express and quantify the uncertainty with which the random variable X takes its specific values, it is given a probability distribution. A probability distribution can be visualized as the ordered sequence, from smallest to greatest, of all of the values that the variable can hypothetically take, each value being assigned the probability of it occurring.

Before developing this concept further, we should mention that it is very useful to be able to summarize probability distributions with a mathematical expression or formula, capable of linking every x value of X to its probability of occurring. This mathematical expression is called a **function** and it is generally indicated by $f(x)$. Once the mathematical expression is known, it is possible to illustrate the function graphically by placing the x values that the variable X can take on the horizontal axis (abscissa), and the corresponding $f(x)$ values on the vertical axis (ordinate). By graphically representing all pairs of values (x, $f(x)$), the curve is obtained.

If we take the frequentist approach and assume we can observe the entire population, the probability of each of the values that a random variable can take in this population is equal to the relative frequency of this value. Depending on whether the random variable is discrete or continuous (see section 1.3.1), its probability distribution will also be discrete or continuous. By convention, the probability distributions of categorical or discrete variables are generally indicated with the letter p, while those of continuous variables, with the letter f.

To introduce **discrete distributions** we shall start with a very simple experiment consisting of three coin tosses. We define the end-point (X) of this experiment as *the total number of heads in three independent throws of a coin*, assuming that the coin is not loaded, i.e. head and tail have the same probability of occurring, equal to 0.5. This is a discrete variable, because its values are whole numbers. Figure 5.1 illustrates all of the different values that the variable X can take, the probability of each value (given by the ratio between the number of cases favorable to the event "head" and the total number of cases), and the graphic representation of the two sets of data.

All possible results of 3 tosses	Probability of each result	Values that X can take	Probability distribution of X
1. T,T,T	1/8		
2. T,T,H	1/8		
3. T,H,T	1/8	0 (result # 1.)	1/8
4. H,T,T	1/8	1 (results # 2.,3.,4.)	3/8
5. T,H,H	1/8	2 (results # 5., 6.,7.)	3/8
6. H,T,H	1/8	3 (result # 8.)	1/8
7. H,H,T	1/8		
8 H,H,H	1/8		

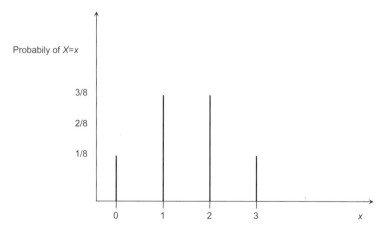

Figure 5.1. Probability distribution of the random discrete variable "number of heads in three independent tosses of a coin"

The graphic representation is obtained by placing the ordered values of X (from smallest to greatest) on the horizontal axis, and the relative frequency with which each value occurs in the population on the vertical axis (note: in this case the population is represented by the 8 possible outcomes). The result is a bar diagram, graphically representing the probability distribution of the variable X in the population. The variable used in the example is a particular case of the random variable $X=$ *number of successes in N independent tests*, where N can take whole values 1,2, ... and the probability of success is π. By setting N=3 and π=0.5 we obtain the case used in the example above. The **distribution** of this variable is called **binomial** and can be represented with graphs similar to the one in Figure 5.1, the shape depending on the values of N and π. This kind of distribution varies between 0 and N, where N can be any positive whole number.

It is important to stress that in discrete distributions, the ordinate of each value represents the probability of that value.

To introduce **continuous distributions** we will consider the random variable X = *diastolic blood pressure (DBP) in the population*. This variable is continuous because the values it can take are a continuum without any restriction. In constructing its probability distribution let us proceed step by step. We shall apply an empirical method, starting with a small group. We measure DBP in a group of 100 individuals, then order the 100 values from the smallest to the greatest and finally group them in intervals of 5 mmHg. We can represent the probability distribution of DBP for this group of individuals with a histogram in which the 5 mmHg intervals are on the horizontal axis and each interval is associated with a rectangle, the basis of which is the interval itself and the area of which is the relative frequency of the interval, as shown in Figure 5.2, part a.

We shall now expand the sample from 100 to 1000 individuals and group the DBP values in smaller intervals, for example of 2 mmHg width. Repeating the procedure described above, we obtain the histogram shown in Figure 5.2, part b.

If we were to repeat the same procedure many times, each time in a larger group of individuals and using smaller intervals, the histogram would have narrower and narrower "steps", progressively approximating a continuous curve. The final stage, that of a curve without "steps", indeed a continuous curve, is the probability distribution of the variable DBP in the population (see Figure 5.2, part c), called **probability density distribution** or **probability density function**.

An example of this distribution is the **normal** or **Gaussian distribution**, previously mentioned in section 1.3.1 and shown in Figure 1.1. This distribution varies between $-\infty$ and $+\infty$ (where the symbol ∞ stands for infinite).

It is important to note that the probability distribution (discrete case) and the probability density function (continuous case) are theoretical. They refer to hypothetical populations, which cannot be actually observed.

In the example above, we started with empirical probability distributions, calculated on larger and larger samples. We then had to make a conceptual leap, and to imagine an infinitely large sample and infinitely small intervals in order

Part a)

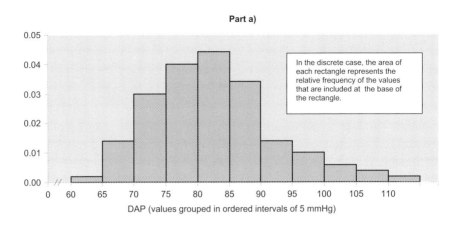

DAP (values grouped in ordered intervals of 5 mmHg)

Part b)

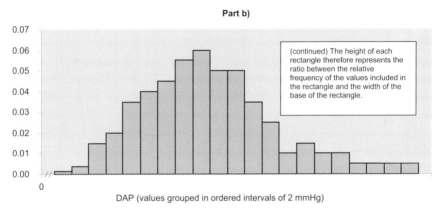

DAP (values grouped in ordered intervals of 2 mmHg)

Part c)

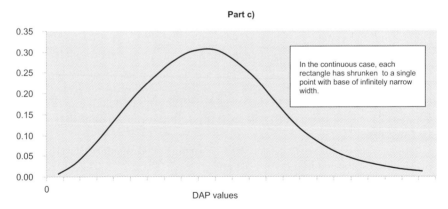

DAP values

Figure 5.2. Probability density function of the continuous random variable diastolic blood pressure (DBP) in the population

to get to the concept of probability density function. Empirical distributions are approximations of theoretical distributions: the larger the sample, the closer the approximation.

The set of probability distributions or density functions defined by a given function are called a **family**. For example, the curves shown in Figure 1.1 are characterized by the same mathematical expression,

$$f(x) = \frac{1}{\sigma\sqrt{2\pi}}\exp\left[-\frac{1}{2}\left(\frac{x-\mu}{\sigma}\right)^2\right]$$ thus belong to the family of normal distributions.

Note: in this expression π represents a mathematical constant approximately equal to 3.14 and the expression $\exp\left[-\frac{1}{2}\left(\frac{x-\mu}{\sigma}\right)^2\right]$ is approximately equal to

$\dfrac{1}{2.72^{\frac{1}{2}\left(\frac{x-\mu}{\sigma}\right)^2}}$. Also note that in the arithmetical notation the formula ab means a multiplied by b, i.e. the multiplication sign is omitted.

To characterize a particular distribution within a family, the so-called parameters are needed. Parameters are quantities which, by taking different values, determine variations of the shape, the width and/or the position of the specific curve within the family. If we take the family of normal distributions as an example, there are two parameters: the mean, indicated by μ, and the variance, indicated by σ^2. By varying these, we can obtain the entire family of normal distributions. Likewise, to identify a specific distribution we only need to specify the values of μ and σ^2: μ defines the center of the distribution, therefore determines the position of the bell-shaped curve, while σ^2 defines the spread of the observations around the center, therefore determines the width of the bell. These concepts are shown in Figure 1.1. The normal distribution characterized by the pair of parameters $\mu=0$ and $\sigma^2=1$ is called **standard normal distribution** and its mathematical expression is $f(x) = \dfrac{1}{\sqrt{2\pi}}\exp\left(-\dfrac{x^2}{2}\right)$.

The family of binomial distributions also has two parameters: the number of tests, N, and the probability of a successful result, indicated by π. By changing these, we can obtain the entire family of binomial distributions, while to identify a specific distribution we need to specify the values of N and π.[1]

---

1. The binomial distribution has the following expression: $p(X=x) = \dbinom{N}{x}\pi^x(1-\pi)^{N-x}$ where, $\dbinom{N}{x} = \dfrac{N(N-1)(N-2)...1}{[x(x-1)....1][(N-x)(N-x-1)...1]}$, the so-called binomial coefficient, represents the number of different cases in which x successes can occur in N tests, that is, the number of groups of x successful outcomes that can be formed with N elements, so that each group differs from the other by at least one element. It is a distribution used in the medical field when dealing with dichotomous end-points (see section 5.4.2).

Whereas in the case of a discrete distribution, the probability of each value is represented by its level on the ordinate, in the case of a continuous distribution, the probability of each single value is always equal to zero. The ordinates of the probability density function are not probabilities, but probability densities. It is possible, though, to calculate the probability of sets of values included in a given interval, for example all of the values included between a given lower extreme, x_{inf} (inf = inferior) and upper extreme, x_{sup} (sup = superior). These probabilities are represented by the corresponding "area under the curve", delimited at the base by the section of the abscissa between x_{inf} and x_{sup}, at the sides by two vertical lines intersecting x_{inf} and x_{sup} and at the top by the segment of the probability curve included between the two vertical lines. In mathematics, the measure of this area is called an **integral**. For example, considering the standard normal curve shown in Figure 5.3, the area under the curve of the section between x_{inf} = -1.96 and x_{sup} = +1.96 is 0.95. This area represents the probability of the values included in the base of the area, namely of the values between –1.96 and +1.96.

In order to get an intuitive idea of why, in continuous distributions, the probabilities of the single values are zero, while those of the areas are measurable and different from zero, the reader can think of a density measurement in the medical field, for example the number of malignant cells per unit of tissue area. If the unit of tissue area considered is infinitesimal, the number of cells is zero; however, as soon as the unit of tissue area becomes different from zero, even if still very small, the number of cells counted can be different from zero. Something very similar happens with probability density.

Both for discrete and continuous distributions, the total area under the curve is 1, because the probability of the variable X assuming a value included in the interval of all of its possible values is 1 (100% of the probabilities).

For both kinds of probability distribution, knowledge of the mathematical expression of the curve makes it possible to calculate the areas of specific sections of the curve. As we will see later, this is of fundamental importance to performing statistical tests. In practice, instead of the mathematical expression of the curve, probability tables are often used containing pre-calculated areas for sections of interest. The probability table for the standard normal curve is enclosed in the appendix as an example. This table reports the areas included between the values of x_{inf} =0 and x_{sup}= any positive value up to 3.99. Using this table, we can find the areas included between any two values by taking advantage of the symmetry of the curve with respect to the zero value (because of this property, the area of half of the curve is 0.5 and any area between x_{inf} =0 and x_{sup} =+z is equal to the area between x_{inf} =-z and x_{sup} =0). For example, if we want to use this table to calculate the area included between the values of x_{inf} = -1.96 and x_{sup} = +1.96, we first find the value 1.96 by taking together the value 1.9 in the first column and the value 6 (the second decimal of interest) in the header. At the intersection of these two values, we find 0.475, which is the area included between x_{inf} =0 and x_{sup} = +1.96. The area that we are interested in can then be obtained by multiplying 0.475 by two (because of the symmetry of the normal curve, the area between $x_{inf} = -1.96$ and $x_{sup} = 0$ is equal to that between $x_{inf} = 0$ and $x_{sup} = +1.96$): the result is an area equal to 0.95.

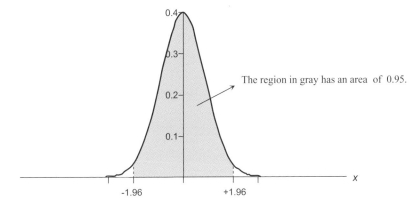

The region in gray has an area of 0.95.

Figure 5.3. Normal distribution with a mean of 0 and a standard deviation of 1 (standard normal curve)

For simplicity we will use the term probability distribution for both discrete and continuous distributions, except when doing so would cause confusion.

5.1.3. Normal or Gaussian Distribution

The reason why we have given so much attention to the normal distribution is that it is frequently used in the biomedical field. The reasons can be summarized as follows.

- Empirically, the distribution of many outcome variables in the biomedical field approximates the shape of this theoretical distribution. Examples of such variables include the levels of many substances in the blood (cholesterol, uric acid, etc.), systolic and diastolic blood pressure in the general population, body weight, walking distance on a treadmill with variable slope, and many more.
- In many other cases, even if the shape of the empirical distribution is not normal, it is possible to "normalize" it, that is to make it approximately normal, with simple transformations of the data, for example by applying a logarithmic transformation. Examples of such values are pain measured with a visual analog scale (VAS), walking distance assessed on a treadmill with fixed slope, etc.
- Finally, the theorem of central limit ensures that for large samples, whatever the distribution of the variable X, the distribution of the sample mean $\bar{X}$ (and consequently of the difference between the means of two independent samples) will tend to approximate the normal distribution, the more so the bigger the sample size.

The statistician should be the one to answer questions like "how large should a sample be to reasonably assume that the variable X or the sample mean $\bar{X}$ have a normal distribution?", because, unfortunately, there is no straightforward recipe one can apply. When the original variable X is not normally distributed, samples well over 100 may be required for the distribution of $\bar{X}$ to approximate a normal distribution.

Usually, the normal distribution is used to describe continuous variables with a symmetrical distribution, bell shaped, i.e. in which the observations have the same probability of being above or below the mean and a higher probability of being close to the mean than far from it.

It is important to point out that the normal distribution has a central role in statistics, in the sense that many techniques are based on this distribution. However, this does not mean that all methods of statistical analysis are based on the normal distribution. On the contrary, statistical analyses can be performed with many other kinds of distribution, although often more complex calculations are required.

5.2. Basic Concepts of Inference

Inference is a very broad area of statistics on which thousands of books and articles have been written. In section 2.1, we briefly defined it as the set of operations allowing conclusions made on a sample to be extended to the entire population from which the sample was taken.

The branch of statistics concerning the conditions under which this "jump" from sample to population is valid is called **inferential** or **inductive statistics**, as opposed to **descriptive statistics** which focuses on describing or summarizing a given group, without drawing conclusions on the underlying population.

We will start with an experiment in only ***one sample***, a single group of patients to whom the experimental treatment is administered. Generally, this kind of experiment is performed to assess the treatment effect expressed as a difference between before and after treatment (in chapter 8 we will discuss the limitations of such a choice). To simplify matters, we will use only two measurements to evaluate the effect of a compound on a hypothetical population affected by intermittent claudication: each patient will have the walking distance measured in a standardized way on a treadmill with variable slope, before the start and immediately after the end of treatment. The end-point is the difference between the measurement at the end of treatment and that at baseline. We shall indicate this end-point with X and assume that an appropriate group indicator for this end-point is the mean (see chapter 4). We indicate with μ the mean calculated on the whole hypothetical population of patients undergoing the treatment of interest. In the terminology of statistical inference, μ is a parameter. Since we cannot measure every unit constituting the population, we cannot truly "calculate" this mean. What we can do is "estimate" it, using a sample taken from the population. We are not interested in this sample as such. We are only interested in it insofar it allows us to estimate the result we would obtain if it were possible to perform the same experiment on the entire population.

To be able to extend the results observed on the sample to the underlying population, the former must be representative of the latter, that is, every type of subject (experimental unit) composing the population must be proportionally represented in the sample. The method generally used to obtain a representative sample is that of choosing the experimental units of the sample randomly from the population. This method ensures that any difference between the units included in the sample and those not included will only be due to chance; thus there will be no "systematic" difference between the two groups (see section 1.3.2) with respect to known and unknown factors, that could potentially be correlated with the object of the study, in our case the treadmill walking distance. One might wonder why it is necessary to randomly extract the experimental units from the population. If we were to proceed systematically, rather than randomly, we could make sure that every type of subject represented in the population is properly represented in the sample. The problem is that, to do so, we would need to know the composition of the population. But, since in most cases we do not know it, we cannot develop a rational method to ensure representativeness. Thus we delegate the task to chance, which is the best tool when there are unknown factors (we will come back to this topic in chapter 9, when we discuss randomization). Besides the sampling method, it is intuitive that the size of the sample must also play an important role. All other conditions being the same, the larger the sample relative to the population, the more likely it is that the units included in the sample are representative of all the units of the population.

It is equally intuitive that even in a very large and representative sample, we cannot expect to get exactly the same result for the chosen end-point that we would get in the whole population, if it were possible to evaluate all its units. Statistical inference must take into account this element of variability. In the example above, we estimate μ, the mean of the end-point X (where X = difference between walking distance at the end of the treatment and that at baseline) in the population of subjects treated with the compound of interest, by using the mean of the same end-point in the sample, which we indicated with $\bar{X}$. We cannot expect that in every sample $\bar{X}$ is identical to μ.

Before continuing, we must introduce the case of **two or more samples.** Inference problems with two or more samples are in fact much more frequent in clinical research than those with just one sample. In this context, inference problems often consist of verifying whether it is legitimate to extend to the underlying populations the difference in response observed between two or more groups (samples) of experimental units (patients or healthy volunteers), each undergoing a different treatment (in each group the response must be summarized by an appropriate group indicator such as the mean, the median, etc.).

Let us imagine that we want to compare k treatments, where k is greater than or equal to 2. If k identical populations affected by the disease of interest were available and we could treat all of the units in each of these populations with one of the k treatments, we would not need statistical inference. Having treated the k populations with the different treatments, we could measure the response in all of the units, summarize the observed results for each population with an appropriate statistical indicator, for example the mean of the response (if it is quantitative) or the proportion of a certain type of event (if the response is dichotomous) and finally numerically compare the values of these indicators. Assuming that the best response is the greatest one (as is the case with walking distance), the best treatment would be the one for which the value of the indicator is greater.

It is obvious however that, in the vast majority of cases, we cannot treat all of the units of the k populations. What we can do is to extract from each population a sample of units and observe the results at the end of the treatment. What is done, in practice, is to extract a sample from the overall population affected by the disease of interest and randomly assign (through randomization, see chapter 9) its units (subjects) to the k treatments of interest. From a methodological point of view, this is equivalent to considering k populations, each hypothetically treated with one of the treatments, and extracting from each one a sample for the study.

For simplicity, we will assume that there are only two groups to be compared and that the two treatments are an active compound (which we will indicate with A) and a placebo (which we will indicate with P). We will also assume that the end-point X is the walking distance measured at the end of the study, with mean equal to μ_A in the population treated with A and mean equal to μ_P in the population treated with P. We would like to be able to calculate μ_A and μ_P and ultimately the difference $\delta_\mu = \mu_A - \mu_P$, but since we cannot treat and measure the whole populations treatable with A and P, we measure the end-point X in each unit of the two samples and calculate the means of these measurements in each group. We indicate with $\bar{X}_A$ and $\bar{X}_P$ the means of the samples A and P respectively, and with them we attempt to estimate μ_A and μ_P.

As with one group it was unreasonable to expect that $\mu = \bar{X}$ in every sample, with two groups it is unreasonable to expect that $\mu_A = \bar{X}_A$ and $\mu_P = \bar{X}_P$ (or, equivalently, that $\mu_A - \mu_P = \bar{X}_A - \bar{X}_P$) for every pair of samples.

Using the terminology of statistical inference, the difference between the two population means ($\delta_\mu = \mu_A - \mu_P$), which expresses the true treatment effect, is the unknown quantity we must estimate. The difference between the sample means ($d_\mu = \bar{X}_A - \bar{X}_P$) is the **estimator** or **statistic** (in fact, it is one of the possible estimators of δ_μ). In clinical terms, we defined δ_μ as the signal (see chapter 4). The single value for d_μ observed in the sample, indicated with d_{obs}, is called the sample value of the statistic or the **estimate** of δ_μ.

In summary, parameters are indicated with Greek letters, estimators with lower-case letters (with the exception of the sample mean which is indicated with $\bar{X}$), while subscripts are used as an aid to the reader: for example, the symbol δ_μ reminds one that the population difference in question relates to means (i.e. $\mu_A - \mu_P$), while the symbol d_{obs} reminds that the difference is between "observed" values. Finally, by convention, the estimate of a parameter is indicated with the sign $\wedge$ above the letter indicating that parameter, therefore, in our case, we could use the symbol $\hat{\delta}_\mu$ to indicate the estimate of δ_μ. Therefore, using these conventions we have $\hat{\delta}_\mu = d_{obs}$.

To verify whether the observed difference in response between the two samples, each receiving a different treatment, can be extended to the underlying populations, we must answer the following questions:

1. Is the observed difference due to chance (seen as a set of accidental factors)?
2. If we accept that the difference is not due to chance, is it really caused by the treatments?
3. If we accept that the difference is caused by the treatments, is it clinically relevant?

One must refer to the **theory of hypothesis testing** to answer question 1 and to the **estimation theory** to answer question 3, whereas question 2 cannot be answered using statistical methods. Indeed, the possibility exists that the observed difference, even if not due to chance, is not due to the treatments, but to a bias, i.e. to a repeated, systematic error which always occurs in the same direction and consequently always favors the same group, independently of the treatment (see chapter 1). Statistical methods can only give some indication regarding the presence of bias, but cannot answer question 2 in a definitive way (see also section 9.1). A more complete and reliable answer to this question can only be given through a correct planning and conduct of the study: only in this way can one be reasonably certain that the observed result is not affected by bias.

Statistical inference encompasses both the problem of hypothesis verification and that of estimation, and it cannot be separated from the planning of the study.

5.2.1. Hypothesis Testing and Statistical Formulation of the Medical Question

The traditional instrument for **hypothesis testing** is the statistical test.

The reasoning behind hypothesis testing starts with the formulation of the so-called **null hypothesis** on the difference between the two treatments under study. Typically, the null hypothesis represents the opposite of what we are hoping to demonstrate with the experiment. The reason for this will be clarified later (see section 5.5.1). Going back to the example of walking distance, where we hope to demonstrate that μ_A is greater than μ_P (i.e. that the active compound induces an improvement in walking distance compared to placebo), the null hypothesis (identified with H_0) is:

$$H_0 : \mu_A = \mu_P$$

or, expressed in terms of the difference between μ_A and μ_P (that is, in terms of δ_μ):

$$H_0 : \delta_\mu = 0$$

In other words, the null hypothesis states that there is no difference between the mean effect of A and that of P on the walking distance measured at the end of the treatment, that is to say that A is an ineffective treatment.

The so-called **alternative hypothesis** (H_1) is formulated to complement the null hypothesis, so that if one is not true, the other must be.

The alternative hypothesis can be one of two types. If one assumes that the presumed active treatment can be either better or worse than the placebo, both possibilities must be considered in the alternative hypothesis. In this case the alternative hypothesis is:

$$H_1 : \ \delta_\mu \neq 0$$

This hypothesis is called **bidirectional**.

If instead, one does not admit that the presumed active treatment could be worse than the placebo, the alternative hypothesis in our example becomes:

$$H_1 : \ \delta_\mu > 0$$

This hypothesis is called **unidirectional**. Note that in this case the entire part of the scale which includes values less than or equal to zero favors the null hypothesis and goes against the alternative hypothesis.

Naturally, in a different situation superiority of the active treatment over placebo can be translated into a mean value for the active treatment that is less than that of the placebo (for example, blood pressure for an antihypertension treatment must decrease). In this case the alternative hypothesis becomes:

$$H_1 : \ \delta_\mu < 0$$

In clinical trials, even when the comparison is made with a placebo, it is generally necessary to allow not only for the possibility that the new treatment is efficacious (that is, better than the placebo), but also for the possibility that the new treatment causes more harm than good (that is, it is actually worse than the placebo). Therefore, in general, the alternative hypothesis must be bidirectional. This approach is almost always required by the regulatory authorities for phase III pivotal studies (see chapter 12). The need for a bidirectional alternative hypothesis is intuitive when both treatments under comparison are presumed to be active, less so when the control group is treated with a placebo. For example, let's assume that the experimental treatment is a new antibiotic against urinary tract infections and the end-point of the study is the number of bacteria per mL of urine in a sample obtained at the end of the treatment. It is certainly unlikely that the new antibiotic will increase the concentration of bacteria compared to placebo. Therefore one would be inclined to consider the unidirectional hypothesis acceptable. However, the possibility that the experimental treatment turns out to be worse than placebo does exist. The experimental treatment could create conditions that favor bacterial growth, for example, by reducing bladder motility and consequently inducing urine retention, which in turn could enhance bacterial growth. Therefore, even in this case, the bidirectional alternative hypothesis seems to be the more prudent approach.

We have dwelled on this issue because it has many practical repercussions. As will be discussed in chapter 6, the test for a bidirectional alternative hypothesis is more conservative in statistical terms than the test for the corresponding unidirectional hypothesis, assuming all other conditions are equivalent. Very briefly, "more conservative" means either that more patients are needed if we want to have the same degree of certainty of being able to demonstrate a difference between the treatments when it exists, or that, with the same number of patients, we must accept a lower degree of certainty. It is for this reason that the researcher, almost inevitably convinced of the superiority of one of the treatments under comparison, is often strongly tempted to use a unidirectional alternative hypothesis. Unfortunately, we must say it once more, surprises in the field of clinical research are frequent. Therefore, it is almost always preferable, no matter how inconvenient, to perform tests with bidirectional alternative hypotheses.

In summary, a typical system of bidirectional hypotheses in clinical trials is the following:

$$H_0 : \quad \delta_\mu = 0 \text{ (null hypothesis)}$$

$$(5.1)$$

$$H_1 : \quad \delta_\mu \neq 0 \text{ (alternative hypothesis)}.$$

To simplify our example, we will use the unidirectional alternative hypotheses system:

$$H_0 : \quad \delta_\mu = 0 \text{ (null hypothesis)}$$

$$(5.2)$$

$$H_1 : \quad \delta_\mu > 0 \text{ (alternative hypothesis)}.$$

In this case, the entire part of the scale which includes values less than or equal to zero favors the null hypothesis and is against the alternative hypothesis. This is equivalent to saying that we consider $H_0 : \quad \delta_\mu \leq 0$. However, for operational purposes it is sufficient to consider that the null hypotheses is $\delta_\mu = 0$.

We will see in sections 5.5.1 and 5.6.1 how to test these hypotheses with the frequentist and the Bayesian approaches, respectively.

5.2.2. *Statistical Estimation as the Tool for Evaluation of Clinical Relevance*

As was stated above, the conclusion that a difference between treatments is not due to chance (as determined by the statistical test) and that it is due truly to the treatments (i.e. not to bias) does not necessarily imply that such difference is clinically relevant. Indeed it is possible that the result of a study is judged as not due to chance, thanks to an appropriate statistical test (answer "no" to question 1 of section 5.2) and as truly due to the experimental treatment, thanks to a sound design and conduct of the study (answer "yes" to question 2), but nevertheless such result is judged as clinically irrelevant (answer "no" to question 3). In chapter 4, we have seen that it is necessary to define, during the planning phase of the study, the threshold of clinical relevance, that is, the minimum difference between treatments that can be considered clinically relevant. As we will see in chapter 6, this value is used to calculate the minimum number of subjects required to reject the null hypothesis in the presence of a difference between treatments equal to or greater than the threshold of clinical relevance.

Once we have demonstrated at the end of the study that the observed difference between the treatments is not due to chance, how do we know if the difference is clinically relevant or not? The answer to this question is in two steps: first, one needs to determine how large the observed difference between the treatments is, and then judge whether this is relevant.

The **estimation** theory is instrumental in addressing the first step: "how large is the observed difference between the treatments?" It is a matter of estimating $\delta_\mu = \mu_A - \mu_P$.

As we said, the value of $d_\mu = \bar{X}_A - \bar{X}_P$ in the observed sample is called estimate of δ_μ or, more precisely, **point estimate** of δ_μ, meaning that it is the "best suggestion" for the value of the unknown quantity δ_μ that we wish to estimate. To complement to the point estimate, of great interest is the **interval estimate**, which gives us a range of possible values for the quantity to be estimated. It is intuitive that such interval includes the corresponding point estimate and that the narrower the interval around the point estimate, the better (i.e. it can replace the interval estimate). In other words, the width of the interval is related with the precision of the estimate (see section 1.3.2).

Once the difference is estimated, we must decide if it is clinically relevant. The one approach we must not take is the following: conduct a simple numerical comparison between the point estimate obtained in the study and the predefined minimum clinically relevant difference; then reject the efficacy of the new treatment if the former is numerically worse than the latter (in our example of walking distance, worse equals shorter distance walked) (see [20] and [75]). The reason why such an approach is wrong is that it does not take into account the variability of the point estimate. In fact, the issue is quite controversial, going beyond the purpose of this book. The most frequently used approach is that of basing the decisions concerning clinical relevance on the interval estimate.

In sections 5.5.2 and 5.6.2 we will see how the estimates of the treatment effect are obtained with the frequentist and Bayesian approaches respectively.

5.3. Statistical Inference in the Frequentist and the Bayesian Approaches

In statistics, two main inference methods exist: the frequentist one, based on the frequentist definition of probability and the Bayesian one based on the subjective definition of probability (see section 5.1). It should be noted that in both camps a variety of approaches exist, ranging from the purist stand to positions bordering on the opposite side. Therefore, the reader must be aware that what we are presenting here is a hyper-simplification of the two approaches.

In the **frequentist approach** the inspiring principle is that of repeated sampling, which assumes that the experiment is repeated an infinite number of times under identical conditions. The statistical procedures are evaluated with reference to this hypothetical series of repetitions of each experiment, during which it is assumed that the conditions are unchanged, including the effect of the treatment under study. This treatment effect is the unknown parameter (see section 1.3.1) to be estimated, which is considered a fixed quantity (mathematical constant) throughout the hypothetical repetition of the experiment.

With this approach, the results from the sample, which once observed are fixed, are summarized into a suitable estimator. The value that this estimator takes in the sample we studied is treated as one of the possible results that could be obtained in the hypothetical, infinite repetition of experiments, all identical to the one actually performed. Therefore, the estimator used to summarize the observed sample results is given a probability distribution (called sample distribution of the estimator - see section 5.5.1), expressing the uncertainty relative to the values that the estimator can assume with different samples. Vice versa, the unknown parameter, even though uncertain (because unknown), is not given a probability distribution, since its true value, although unknown, is considered fixed.

Going back to the hypothesis systems (5.1) and (5.2), in the frequentist approach, δ_μ represents the "true" difference between the two treatments, which is the unknown parameter of interest, seen as a fixed quantity, while d_μ represents the estimator of the true effect and is seen as a quantity that varies with each different sample, i.e. a random variable with its own probability distribution.

Example. Let us return to the example of the distance walked by patients with intermittent claudication to illustrate the frequentist reasoning described above. The researcher randomly extracts a sample of n_A patients from the population of patients treated with A and a sample of n_P patients from the population of patients treated with P (or randomly extracts a sample of $n_A + n_P$ subjects from the population of untreated patients with intermittent claudication and then randomly assigns them to A or P - the two procedures are analogous from a probabilistic point of view).

Once the sample is obtained (we shall call it sample number 1), the researcher measures the walking distance in each of the patients treated with A and with P, each time rigorously adhering to the conditions of the experiment. These values are metaphorically extracted from the (theoretical) underlying populations of walking distances of all patients with intermittent claudication treated with A and of all those treated with P.

From sample 1 the researcher obtains a mean $\bar{X}_{obs\_A\_1}$ for the group A and a mean $\bar{X}_{obs\_P\_1}$ for the group P, with a difference d_{obs_1}. This result is seen as one of the possible outcomes of the variable d_μ, namely the outcome obtained in experiment 1. The result is treated in the theoretical context in which the experiment is repeated an infinite number of times, that is, imagining that at the end of the first experiment, a second experiment (on sample number 2) is performed under identical conditions, with identical sample size, obtaining as a result the difference between $\bar{X}_{obs\_A\_2}$ and $\bar{X}_{obs\_P\_2}$, equal to d_{obs_2}. Proceeding in the same way, one can imagine obtaining a series of values d_{obs_3}, d_{obs_4}, d_{obs_5}... that continues in a hypothetical series of identical experiments until a very large number - which can be approximated to infinite - of differences d_{obs} between $\bar{X}_A$ and $\bar{X}_B$ is reached (all of the possible outcomes of d_μ). Each of these differences d_{obs} is an estimate of δ_μ and, in general, will differ from the other estimates. However, all the possible estimates will be distributed around the value of the true mean difference d_μ, which could be calculated if it were possible to observe the entire population.

All of the hypothetical results obtained for d_μ can therefore be "described" by its probability distribution, also referred to as "sample distribution" of d_μ (because it is generated from the variation of the hypothetical samples), which has mean δ_μ (we will return to this topic in section 5.5.1).

In our example, we started from the difference of means and then we obtained the sample distribution of the difference of means. Naturally, we can also build a sample distribution of the differences of medians, modes, etcetera. The challenge is to find the mathematical expression (function) describing this probability distribution. A very important probabilistic property is that, when the distribution of the end-point is normal, the sample distribution of the difference of means is also normal and has properties that are crucial for performing statistical tests with the frequentist approach (see Table 5.7 and section 5.1).

The inspiring principle of the **Bayesian approach** is that all unknown quantities can be assigned a probability. In other words, every type of uncertainty can be represented in probabilistic terms. In this approach, probability is not an objective property of the events (simply stated, it is not obtained from their relative frequency) as for the frequentist approach, rather it is the expression of an evaluation of the event made by the researcher on the basis of the information available to him/her.

In the Bayesian approach there are two phases in each experiment: the pre-experimental one (*a priori*), where the results have not yet been obtained, and the post-experimental one (*a posteriori*), where the results are available. In the pre-experimental phase, the inference method based on the Bayesian approach requires that both the unknown parameter (i.e. the true effect of the treatment) and the set of all possible sample results, unknown *a priori*, be treated as random variables and therefore be given their own probability distribution. The probability distribution of the parameter is called "*a priori* distribution". In the post-experimental phase, the sample result, summarized by an appropriate group indicator, is not considered the outcome of a random variable, since there are no more elements of uncertainty associated with it (in the Bayesian approach there is no such thing as repeated sampling). Instead, the unknown parameter, for the very reason it is unknown, continues to be considered a random variable, with its own probability distribution. This will be different from the *a priori* one, since it will have been modified by the information obtained from the experiment just performed. It is called "*a posteriori* distribution" of the parameter (see section 5.6.1). Bayesian scientists use this distribution to test the hypothesis under study and to estimate the unknown parameters.

Returning again to the hypothesis systems (5.1) and (5.2), in the Bayesian approach, δ_μ expresses, as in the frequentist one, the "true" difference between the two treatments. However, since δ_μ is unknown, it is also uncertain and therefore, differently from the frequentists, it is considered a random variable. Vice versa, the sample estimator d_μ is a known quantity once the results of the samples are observed, and therefore is fixed.

Example. We are back to the example of the walking distance covered by patients with intermittent claudication. The parameter δ_μ is the (unknown) difference between the mean walking distances in the populations treated with A and P, respectively. Before performing the experiment, the researcher defines the *a priori* probability distribution of δ_μ, which expresses the degree of uncertainty about this parameter in the pre-experimental phase, taking into account all of the knowledge available up to that moment on δ_μ. Then, the researcher performs the experiment and obtains a sample result, that is, a set of $n_A + n_P$ observations, with mean $\bar{X}_{obs\_A}$ in the group treated with A and mean $\bar{X}_{obs\_P}$ in the group treated with P, and with difference d_{obs} between these means. The sample result is considered known, while what is still unknown, therefore uncertain, is the parameter δ_μ. However, this uncertainty is modified by the result of the experiment compared to what was known *a priori* and it is expressed by a new probability distribution, the *a posteriori* one.

Historically, in the field of biomedical research the frequentist approach has taken a much stronger foothold than the Bayesian approach. Only recently has the Bayesian approach started to appear in medical publications, offering a solution to specific problems of applied methodology that had no convincing solution within the frequentist approach. Nevertheless, the Bayesian methods are today mostly limited to the analysis of phase I and phase II studies (see chapter 12), because they are generally not accepted by the regulatory authorities for the analysis of phase III pivotal studies. However, there are many signs suggesting that health authorities will be more open to Bayesian methods in confirmatory studies in the future (see for example FDA Draft Guidance for the use of Bayesian Statistics in Medical Device Clinical Trials, in www.fda.gov).

Because of the pragmatic approach of this book, in most cases we base our discussion on the frequentist approach.

5.4. Two Digressions: Measures of Variability and Likelihood Function

5.4.1. Measures of Variability

As repeatedly stated, the root problem of biomedical research is that observations are affected by variability. As a consequence, conclusions must be drawn under conditions of uncertainty. Even though variability has a central role in the planning, analysis and interpretation of the results of biomedical studies, in this chapter we are rather vague about the statistical methods for dealing with it, both in hypothesis testing and in estimation. We have taken this approach to simplify the discussion, since we have chosen to favor logical aspects over computational ones.

Nevertheless, some clarification on the most common measures of variability is essential, not least because medical publications are often confusing in this area.

The variability of the observations can be expressed by different indicators, depending on the shape of the probability distribution of the end-point of interest.

- For distributions symmetrical with respect to the mean, including the normal distribution, the most frequently used indicators are the **variance** and the **standard deviation (SD)**.
- For distributions asymmetrical with respect to the mean, the **distance between percentiles** is generally used, for example that between the 25th percentile (also called the first **quartile**) and the 75th one (also called the third quartile).

As we will see below, the **standard error (SE)** does not quantify the variability of the observations. However, it is often erroneously used for this purpose.

These measures of variability can be applied to the population and to the sample. Table 5.2 illustrates the formulas for calculating these indicators and for each gives a brief explanation.

Experimental data are often summarized by a pair of values: a measure of the central tendency (for example, mean, median, mode) and a measure of variability (for example, standard deviation, distance between percentiles). When data come from a symmetrical distribution, they are generally summarized in terms of $mean \pm SD$ (SD has the same order of magnitude of the observations, while σ^2 has an order of magnitude equal to the square of the observations). Unfortunately these data are often erroneously summarized in terms of $mean \pm SE$ (see below). When the data come from an asymmetrical distribution, they are generally summarized in terms of median and distance between the 25th and 75th percentile. In this case, the median is often preferred to the mean because the median is not affected by extreme values, which in asymmetrical distributions tend to predominate in one of the two tails. In other words, for asymmetrical distributions, the median is a better measure of central tendency than the mean.

Table 5.2. Indicators of variability of a random variable (the sign ∧ indicates sample estimate)

Indicator	Population size = N, where N can be ∞	Sample size= n (subjects extracted from the N subjects of the population)	Explanation
Variance	***Discrete Variables:*** $$\sigma^2 = \frac{\sum_{i=1}^{N}(x_i - \mu)^2}{N}$$ (where x_i, which takes a different value with each value of the subscript i, indicates the N values of X in the population)	$$\hat{\sigma}^2 = \frac{\sum_{i=1}^{n}(x_i - \overline{X})^2}{(n-1)}$$ (where x_i, which takes a different value with each value of the subscript i, indicates the n values of the sample)	The variance of a discrete random variable is calculated starting from the sum of the squares of the differences between each observation and the mean. This sum is then divided by the number of units (N) in the case of the population or by the number of unit minus one (n-1) in the case of the sample. The denominator (n-1) is used instead of n to obtain an estimator with better statistical properties.
	Continuous Variables: the calculation uses the integral and is based on the density function		The variance of a continuous random variable in the population has the same meaning as that of a discrete random variable but it is calculated with the integral, based on the density function of the variable of interest.
Standard Deviation	$\sqrt{\sigma^2} = \sigma$	$\sqrt{\hat{\sigma}^2} = \hat{\sigma}$	The standard deviation is the square root of the variance. The standard deviation of the sample is often indicated with S, instead of $\hat{\sigma}$.
Distance between the 25ᵗʰ and 75ᵗʰ percentile	$P_{75} - P_{25}$	$\hat{P}_{75} - \hat{P}_{25}$	The **percentiles** are the values dividing the ordered sequence of values of a random variable from the smallest (extreme left of the horizontal axis) to the largest (extreme right of the horizontal axis) into 100 equal parts. Therefore, for example, the 25ᵗʰ percentile is the value that has 25% of the ordered values to its left.
Standard Error of the sample mean		$\dfrac{\hat{\sigma}}{\sqrt{n}}$	$SE = \sigma/\sqrt{n}$ is the standard deviation of the probability distribution of the sample mean, calculated on an infinite number of repeated samples, each of n observations. It is not an indicator of the population, therefore it has been omitted from the second column.

With regard to the standard deviation, when the observations have an approximately normal distribution, about 68% of the observations are included in the interval *mean ± 1 SD* and about 95% are included in the interval *mean ± 2 SD*. For example, if we have a normally distributed variable from which we extract a sample of $n=16$ subjects and obtain $\hat{\mu} = \overline{X} = 100$ and $\hat{SD} = 50$, about 95% of the observations are included in the interval 0 to 200.

The standard error of the sample mean (SE) does not quantify the variability of the observations but rather the precision with which the sample mean estimates the true mean of the population. SE is in fact the standard deviation of the probability distribution of the sample mean. Therefore, assuming that the sample distribution of the mean is normal, the expression *mean ± 1 SE* tells us that there is about a 68% probability that the real mean of the population from which the sample was extracted will fall within this interval, and this probability increases to about 95% for the interval *mean ± 2 SE*. As we will see in section 5.5.2, the intervals *mean ± 1 SE*, *mean ± 2 SE*, ... are called confidence intervals of the mean, at different confidence levels. In the previous example, $\hat{SE} = 50/\sqrt{16} = 12.5$. Therefore the 95% confidence interval of the mean is 75 – 125, often written as (75; 125) (see section 5.5.2).

In conclusion, *SD* must be used to summarize the observed data, not *SE*. *SE* is used more frequently than *SD* because it is much smaller, thus it makes the data look less variable. Clearly this approach is misleading and exploits the fact that many scientists confuse *SD* with *SE*.

To avoid confusion, we suggest that data be summarized by indicating *mean, SD* or *mean (SD)*. The ± sign should not be used in this context, rather it should be reserved for the confidence interval of the mean (see again section 5.5.2).

We need to make one more step before the end of this digression. So far, we have only considered the case of one population and one sample, whereas in the rest of the chapter we discuss the case of difference between means, which implies two populations and two samples. What was stated above concerning SD and SE is also valid in the case of two samples from two populations, but obviously the formulas must be modified. These modifications are shown in Table 5.3, in which it is assumed that the two random variables have the same variance. The assumption of equal variance in the underlying populations is called **homoscedasticity.** It is commonly assumed in statistical tests, mainly by the frequentists.

In clinical experiments, the interest of the researcher almost always focuses on the treatment effect, quantified in terms of mean, median, mode or other parameter of central tendency. In this context variability is a **disturbance** or a **nuisance parameter** in the sense that the conclusion on the parameter of interest is hindered by the presence of this second unknown parameter. However, this parameter is necessary for the statistical formulation of the problem to reflect reality.

Table 5.3. Indicators of variability of the difference between two independent random variables with identical variance σ^2 (the symbol $\wedge$ indicates sample estimate)

Indicator	Two populations A and P (*)	Two samples A and P (*) (sample sizes n_A and n_P)	Explanation
Variance	$2\sigma^2$	$2\hat{\sigma}^2$ where: $\hat{\sigma}^2 = \dfrac{(n_A-1)\hat{\sigma}_A^2 + (n_P-1)\hat{\sigma}_P^2}{(n_A + n_P - 2)}$	Given two independent random variables, their difference is itself a random variable, with variance equal to the sum of the variances of the two initial variables, i.e. equal to $2\sigma^2$ if these variables have equal variance. Under this assumption, each of the two samples generates an estimate of σ^2 and the best estimate of this parameter is the weighted mean of the two estimates, where the weights are the respective sample sizes minus 1 (see table 5.2).
Standard deviation	$\sqrt{2\sigma^2} = \sigma\sqrt{2}$	$\sqrt{2\hat{\sigma}^2} = \hat{\sigma}\sqrt{2}$ where: $\hat{\sigma} = \sqrt{\dfrac{(n_A-1)\hat{\sigma}_A^2 + (n_P-1)\hat{\sigma}_P^2}{(n_A + n_P - 2)}}$	The standard deviation is the square root of the variance.
Distance between the 25th and 75th percentile	$P_{75} - P_{25}$	$\hat{P}_{75} - \hat{P}_{25}$	The percentiles are the values dividing the sequence of ordered differences between the two random variables into 100 equal parts. To obtain the sample estimate, the differences between all possible pairs of values observed in the two treatments must be calculated and then ordered from the smallest to the greatest. The percentiles are calculated on these ordered differences.
Standard error of difference between two sample means	$\sqrt{\left(\dfrac{\hat{\sigma}^2}{n_A} + \dfrac{\hat{\sigma}^2}{n_P}\right)} = \hat{\sigma}\sqrt{\dfrac{(n_A+n_P)}{n_A \times n_P}}$ where: $\hat{\sigma} = \sqrt{\dfrac{(n_A-1)\hat{\sigma}_A^2 + (n_P-1)\hat{\sigma}_P^2}{(n_A + n_P - 2)}}$	$SE = \sqrt{\left(\dfrac{\sigma^2}{n_A} + \dfrac{\sigma^2}{n_P}\right)}$ is the standard deviation of the probability distribution of the difference between two sample means, calculated on pairs of independent samples, each of n_A and n_P observations, coming from two populations. It is not an indicator of the difference of two populations, therefore it has been omitted from the second column.

(*) From a methodological point of view, extracting a sample from the untreated population and randomly assigning its units to two treatments A and P is equivalent to considering two independent populations, each hypothetically treated with A or with P and extracting from each population a sample for the study. Therefore the difference between two random variables can be referred to both one population and two populations.

5.4.2. Likelihood Function

The likelihood function is an inferential instrument used by both frequentists and Bayesians. In this book, we will only use it for the Bayesian approach. However, we decided to introduce it at this point to avoid it being considered as an instrument used exclusively by the Bayesians.

We shall start with the easier case of a discrete end-point. Let us consider a given end-point having a given probability distribution. Before the study is carried out, the results for the units of the sample are unknown, i.e. random variables and, therefore, each of them has a probability distribution, which is the probability distribution of the end-point. If we consider the entire sample as the set of n random variables, it will also have its own probability distribution. Before the study is carried out, the probability distribution of the end-point is a function of both the unknown parameter and the possible *a priori* results for the sample. Once the study is conducted and the results (i.e. the values of each unit of the sample) are known, the probability distribution of the end-point remains a function of the unknown parameter only. This function, called **likelihood function**, often indicated with $L(parameter)$, is not a true probability distribution but it is similar to one. It expresses the probability that existed *a priori* (i.e. before carrying out the study) of selecting the sample values that were actually observed in the study: depending on the unknown value of the parameter, there is a different probability of actually observing in the study the same given set of values. The concept can also be expressed in reversed terms: the likelihood function expresses the likelihood of the different values of the parameter, given the result obtained in the experiment. Hence the name likelihood function. The values that it can assume can be interpreted as a system of weights, expressing the degree of agreement between each possible value of the parameter and the empirical observation. Since these are weights, what counts are the ratios, not the absolute values. Assuming we want to attribute a relative preference to two values of the unknown parameter, say v_1 and v_2, this preference is determined by the ratio of the likelihoods $L(v_1)/Lv_2)$ (we shall assume that the denominator is not equal to zero).

Since the likelihood ratio does not change if both terms are multiplied by the same constant, assuming the constant is positive and independent of the parameter, what matters in comparing different values of the parameter is the likelihood function, whatever the multiplicative constant. It should be noted that, even if every value of $L(parameter)$ is characterized by a probability distribution, the likelihood function itself is not a probability distribution, because it does not change with changes of this multiplicative constant, which is independent on the parameter (i.e. the area under the curve of the likelihood function is not necessarily equal to 1).

Let us try to clarify this concept with an example. A new treatment can have a positive effect (*success*) or a negative effect (*failure*). The end-point X in this case is a dichotomous variable. We shall assign the value 1 to each *success* and the value 0 to each *failure*. The probability of the treatment being a *success* in a single patient, which we will indicate with π, is the unknown parameter on which the interest of the researcher is focused. It can be seen as the proportion of *successes* in the hypothetical population of all patients receiving the new treatment. If the probability of a *success* is π, then the probability of a *failure* is ($1-\pi$). To estimate π, this treatment is tested on n patients. For simplicity let us assume $n=4$ (such a small sample is used just to simplify the example: it is obviously an under-sized experiment!). With this assumption, the sample result is given by the set of four values (x_1, x_2, x_3, x_4), each of which can be 1 (*success*) or 0 (*failure*). To indicate the total number of *successes* in the four subjects of the sample we can use the notation $\sum_{i=1}^{4} x_i$ (where the symbol $\sum$ means sum), which can take values 0, 1, 2, 3, 4. The number of *failures* will be given by $4 - \sum_{i=1}^{4} x_i$. The probability of obtaining $\sum_{i=1}^{4} x_i$ *successes* in four tests, i.e. in the four subjects, is given by:

$$P(x) = \binom{4}{\sum_{i=1}^{4} x_i} \pi^{\sum_{i=1}^{4} x_i} (1-\pi)^{(4-\sum_{i=1}^{4} x_i)}$$

This is the binomial probability distribution, introduced in section 5.1.2 (see note 1)

In Table 5.4 all of the possible results of our experiment on four patients are listed, while only some of the possible values of π (each representing a hypothesis) are indicated, namely $\pi = 0.25$, $\pi = 0.50$ and $\pi = 0.75$.

The probabilities reported in Table 5.4 have been calculated assuming that the probability of a *success* is π and that of a *failure* is ($1 - \pi$), and that the tests on the subjects are independent of one another. With these assumptions, the probability of obtaining $\sum_{i=1}^{4} x_i$ *successes* and $4 - \sum_{i=1}^{4} x_i$ *failures* is obtained by multiplying their respective probabilities[2] (the formula $\pi^{\sum_{i=1}^{4} x_i} (1-\pi)^{(4-\sum_{i=1}^{4} x_i)}$ was used).

---

2. Given two independent events E1 and E2 (i.e. the knowledge of the event E1 does not change the probability of the event E2, and vice versa), the probability of both events occurring is given by the product of the probabilities of each event occurring.

Table 5.4. All possible experimental results and some possible values of π for an experiment with a binary end-point on $n = 4$ patients

All possible results	Number of successes	Probability of the result if:		
(x_1, x_2, x_3, x_4)	$\sum_{i=1}^{4} x_i$	$\pi = 0.25$	$\pi = 0.50$	$\pi = 0.75$
0 0 0 0	0	0.3164	0.0625	0.0039
0 0 0 1	1	0.1055	0.0625	0.0117
0 0 1 0	1	0.1055	0.0625	0.0117
0 1 0 0	1	0.1055	0.0625	0.0117
1 0 0 0	1	0.1055	0.0625	0.0117
0 0 1 1	2	0.0352	0.0625	0.0352
0 1 0 1	2	0.0352	0.0625	0.0352
0 1 1 0	2	0.0352	0.0625	0.0352
1 0 0 1	2	0.0352	0.0625	0.0352
1 0 1 0	2	0.0352	0.0625	0.0352
1 1 0 0	2	0.0352	0.0625	0.0352
0 1 1 1	3	0.0117	0.0625	0.1055
1 0 1 1	3	0.0117	0.0625	0.1055
1 1 0 1	3	0.0117	0.0625	0.1055
1 1 1 0	3	0.0117	0.0625	0.1055
1 1 1 1	4	0.0039	0.0625	0.3164
Total	1.0000	1.0000	1.0000	1.0000

These data can be summarized as shown in Table 5.5 by grouping the results leading to the same number of *successes* and summing the corresponding probabilities[3].

In summary, Table 5.5 (and likewise table 5.4) illustrates how the binomial probability distribution described above changes with all possible *a priori* results and some values of π (as said, for simplicity only few are presented).

We have now completed the experiment. The values of x_1, x_2, x_3, x_4 become known, therefore constant. Therefore, the distribution illustrated in Tables 5.4 and 5.5 is a function of the parameter π only. In other words, once the experiment is performed, one row in the table is "chosen" i.e. becomes fixed and the function represented in it can vary only relative to the columns, that is, relative to π. What we obtained is the likelihood function for our experiment. Let us indicate it with $L(\pi)$ to highlight that it is a function of the parameter π.

---

3. The probabilities listed in table 5.5 can be obtained directly by using the entire expression of the binomial distribution. The binomial coefficient $\binom{4}{\sum x}$ represents the number of different ways in which $\sum_{i=1}^{4} x_i$ *successes* can occur in four tests. For example, with four tests there are six different ways to obtain the result "2 *successes*" and the binomial coefficient is $\binom{4}{2} = \dfrac{4 \times 3 \times 2}{2 \times 2} = 6$.

Table 5.5. Summary version of Table 5.4 obtained by grouping the results with the same number of *successes* (*)

Number of successes	Probability of the result if:		
$\sum_{i=1}^{4} x_i$	$\pi = 0.25$	$\pi = 0.50$	$\pi = 0.75$
0	0.3164	0.0625	0.0039
1	0.4219	0.2500	0.0469
2	0.2109	0.3750	0.2109
3	0.0469	0.2500	0.4219
4	0.0039	0.0625	0.3164
Total	1.0000	1.0000	1.0000

(*) See also note 3. The apparent inconsistencies between this table and Table 5.4 are due to rounding

Assuming, for example that we have performed the experiment and obtained the result (1, 0, 0, 1), that is, two *successes* and two *failures*, the likelihood function is:

$$L(\pi) = \binom{4}{2} \pi^2 (1-\pi)^2$$

The values of this function (illustrated in the row of Table 5.5 corresponding to the result "2 *successes*") can be interpreted as follows: 0.2109 is the likelihood of the value 0.25 of the parameter, indicating that, if the value of the parameter was 0.25, before starting the experiment we would have had a probability of about 20% (precisely 0.2109) of obtaining the result we actually obtained. The other values can be interpreted in the same way.

We now move on to estimating π. Common sense would tell us to estimate the proportion of *successes* in the population with the proportion of *successes* observed in the sample, that is with $p = \sum_{i=1}^{4} x_i / 4$, which in our experiment is 2/4=0.5. Let us forget this solution for a moment and use the likelihood function as an instrument to estimate π.

A "reasonable" value of π appears to be the one for which the likelihood function is greatest. Indeed, choosing the value of $\hat{\pi}$ for which $L(\pi)$ is maximum to estimate π is the same as choosing the hypothetical value of the population which, in the pre-experimental phase, would have generated the observed sample with the highest probability. The value $\hat{\pi}$ for which $L(\pi)$ is maximum is called the **maximum likelihood estimate** of π. This estimate is obtained with a mathematical procedure for the maximization of functions (the mathematical calculus is carried out through the so-called derivatives). Applying this method to our experiment, we obtain $\hat{\pi} = 0.50$. Note that the maximum likelihood estimate of π is the observed frequency of successes, that is, it coincides with the solution suggested by common sense (that of estimating a parameter with the corresponding sample indicator). Such correspondence between the maximum likelihood estimate and the estimate of common sense occurs often, but not always.

So far the frequentist and Bayesian approaches do not differ. However, the manner in which the frequentists and Bayesians employ the likelihood function to conduct the inferential analysis is different. It is clear that the inferential analysis cannot finish in this way: the estimate $\hat{\pi}$ will never be identical to the true value of π; therefore it is necessary to accompany $\hat{\pi}$ with an interval estimate. Furthermore, once a value for π (or an interval of values) has been hypothesized, it is necessary to proceed with the hypothesis testing, which allows us to find out whether the difference between the estimated value and the hypothesized value can be explained by chance or not. The likelihood function is used to this end differently in the two approaches.

Bayesians, when faced with the result (1,0,0,1), will consider only the corresponding row of Table 5.5 (or 5.4). Thus, they will only use the likelihood function for the observed sample to perform all of the inferences on the parameter. The Bayesian approach is a so-called **conditional approach**, because the inferential reasoning is conditioned to the result of the experiment.

On the contrary, frequentists base their approach on the principle of **repeated sampling**, i.e. they see the estimates as outcomes of random variables, which vary with every possible result *a priori*. When faced with the same result (1,0,0,1,) and once the maximum likelihood estimate $\hat{\pi} = 0.50$ is obtained, the frequentists ask themselves how this estimate changes as the possible samples change. It is clear that different sample results would have led to different likelihood functions. Therefore, the likelihood function is considered a function not only of π but also of X. Once this function is maximized with respect to π, the maximum likelihood estimate remains a function of X only. In the example, the

likelihood function is $L(\pi, x) = \begin{pmatrix} 4 \\ \sum_{i=1}^{4} x_i \end{pmatrix} \pi^{\sum_{i=1}^{4} x_i} (1 - \pi)^{(4 - \sum_{i=1}^{4} x_i)}$. If we maximize it

with respect to π, we obtain $\hat{\pi} = \sum_{i=1}^{4} x_i / 4$, i.e. the estimator of maximum like-

lihood, considered a random variable which will be different with every one of the possible samples. It is as if in Table 5.5 (or 5.4) the frequentists, once the maximum likelihood estimate $\hat{\pi} = 0.50$ is obtained, considered only the column corresponding to this estimate, i.e. a different likelihood for each sample result. In reality, the frequentists go back to using the sample distribution of the estimator to complete the inferential analysis.

In the introduction of this section we said that, since the values of the likelihood function can be interpreted as weights, nothing would change if we multiply all of them by any positive, parameter-independent constant. In light of this observation, we can rewrite the likelihood function for our experiment as:

$$L(\pi) = const \; \pi^2 \, (1 - \pi)^2$$

where the term "*const*" encompasses all of the components in which the parameter does not appear, that is, it indicates any positive constant. For example, the values of the row (1,0,0,1) of Table 5.4, which are values of $L(\pi)$ with *const*

= 1 (each row represents only one of the possible results) and the values of the row "2 *successes*" of Table 5.5, which are values of $L(\pi)$ with *const* = 6 (the possible ways in which 2 *successes* can be obtained in 4 attempts), express the same likelihood function. It is easy to verify that the ratio between the likelihoods corresponding to any pair of values of π is the same in the two tables (aside from rounding off of values).

So far we have considered an experimental setting characterized by a dichotomous end-point (an example of a discrete variable), one sample and a very small sample size. It is simple to extend the reasoning to any sample size n, and relatively simple to extend the reasoning to the comparison between two samples. We will not do so because we do not believe it would help to grasp the basic concepts any better and because this chapter is already too long!.

However we will briefly touch upon continuous variables. What was said concerning the likelihood function for discrete variables is also valid for continuous variables. However, it is necessary to include a small modification, due to the fact that the continuous variable does not have a probability distribution but a probability density function. In the case of a continuous variable, the likelihood function derives from the probability density function of the end-point. Assuming, for example, a normally distributed density function with parameters μ and σ for the end-point of interest and a sample of n subjects, each observation of the sample (i.e. each x) is an expression of the same normal density function. Since all of the sample observations are independent of one another, the likelihood function is based on the product of n normal density functions, all having the same parameters μ and σ. Once the sample is obtained, this product will be a function only of the parameters, that is, it will be the likelihood function. In this case, such a function represents the density of probability which existed *a priori* (i.e. before conducting the experiment) of observing the values of the sample that were actually observed as the outcome of the experiment. In section 5.6.1 we will introduce the likelihood function for two independent samples extracted from normal populations.

An approach to inferential statistics based on the concept of likelihood and on the methods related to it can be found in a book by Azzalini [7], which however requires a sound basis of mathematical analysis and probability theory.

5.5. Frequentist (Classical) Analysis of a Clinical Trial

Throughout this section, we always make the assumption that the groups under comparison are not affected by bias, thanks to a good planning and execution of the study.

5.5.1. Hypothesis Testing: the Frequentist Solution

Having completed a study on a pre-selected sample and obtained the values $x_{1\_A}, x_{2\_A}, ..., x_{n_A\_A}$, for the group treated with A, and the values $x_{1\_P}, x_{2\_P}, ..., x_{n_P\_P}$, for that treated with P, we wish to verify the unidirectional hypothesis system (5.2).

Table 5.6. Symbols used in this section

Symbol	Meaning
$\delta_\mu = \mu_A - \mu_P$	Difference between the (true) means of the populations treated with A and P
$d_\mu = \bar{X}_A - \bar{X}_P$	Difference between the sample means, i.e. sample estimator of δ_μ
$d_{oss} = \hat{\delta}_\mu$	Value observed for the estimator d_μ in the specific sample, i.e. estimate of δ_μ
d_μ^*	Test statistic for the comparison of means
d_{oss}^*	Value observed for the test statistic d_μ^* in the specific sample

Since in our example the inference concerns the mean, we calculate the two sample means, $\bar{X}_{obs\_A}$ (for the group treated with A) and $\bar{X}_{obs\_P}$ (for the group treated with P), with a difference $d_{obs} = \hat{\delta}_\mu$.

In this section we will use a series of symbols, in part introduced previously, in part described later. For the reader's convenience, we have summarized them in Table 5.6.

The frequentist inferential reasoning. The inferential reasoning in the frequentist approach starts from the initial assumption that the null hypothesis is true, that is, in our example, that there is no difference, at the population level, between the presumed active treatment and the placebo.

If the null hypothesis is true, any difference between the two sample means observed in the study can only be due to "chance", a term with which we indicate the complex of fluctuations due to biological variability and to variability in measurement, which we cannot control and are independent of the treatment (see chapter 1 and section 2.4).

On the basis of these considerations we ask the fundamental question of the frequentist inference:

"If the null hypothesis is true (that is, there is no difference between treatments in the populations from which the samples are extracted), what is the probability of obtaining by chance a difference between the treatment groups equal to or greater than the one we have observed in our study?"

If this probability is "sufficiently small", we reject the null hypothesis and accept the alternative hypothesis that there is a difference between the treatments. If instead this probability is not "sufficiently small", we accept the null hypothesis and conclude that there is not enough evidence to claim a difference between the treatments. According to some statisticians, the expression "to accept the null hypothesis" is not correct, since we can only "not reject the null hypothesis", that is, we can only conclude that we do not have enough evidence to reject it. According to others, the two expressions are equivalent. We will not make any attempt to go to the heart of the matter, but for the sake of simplicity we will talk about "acceptance" of the null hypothesis.

This type of reasoning will appear very strange indeed to those that are new to scientific logic. In fact, it is identical to the reasoning of the "reductio ad absurdum" (Latin for "reduction to the absurd"), typical of the demonstration of geometry theorems: one proposes a hypothesis, then demonstrates that such hypothesis is impossible (in our case it is very improbable), and consequently accepts the alternative hypothesis. The fact that the null hypothesis is opposite to our interests is the result of a conservative mindset, typical of scientific investigation: the conceptual starting point is the "truth of today", as we know it before the experiment. In the case of a study of a new treatment versus placebo, the starting point is that the new treatment does not exist; therefore, the "truth of today" is that there is no difference between it and placebo. To accept the "alternative truth" that the new treatment exists, that is to say, that it is better than the placebo, it is necessary to firmly disprove the "truth of today" (the null hypothesis). This approach is common to other types of investigation. For example, in many judiciary systems, the suspect is considered innocent until proven guilty.

A threshold value remains to be established to quantify a probability as "sufficiently small". Based on this value, commonly called **threshold of statistical significance,** the null hypothesis will be rejected or accepted. Its choice is absolutely arbitrary, even though two values have been consecrated by their continual use over time: 0.05 (5%) used in the majority of cases and 0.01 (1%) used less frequently, when one wishes to be more conservative.

If we adopt 0.05 as the threshold of statistical significance, the inferential reasoning takes the following form. If the probability of obtaining the difference between the groups observed in the study or an even greater one totally by chance (i.e. in the absence of any treatment effect) is 0.05 (5%) or less (i.e. this outcome occurs once in every 20 hypothetical experiments identical to the one just performed, or even less frequently), then we conclude that such probability is "sufficiently small" to rule out chance. In other words, we conclude that the observed difference cannot be explained by a chance effect. Thus something else must be responsible for the effect: this something else can be either the treatment or some form of bias. As we are assuming that bias can be reasonably ruled out in our experiment (see above), the observed difference must be due to treatment. Therefore, we reject the null hypothesis and accept the alternative one. The probability we are talking about is the famous "p-value", which will be discussed below (we hope the reader will easily link the reasoning described here to the operational mechanism of the test, described later).

In choosing 0.05 as the threshold of statistical significance, we accept the risk of erroneously rejecting the null hypothesis when it is in fact true once in 20 times. If we use a significance threshold of 0.01, the risk of such an error will be lower, namely once in 100 experiments; still it will exist. To erroneously reject the null hypothesis, that is, to claim that there is a difference between the treatments when in truth there is none, is defined as a **type I error**. In other words, a type I error is a **false-positive** result. The probability of making such an error is usually indicated with α. In the planning phase of the experiment, a value of α is arbitrarily established, representing the risk one is willing to run of obtaining a false-positive result. This value is indeed the threshold of significance introduced above.

If instead the probability of obtaining by chance a difference equal to or greater than that observed in the experiment is higher than 0.05, then we conclude that chance remains a plausible explanation. Therefore, we accept the null hypothesis.

Also in this case, there is the risk of making a mistake. Here the potential error is of erroneously accepting the null hypothesis, that is, of declaring that there is no difference between the treatments when in fact there is one . This is defined as a **type II error**. In other words, a type II error is a **false-negative** result. The probability of making such an error is usually indicated with β. In the planning phase of the experiment, just as we do for α, we chose an arbitrary value for β, that we consider an acceptable risk of false-negative result. A commonly accepted value of β is 0.2 (20%), which means that we accept that such an error will be made once every five hypothetical experiments identical to the one just performed. Generally, β is set at a higher (i.e. less conservative) level compared to α, because the consequence of erroneously rejecting an effective treatment is considered less dangerous than that of erroneously accepting a treatment that is not effective. However, there are situations where the opposite is true, a false-negative having worse consequences than a false-positive. In these cases it is appropriate to be more conservative with β than with α (we will see shortly why, given a fixed sample size, it is not possible to be conservative with α and β at the same time). We urge the reader to ponder the reasoning behind certain assumptions and not to accept dogmatically the "standard" choices.

The quantity $1 - \beta$ is commonly referred to as the **power** of the test. It represents the probability of claiming, based on the results observed in the study, that there is a difference between treatments, when there actually is one in the population. Therefore, the power is the probability of drawing the correct conclusion. In the presence of a type II error equal to 0.2 (20%), the power of the study is 0.8 (80%). This means that, assuming we can repeat the study a great number of times under identical conditions, we will be able to demonstrate a difference between the treatments, when it really exists, eight times out of 10. On the other hand, in two out of 10 repetitions, the study will conclude in favor of the null hypothesis, even when a difference between the treatments actually exists in the underlying populations.

The choice of the values of α and of β comes at a cost. The cost is in the number of subjects required to perform the experiment. As we will see in chapter 6, all other conditions being equal, the smaller the values we set for α and β, the larger is the sample required to detect a given difference between treatment groups. Furthermore, for a fixed sample size, α and β are linked: if α decreases, β increases and vice versa (see chapter 6). This linkage makes it practically impossible to simultaneously protect the study from both types of error, by choosing very small values for both α and β, as this would cause an unrealistic increase in the sample size of the study.

The mechanism of the frequentist test. Let us now move on to the mechanism for calculating the probability at the heart of the basic question of frequentist inference: the probability of obtaining by chance a difference between the treatments equal to or greater than the one obtained in the study, when the null hypothesis is true.

Many types of statistical tests exist. The choice of the best statistical test from an operational point of view depends on:
- The type of end-point (see chapter 4).
- The type of distribution of this end-point in the population of interest (see section 5.1.2).
- The design chosen for the study (see chapters 10 and 11).

In this section, we will make no attempt to be specific on the different tests. Instead, we will focus the discussion on the "ingredients" and on the general operational mechanism of the statistical test conducted with the frequentist approach. We will use the example of a continuous end-point, with normal distribution, for which we are interested in the comparison of two means.

The basic ingredients of the frequentist statistical test are:
1. The α significance level (β is taken into consideration only in the planning phase of the trial, in the context of the calculation of the sample size – see chapter 6).
2. A so-called "test statistic".
3. Its "sample distribution".
4. The "region of rejection" of the null hypothesis.

To follow more easily what will be a somewhat long and complex reasoning, it is useful to have a general frame of reference, in which we can then place the details. Here it is. The test statistic tells us how big the treatment effect is compared to the variability of the phenomenon. If we know the sample distribution of the test statistic, we can identify the region of rejection of the null hypothesis, which also depends on the pre-selected hypothesis system (unidirectional or bidirectional). Once we identify this region, we can calculate the p-value. If the calculated p-value is equal to or less than the pre-selected level of significance, we reject the null hypothesis, otherwise we accept it.

"Ingredient" 1: significance level. We have already discussed the significance level.

"Ingredient" 2: test statistic. The **test statistic** is generally a mathematical elaboration of the sample estimator of the treatment effect used in the study. Very often it is the ratio between the sample estimator of the treatment effect and its variability. In figurative terms, it is the ratio between an estimate of the signal and an estimate of the background noise. The test statistic, being a function of the end-point, is a random variable as well as the estimator, and therefore it has a probability distribution.

In our example, the test statistic is a function of the estimator d_μ (which, we remind the reader, is the difference between the sample means, $\bar{X}_A - \bar{X}_P$). More precisely, it is the ratio between d_μ and its variability in the hypothetical succession of identical experiments. This variability is the standard error, which we know from Table 5.3 is equal to $\sqrt{\left(\dfrac{\sigma^2}{n_A} + \dfrac{\sigma^2}{n_P}\right)}$. Let us indicate this ratio with d_μ^*.

Therefore, the test statistic is:

$$d_\mu^* = \frac{\left(\bar{X}_A - \bar{X}_P\right)}{\sqrt{\left(\dfrac{\sigma^2}{n_A} + \dfrac{\sigma^2}{n_P}\right)}} \tag{5.3}$$

d_μ^* is a random variable, as is d_μ and, therefore, has a probability distribution (see "ingredient" 3 below).

The test statistic, intended as the ratio between a difference and its variability, has an intuitive conceptual meaning, and is also operationally useful.

From a conceptual point of view, it is intuitive that, when we compare two quantities, in our example two means, we can establish if their difference is large or small only against a "yardstick" represented by the variability of the phenomenon. A difference of 100 yards has a completely different meaning if the variability is 100 or 1000! The test statistic puts the difference between treatments in the context of its variability.

From an operational point of view, the test statistic obtained with the ratio described above, has a probability distribution that no longer depends on one of the unknown parameters, namely the measure of variability (see below).

"Ingredient" 3: sample distribution of the test statistic. The third ingredient is the **sample distribution of the test statistic**, which is the probability distribution of this statistic. So far, it has not been necessary to make any assumption on the probability distribution of the end-point. However, generally (although not always – see section 5.8) we do need this information in order to know the probability distribution of the test statistic, which in turn is necessary to calculate the area of any region of this distribution. Each area is the probability of the values at the base of the corresponding region (see section 5.1). In particular, the regions we are interested in are the tails of the probability distribution of the test statistic, which represent the probability of obtaining values of the test statistic equal to or more extreme (smaller or greater) than the one observed on the sample. This is the famous **p-value** which allows us to draw the frequentist test to a conclusion, as illustrated at the beginning of this section.

In our example, we assume that the probability distribution of the end-point is normal (but the reasoning is conceptually valid also for other types of assumptions). The assumption of normality of the end-point allows us to conclude that the distribution of d_μ^* is itself normal, with mean δ_μ and standard deviation 1. We reach this conclusion by applying the probability laws on distributions summarized in Table 5.7 below and the laws on variability summarized earlier in this chapter in Table 5.3.

The laws of probability of Table 5.7 can be demonstrated mathematically, but this goes beyond the purpose of this book. To have a graphic idea of these laws, the reader can turn to Figure 5.4.

As shown in this figure, the only unknown parameter in the distribution of d_μ^* is $\delta_\mu = \mu_A - \mu_P$. However, under the null hypothesis H_0 this parameter is also known, being equal to zero. Therefore, the sample distribution of the test statistic d_μ^*, under the null hypothesis, is completely known: it is the standard normal distribution. As this curve is completely known, we can calculate the area under any region of the curve. This area gives us the probability of the interval of values at its base. Therefore, we can calculate the p-value. As stated in section 5.1.2, when a distribution is completely known, we have access to its mathematical expression and to its probability tables. Both allow the computation of the areas (i.e. the probabilities) of interest, which in our case are the tails of the distribution. To know if we must calculate the area of the left tail, the right tail or both tails of the distribution of the test statistic under H_0, we must localize the region of rejection of the null hypothesis (see "ingredient" 4).

"Ingredient" 4: region of rejection of the null hypothesis. The fourth and last ingredient is the **region of rejection of the null hypothesis.** It is the

Table 5.7. Probability laws for a normally distributed random variable

a. When the probability distributions of two independent random variables X_A and X_P are normal, with means μ_A and μ_P, respectively, and identical standard deviations σ, the probability distribution of their difference $X_A - X_P$ is itself normal, with mean

$\delta_\mu = \mu_A - \mu_P$ and standard deviation $SD = \sqrt{2\sigma^2}$.

b. When the probability distribution of a random variable X is normal, with mean μ and standard deviation σ, the mean $\bar{X}$, calculated on n units extracted from X, is itself a random variable (in the frequentist approach) with normal distribution, with mean μ

and $SD = \sqrt{\dfrac{\sigma^2}{n}}$.

c. Combining the laws a. and b., it follows that, when the probability distributions of two independent random variables X_A and X_P are normal, with parameters described in a., the distribution of the difference of two means $\bar{X}_A - \bar{X}_P$, calculated on n_A and n_P units extracted from X_A and X_P respectively, is still normal, with mean $\delta_\mu = \mu_A - \mu_P$

and $SD = \sqrt{\left(\dfrac{\sigma^2}{n_A} + \dfrac{\sigma^2}{n_P}\right)}$.

d. If, instead of the random variable $d_\mu = \bar{X}_A - \bar{X}_P$, we consider the variable d_μ^* described in (5.3), this has a normal distribution with mean $\delta_\mu = \mu_A - \mu_P$ and standard deviation . $SD = 1$.

region of the values of the test statistic for which the null hypothesis is rejected. The localization of this region depends on three factors: the type of alternative hypothesis, i.e. whether it is unidirectional or bidirectional (for the former, the direction must also be specified), the type of test statistic and the level of significance. In our example, if we adopt the unidirectional system (5.2) with the alternative hypothesis H_1: $\mu_A > \mu_P$, then under the null hypothesis H_0, the region of rejection is located only in one tail of the probability distribution of the test statistic, namely in the right tail, since high values of the test statistic lead to the rejection of the null hypothesis. In this case, assuming that we perform a test with a 5% significance level, the region of rejection of the null hypothesis is given by the right tail of the distribution of d^*_μ under H_0, which has an area of 0.05, while the p-value to be calculated is the area of the tail of the same distribution to the right of d^*_{obs}. If instead we adopt the hypothesis system (5.1) with alternative hypothesis H_1: $\mu_A \neq \mu_P$, the region of rejection is located in both tails (see below).

In the medical literature it is an established convention to call **two-tailed test** the test performed with a bidirectional alternative hypothesis, and **one-tailed test** the test performed with a unidirectional alternative hypothesis[4].

Having defined the "ingredients" of the test, we can now carry it out. Let us suppose we decide to perform a test for the unidirectional hypothesis system (5.2). Since d^*_μ has a standard normal distribution, having obtained from the study its sample value d^*_{obs}, we can apply a process similar to the one described in section 5.1 to find the p-value, with d^*_{obs} in place of x_{inf}. For example, assuming the value of d^*_μ is 1.77, the corresponding p-value is the area between $x_{inf} = 1.77$ and $x_{sup} = +\infty$. We can use the table for the standard normal distribution reported in the appendix to obtain the area between $x_{inf} = 0$ and $x_{sup} = +1.77$, which is equal to 0.4616. We can then calculate the p-value by subtracting this value from 0.5, which is the area of half of the distribution. The result is 0.0384.

Unfortunately there is another complication. For the sake of simplicity, our discussion of "ingredients" 2 and 3 above has been somewhat too superficial. At this stage, the reader can recognize that σ^2 is yet another unknown parameter. Therefore, if it is true that d^*_μ no longer depends on σ^2 ("ingredient 2"), it is also true that we are unable to calculate d^*_μ because we do not know σ^2. Consequently, it is not true that the distribution of d^*_μ is completely known under the null hypothesis, nor is it true that it is a standard normal distribution ("ingredient" 3). To solve these problems it is necessary to estimate σ^2 as well

---

4. Strictly speaking, statistical tests are defined as one- or two-tailed depending on where the region of rejection of the test is located. In other words, it is not necessarily guaranteed that a unidirectional alternative hypothesis will generate a one-tailed test and a bidirectional alternative hypothesis a two-tailed test. Whereas in the case of the test discussed here, such correspondence exists, in other cases, such as the so-called F test (which is carried out in the analysis of variance, not treated in this book), it does not exist: the F test for a bidirectional alternative hypothesis is a one-tailed test. However, in medical statistics it is customary convention to define the test as one- or two-tailed depending on whether the alternative hypothesis is unidirectional or bidirectional.

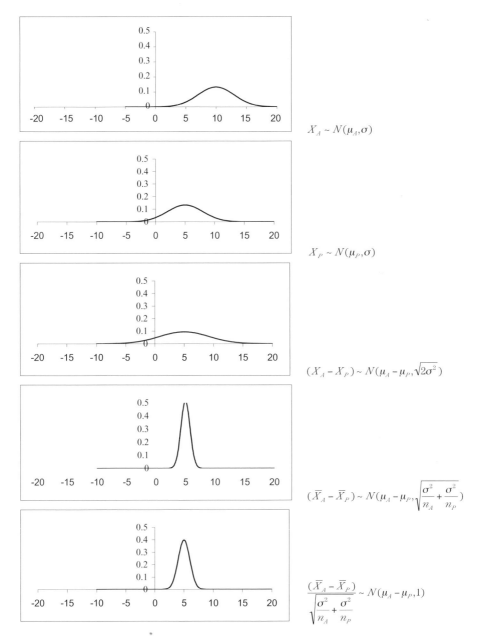

Figure 5.4. Relationship among different normal distributions (for the example in the graph: $\mu_A = 10$; $\mu_P = 5$; $\sigma = 3$; $n_A = n_P = 30$)

from the data obtained from the sample. In addressing inferential problems, the frequentists generally assume that the two samples under comparison have the same variance, i.e. $\sigma_A^2 = \sigma_P^2 = \sigma^2$, an assumption we have made from the start (see Table 5.3). The reader will guess that this assumption of equal variance (called homoscedasticity) can sometimes be problematic. This issue, even though important, goes beyond the limits that we have set for this book. Under the condition of homoscedasticity, both samples can give an estimate of σ^2. This estimate is used to calculate d_μ^* (see again Table 5.3). Once σ^2 is estimated, what was stated above for "ingredients" 2 and 3 is again true. The only difference is that, because we have estimated σ^2 from the data of the sample, the distribution of d_μ^* is no longer normal, as stated above, but it is of the **Student's t** type. Here we ask the reader to make a leap of faith, because a deeper discussion of this distribution requires knowledge of probability calculus exceeding the level assumed for this book. However, the key point here is not that of describing the mathematical expression of the sample distribution of the test statistic, but is that of understanding that the test statistic is completely known under the null hypothesis. Probability tables also exist for the Student's t distribution, conceptually similar to the one for the standard normal distribution, but more laborious to use, because, in order to find the p-value of interest, the sample value of the test statistic is not sufficient. It is necessary to calculate another parameter, the so-called degrees of freedom, which depends on the size of the sample[5]. For large samples, as mentioned in section 5.1.3, the Student's t distribution approximates the normal distribution.

Execution of the frequentist test. To have a graphic idea of the operational procedure, the reader can refer to Figure 5.5, which illustrates the performance of the test for the unidirectional hypotheses system (5.2), assuming that the end-point (in the example, the walking distance measured at the end of the treatment) has a normal distribution.

---

5. The shape of the Student's t distribution is similar to that of the normal distribution. However, for small samples it shows more dispersion around the mean, since the use of $\hat{\sigma}$ in place of σ introduces a higher degree of uncertainty. As the sample size increases, the Student's t distribution approximates more and more the normal distribution. Therefore, the shape of the Student's t distribution depends not only on the mean and the standard deviation, but also on the size of the sample. However, the dependency of the Student's t distribution on the sample size is indirect, via the so-called degrees of freedom, which are the number of observations free to vary in the sample. These are equal to the difference between the number of observations and the number of constraints or relations among them. For example, if we extract a sample of 3 units so that $x_1 + x_2 + x_3 = 3\bar{x}$, we will have 2 degrees of freedom because only 2 of the 3 variables can assume any value (the third value must be such that, when added to the other two, gives $3\bar{x}$). Likewise, going back to our example, this notion can be explained as follows: at the start we have n_A observations in the group A and n_P in the group P; however, in each of the two samples we loose one degree of freedom when we calculate the mean, so that $(n_A - 1)$ and $(n_P - 1)$ degrees of freedom remain, in the two groups respectively $((n_A + n_P - 2)$ in total), to estimate the standard deviation.

Figure 5.5 shows the sample distribution of the test statistic d_{μ}^{*}, which we know by now has a Student's t probability distribution (but this detail is not crucial). In particular, the curve on the left side of the figure is the sample distribution of d_{μ}^{*} assuming the null hypothesis is true (i.e. that $\delta_{\mu} = 0$). The curve on the right side represents one of the possible distributions of d_{μ}^{*} under the alternative hypothesis (the selected one corresponds to the smallest difference considered clinically relevant – see chapter 6). Once the experiment is carried out and the data are obtained, we calculate first the value d_{obs} (that is, the value taken by d_{μ} in our sample) and then the ratio between this and the estimate of the standard deviation of its sample distribution (the standard error), that is, d_{obs}^{*}. As shown in Figure 5.5, the probability of obtaining a value equal to or greater than d_{obs}^{*} under the null hypothesis is the area of the tail located at the right of d_{obs}^{*} under the left curve of the figure (the one assuming that the null hypothesis is true). This probability is the p-value.

If the p-value is less than or equal to the significance threshold α (typically 0.05), the result is declared **statistically significant**. This means that it is considered unlikely that differences between treatments equal to or greater than the difference observed in the study could be due to chance. Therefore, the difference observed in the study is judged not due to chance. Vice versa, if the p-value is greater than the significance threshold, the result is not statistically significant.

At this point, the frequentist test is completed. In Figure 5.5 we have illustrated a case in which the test ends with the rejection of the null hypothesis.

We now return to the example at the beginning of the chapter. At the end of the study, the group treated with A achieved a mean walking distance equal to 471.6 meters, while the group treated with P achieved a mean walking distance equal to 404.5 meters. Let us also assume that:

- The alternative hypothesis is $H_1 : \mu_A > \mu_P$ and the test is performed at the 5% significance level (one-tailed).
- The walking distance is measured with a treadmill having variable inclination, therefore its distribution is normal.
- The two samples have sizes $n_A = 54$ and $n_P = 62$.
- There is homoscedasticy and the estimate of σ in the two groups treated with A and P is respectively $\hat{\sigma}_A = 232.65$ and $\hat{\sigma}_P = 204.15$.

With these assumptions, the formulas presented in table 5.3 give us:

$$\hat{\sigma}_A = 217.86$$

$$S\hat{E} = 217.86 \times \sqrt{\frac{62 + 54}{3348}} = 40.55$$

The test statistic takes the value:

$$d^{*}{}_{obs} = \frac{(471.6 - 404.5)}{40.55} = 1.65$$

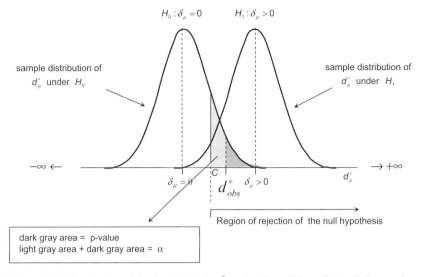

Figure 5.5. Distribution of the test statistic d_μ^* under the null hypothesis (left curve) and under the unidirectional alternative hypothesis (right curve). The distribution of the end-point is assumed to be normal

Using the Student's t distribution tables (not provided), for the one-tailed test, we obtain a p-value of 0.051 (the reader wishing to verify this calculation will need to refer to some other text or software and consider that the number of degrees of freedom for our example is equal to $54 + 62 - 2 = 114$). An approximate p-value can also be calculated by using the normal distribution tables. Since the p-value is greater than 0.05, strictly speaking, the test ends without rejecting the null hypothesis. However, if the unidirectional alternative hypothesis is considered acceptable, a researcher faced with this result (the observed p-value is very close to the threshold of significance) would justifiably have a strong suspicion that treatment A is in truth superior to placebo. As we said, the significance level of 5% is a convention, therefore the difference between the observed p-value (0.051) and the nearest significant p-value (0.05) is negligible. In these "borderline" cases, the researcher's overall conclusion should not be determined by whether our p-value is slightly to the left or to the right of the arbitrary threshold, but rather on a set of considerations, among which are the following:

- What are the characteristics of the confidence interval on the mean difference between treatments? Important are its width and the location of the threshold of clinical relevance inside it (see section 5.5.2).
- How does the result change if we change the assumptions? For example, it would be useful to perform a non-parametric test as well, which does not require assumptions on the distribution of the end-point (see section 5.8).
- How do the secondary end-points behave? It is important to evaluate if they overall confirm or not the efficacy of the treatment under evaluation.

- What results do similar studies give?

It should be noted that similar considerations must be made also in the case of a clearly statistically significant result.

Link between p-value, estimator and test statistic. As a final step, we shall delve deeper into the link connecting the p-value to the values of the test statistic d_μ^* and of the estimator d_μ. We will continue to refer to Figure 5.5 and in particular to the distribution of d_μ^* under H_0. From that figure it can be seen that as the p-values (i.e. the areas of the right tail) get smaller, the values of the test statistic d_μ^* get bigger and vice versa. The same relationship exists between the p-values and the values of the estimator d_μ. Consequently, the question we ask when performing a test can also be formulated as follows: "Is the difference observed between the sample means sufficiently great, compared to its variability, to indicate a real (non-random) difference between the means of the corresponding populations?" If we keep in mind that d_μ^* is the ratio between d_μ and its variability, we should now understand better the statement made in chapter 4, that the object of the statistical test in a clinical trial is that of differentiating the signal (effect of the treatment) from the background noise (effect of chance).

From Figure 5.5, we can also see that a specific value C corresponds to the significance threshold α. This value is called the **critical value of the test**, because to its right we find the region of rejection of the null hypothesis. An alternative way of performing the test is that of calculating d_{obs}^* and C. If the value of d_{obs}^* is to the right of C, i.e. is equal to or greater than C, it falls in the region of rejection of the null hypothesis; consequently the difference between the groups under comparison is statistically significant. This means (we repeat it one more time) that the difference between the sample means is so large that, in the hypothetical repetition of the experiment under the same conditions, such a difference, or an even greater one, would occur in 5% or less of the outcomes, if the two groups were selected from populations with identical means (therefore assuming that the null hypothesis is true).

In the example described above the critical value of the one-tailed test corresponding to a 5% significance level is $C = 1.66$. Since the value of d_{obs}^* is smaller than C ($1.65 < 1.66$), the test is concluded without being able to reject the null hypothesis, but leaving strong suspicion that A is superior to placebo.

In summary, the statistical test for the unidirectional hypothesis system (5.2) can be performed in one of two equivalent ways:

- Using the significance threshold, calculating the p-value and applying the following decisional rule:
  - H_0 is rejected if $p\text{-}value \le \alpha$;

    H_0 is accepted if $p\text{-}value > \alpha$.   (5.4)

- Using the critical value C (known once α is chosen), calculating the test statistic and applying the following decisional rule:
  - H_0 is rejected if $d_{obs}^* \ge C$;

    H_0 is accepted if $d_{obs}^* < C$.   (5.5)

Unidirectional and bidirectional hypothesis testing. What has been discussed up to this point applies to the unidirectional hypothesis system in (5.2) with $H_1 : \delta_\mu > 0$. However, it is simple to extend the reasoning both to the other unidirectional hypothesis system, in which the alternative hypothesis goes in the opposite direction, and to the bidirectional hypothesis system.

When the hypothesis system is unidirectional with $H_1: \delta_\mu < 0$, we can still use the decision rule in (5.4) but we have to keep in mind that the *p-value* refers to the area of the tail opposite to the one to be used for the hypothesis system with $H_1: \delta_\mu > 0$. Alternatively, we need invert the inequality signs and replace C with $-C$ in the decision rule in (5.5), i.e. the rule becomes: H_0 is rejected if $d^*_{obs} \leq -C$ and is accepted if $d^*_{obs} > -C$. A useful exercise for the reader would be to build a figure similar to Figure 5.5, in which the sample distribution under the hypothesis H_1 is to the left of that under H_0. The test is still one-tailed in this case.

When the hypothesis system is bidirectional with $H_1 : \delta_\mu \neq 0$, as in (5.1), Figure 5.6 must replace Figure 5.5. In Figure 5.6 there are two probability distributions of the test statistic under the hypothesis H_1, one to the left and one to the right of the probability distribution under the hypothesis H_0. Furthermore, the decisional rules (5.4) and (5.5) must be modified to take into account that, with the hypothesis system (5.1), a result "far" from 0 (that is, "far" from the null hypothesis of no difference between the population means) in either direction favors the alternative hypothesis. For a test at the 5% significance level ($\alpha = 0.05$), since in this case the region of rejection of the null hypothesis is located in both tails of the distribution of the test statistic d^*_μ under the null hypothesis H_0, each of these tails has an area equal to $\alpha/2 = 0.025$. The test is two-tailed (see note 4).

Considering the decisional rule (5.4), first we calculate the value of d^*_{obs}; next we calculate the area of the tail of the distribution of d^*_μ under H_0 to the right of $|d^*_{obs}|$ ($|d^*_{obs}|$ is the value of d^*_{obs} always with a positive sign) by taking advantage of the symmetry of the sample distribution of d^*_μ (under H_0 the area to the right of d^*_{obs} is equal to the area to the left of $-d^*_{obs}$). Therefore:

- H_0 is rejected if *p-value* $\leq \alpha/2$.
- H_0 is accepted if *p-value* $> \alpha/2$.

(5.6)

The decisional rule (5.5) can also be adapted to this case. For a significance level equal to α, two critical levels C_1 and C_2 must be considered, where C_1 is the point which leaves to its left a surface area of $\alpha/2$ and C_2 is the point which leaves to its right a surface area of $\alpha/2$. Taking advantage again of the symmetry of the distribution of the test statistic d^*_μ, we see that, under H_0, $C_1 = -C$ and $C_2 = +C$. Therefore, the decisional rule becomes:

- H_0 is rejected if $|d^*_{obs}| \geq C$.
- H_0 is accepted if $|d^*_{obs}| < C$.

(5.7)

The decision rule (5.7) states that H_0 is rejected if the computed value of the test statistic is either $\geq C$ or $\leq -C$; otherwise H_0 is not rejected.

In the example illustrated in Figure 5.6 the test ends without rejecting the null hypothesis.

Let us return once more to the example discussed above and repeat the test with a bidirectional alternative hypothesis, again at the 0.05 significance level. Indeed, the bidirectional hypothesis is the appropriate one for our example. The result is $p\text{-}value > \alpha/2$: in fact, $0.051 > 0.025$. Therefore, the test ends again without rejecting the null hypothesis. In this case however, the outcome is more clear-cut compared to the unidirectional case. Obviously, we get the same result by applying the decisional rule (5.7), where the critical value C obtained from the Student's t distribution table is 1.98. Had we used the normal distribution table, C would have been 1.96, which is a good approximation of the value 1.98.

We feel the need to remind the reader one more time that attaining statistical significance only allows the exclusion with reasonable certainty that chance alone can explain the result. Statistical significance does not allow the exclusion of bias and does not allow to conclude that the result is clinically relevant. The effect of the treatment and that of bias cannot be separated from each other through the statistical test described in this section. Statistical techniques helpful in uncovering bias do exist, but their outcomes are always of an exploratory nature. The danger of bias can be minimized only in the planning phase of a study. We will return to the concept of bias and the importance of planning in chapter 9.

We have already talked about the clinical relevance of the result in section 5.2.2. In the next section of this chapter we will discuss the frequentist methods for statistical estimation, which allow assessment of the clinical relevance of a result.

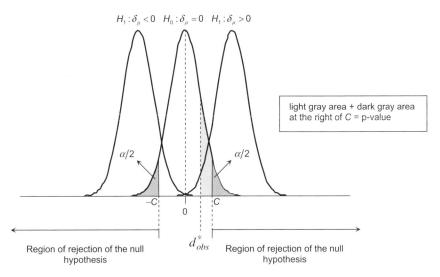

Figure 5.6. Distribution of the test statistic d_μ^* under the null hypothesis (middle) and under the bidirectional alternative hypothesis (right and left). The distribution of the end-point is assumed to be normal

Assumptions for the application of the Student's t test. In concluding this long section, we must point out that the statistical comparison between two treatment groups cannot always be conducted by means of the Student's t test, as some non-statisticians seem to believe!

The correct application of such test requires the following assumptions to be verified:

1. The end-point of interest must be quantitative and normally distributed.
2. The two groups under comparison must have the same variance (homoschedasticity).

If the end-point of interest is not quantitative, it cannot be appropriately summarized by the mean and if the other requirements above described are not fulfilled, the test statistic d_μ^* does not have a Student's t distribution.

A logical reasoning similar to the one developed in this section can still be applied. However, other test statistics, different from d_μ^*, must be chosen and/or other probability distributions, different from the Student's t distribution, must be used.

Concerning the assumptions at point 1, the reader is referred to sections 1.3.1 and 5.1.3.

In case of violations of the assumption at point 2, different solutions exist in the literature which, for lack of space, we will not introduce (see for example [24]). It should be noted however that the Student's t test is robust to violations of the assumption of normality, especially when the distribution of the end-point is not clearly asymmetrical and when the sample size is "reasonably" large (see 5.1.3) and to violations of the assumption of homoscedasticity, especially when the sample sizes of the two groups under comparison are similar. A **test** is defined as **robust** with respect to a particular assumption when the violation of the assumption, within limits, does not result in a loss of validity of the methodology used and consequently does not result in a loss of reliability of the results. In other words, the Student's t test remains valid, within limits, when the variances of the two groups are different.

A very common procedure, when one is not sure whether the assumption of homoscedasticity is appropriate, is that of verifying the equality of the variances using an appropriate statistical test (Fisher's F test). If the result of the test is not significant, the two variances are considered equal and the Student's t test is applied for the comparison of the means. This procedure is commonly used, even if it is not without problems: first of all, there is no guarantee that it will have enough power to detect the difference between the variances under comparison; second, the application of more than one type of test in sequence (in the example, a F-test followed by a t-test) increases the total level of significance (due to a mechanism similar to the one described in section 4.7), which calls for caution in interpreting the overall outcome, without an adequate adjustment for multiplicity.

5.5.2.   Estimation of the Effect: the Frequentist Solution

When analyzing data from clinical trials, one must always report, next to the p-value, the estimate of the treatment effect. This is because statistical significance and clinical relevance are two different concepts. This message is so important and so often ignored by the medical literature that we feel it is useful to stress it one more time: statistical significance, which tells us whether the observed difference is due to chance or not, is linked to the statistical test; clinical relevance, which tells us whether the observed difference is relevant or not for the patient, is linked to the estimate of the treatment effect. An interpretation of the results based on only one of the two aspects would be incomplete and would make it impossible to draw reliable conclusions on the experimental treatment.

A first method for estimating the unknown parameter, that is, the magnitude of the effect of the treatment (the signal), is the point estimate, by which the unknown parameter in the population is estimated with the corresponding sample statistic. This is the method we have used so far, which we will call **method of analogy.** For example, the population mean is estimated with the mean calculated on the sample, the population variance with the sample variance, and so on. A choice of this type seems to satisfy common sense: it is logical and it uses all of the sample observations.

The point estimate by analogy is not the only method to obtain point estimates used by the frequentists. In section 5.4.2 for example, we talked about the maximum likelihood estimates. We refer the reader interested in the topic to other textbooks (for example, [105]). In our example, both the method of analogy and that of maximum likelihood give $\hat{\delta}_\mu = 67.1$.

Regardless of the method used to obtain the point estimate of the parameter of interest, its validity is assessed based on a series of properties desirable for the estimator that generated it. As we know well by now, in the frequentist approach statistical procedures are evaluated with reference to a hypothetical repetition of experiments, performed under the same conditions. It is exactly in these terms that the properties of the different estimators are evaluated. The limits of this book prevent us from discussing further these properties. However, it is important for the reader to remember that not all estimators are equally "valid".

In the frequentist approach, to compliment the point estimate, the **confidence interval** is calculated, generally at 95% level (corresponding to a test with a significance level of 5%), or at 99% level (corresponding to a test with a significance level of 1%). This is a method for estimating the magnitude of the unknown parameter (the effect of the treatment) through an interval, instead of a point.

In the previous section we saw that, if X is a normally distributed random variable, the estimator d_μ is also normally distributed, with mean $\mu_A - \mu_P$ and standard deviation $\sqrt{\sigma^2 / n_A + \sigma^2 / n_P}$ (under the assumption of homoschedasticity).

Therefore the quantity:

$$\frac{(\overline{X}_A - \overline{X}_P) - (\mu_A - \mu_P)}{\sqrt{\sigma^2/n_A + \sigma^2/n_P}}.$$

has a standard normal distribution with mean = 0 and standard deviation = 1.

We also know that the probability of a variable with standard normal distribution falling between the critical values $-C$ and C, where $C = 1.96$, is equal to 0.95, i.e. these two values are such that 95% of the standard normal distribution is included between them, while 2.5% of this area is included in each of the remaining tails (see Figure 5.6, middle curve). To be precise, the interval included between -1.96 and 1.96 is the smallest interval defining an area equivalent to 0.95 on the standard normal distribution.

Expressed in a formula this becomes:

$$\Pr\left\{-1.96 < \frac{(\overline{X}_A - \overline{X}_P) - (\mu_A - \mu_P)}{\sqrt{\sigma^2/n_A + \sigma^2/n_P}} < 1.96\right\} = 0.95$$

With a few algebraic transformations, this expression can be rewritten as follows:

$$\Pr\left\{(\overline{X}_A - \overline{X}_P) - 1.96\sqrt{\sigma^2/n_A + \sigma^2/n_P} < (\mu_A - \mu_P) < (\overline{X}_A - \overline{X}_P) + \right.$$
$$\left. + 1.96\sqrt{\sigma^2/n_A + \sigma^2/n_P}\right\} = 0.95$$

This is equivalent to:

$$\Pr\left\{(d_\mu - 1.96\sqrt{\sigma^2/n_A + \sigma^2/n_P}) < \delta_\mu < (d_\mu + 1.96\sqrt{\sigma^2/n_A + \sigma^2/n_P})\right\} = 0.95.$$

Once the sample is extracted, in place of d_μ we have d_{obs} (the point estimate of δ_μ). Since we are no longer dealing with a random variable, the probabilistic relationship reported above can no longer be interpreted in the strict sense. In other words, when d_{obs} is substituted for d_μ, strictly speaking, we can no longer see this relationship as an event which has a 95% probability of occurring. It is for this reason that we speak of a 95% confidence interval for δ_μ which can be expressed in one of the following two equivalent ways:

$$(d_{obs} - 1.96\sqrt{\sigma^2/n_A + \sigma^2/n_P} \; ; \; d_{obs} + 1.96\sqrt{\sigma^2/n_A + \sigma^2/n_P})$$

or:

$$(d_{obs} \pm 1.96\sqrt{\sigma^2/n_A + \sigma^2/n_P}).$$

Here, again, we face the problem of having to estimate σ^2 from the sample data. Therefore, if the sample is not large, the value 1.96, which is taken from the normal distribution under the assumption that σ^2 is known, must be replaced by the critical C value obtained from the Student's t distribution tables (with a number of degrees of freedom equal to $(n_A + n_P - 2)$).

In the example discussed in the previous section, the 95% confidence interval for δ_μ is $(67.1 \pm 1.98 \times 40.55)$ meters, often written as $(-13.2; 147.4)$ meters, in favour of treatment A.

The procedure described in this section guarantees that, repeating the calculation of the interval on an infinite number of samples, the confidence interval obtained will include the true value of the parameter in 95% of the cases. In other words, we have applied a technique that, in the long run, gives us correct interval estimates 19 times out of 20, that is, with a probability of 95%. For convenience, the property of this procedure is extended to the single interval and therefore this is interpreted by stating that it includes the true and unknown value of the parameter with a 95% probability. Actually, however, the single interval either includes or does not include the true value of δ_μ i.e. it is "certainly right" or "certainly wrong" and there is no way to know which of the two situations we are in.

The confidence interval introduced above is a bidirectional interval. It is naturally possible to build unidirectional intervals. These intervals are limited only on one side. Assuming again a normal distribution, the unidirectional confidence interval at 95%, suitable for the hypothesis system (5.2), has only the lower lim-

it, which is equal to $(d_{obs} - 1.645\sqrt{\sigma^2/n_A + \sigma^2/n_P})$. In this case:

- the critical value C is equal to 1.645, instead of 1.96, because here we are interested in an expression of the type:

$$\Pr\left\{-C < \frac{(\overline{X}_A - \overline{X}_P) - (\mu_A - \mu_P)}{\sqrt{\sigma^2/n_A + \sigma^2/n_P}}\right\} = 0.95$$

- $-C = -1.645$ because the probability that a variable with standard normal distribution falls to the right of this value is 0.95.

Strictly speaking, also in this case we should consider the critical value C obtained from the Student's t distribution. For our example, the critical value C is equal to 1.66 and the unidirectional interval at 95% is given by the set of values > -0.2 meters in favor of treatment A.

The width of the confidence interval depends on the precision of the estimate: the higher the precision (that is, the lower the variability of d_μ), the narrower the width of the interval and vice versa (see also section 5.4.1).

It is important to note that there is a link between a test performed at the 5% significance level to verify a difference between two means and the confidence interval at 95% built on this difference: if the test is statistically significant, the confidence interval does not contain the 0 value and vice versa. Therefore, if we know the confidence interval, we also know whether the result of the test is statistically significant or not (at the level (100-level of confidence of the interval)%), even without actually performing the test. In our example, in the case of the bidirectional hypothesis (5.1), once we know that the 95% confidence interval has limits -13.2 and 147.4 meters, we know that the corresponding two-tailed test at the 5% significance level is not significant. In the case of the unidirectional hypothesis (5.2), once we know that the 95% confidence interval has a lower limit equal to –0.2 meters, we also know that the corresponding one-tailed test is not significant, although it is very close to the limit of significance.

The reader must pay attention to the definition of the confidence interval. Unfortunately, it does not imply that δ_μ has a 95% probability of taking a value included between the extremes of the confidence interval. Such information, of course, would be of much more interest for the researcher. This is due to the fact that in the frequentist approach δ_μ is not a random variable, but a constant value of the population. The confidence interval expresses a probabilistic relationship with respect to the only random variable, which is d_μ. We will return to this point in section 5.7.

5.6. Bayesian Analysis of a Clinical Trial

In this section, as in section 5.5.1, we will make the assumption that the groups under comparison are not affected by bias.

5.6.1. Hypothesis Testing: the Bayesian Solution

As we did in section 5.5.1, we shall start by testing the unidirectional hypothesis system (5.2). We have completed a study on a pre-selected sample and obtained the values x_{1_A}, x_{2_A},....$x_{n_A\_A}$, for the group treated with A and the values x_{1_P}, x_{2_P},....$x_{n_P\_P}$, for the group treated with P. The Bayesian inference, like the frequentist inference, requires knowledge of the probability distribution of the end-point of interest. For our example, we will assume that this distribution is normal.

For the reader's convenience, in Table 5.8 we report and explain the symbols appearing in this section.

The Bayesian inferential reasoning. The Bayesian inferential reasoning unfolds in three key points:
1. The unknown value, i.e. the parameter, is considered variable because uncertain. Therefore, the parameter is assigned a probability distribution, referred to as the **a priori probability distribution.** It reflects the knowledge the researcher has of the parameter of interest before the start of the study. In our example, the parameter of interest is the difference between the means of the two populations, $\delta_\mu = \mu_A - \mu_P$.
2. The results of the experiment are synthesized by the likelihood function, which, as seen in section 5.4.2, expresses the likelihood of different values of the unknown parameter in light of the results obtained, or in other words, the support that the observed results provide to the different hypotheses on δ_μ. Before the experiment is started, the likelihood function is a function of both the values of the sample and the values of the unknown parameter. Once the experiment is performed, the values of the sample are known, i.e. become constants. Thus, the likelihood function remains a function only of the parameter.

3. Combining the initial (*a priori*) probability distribution with the likelihood function, the final probability distribution is obtained, referred to as the **a posteriori probability distribution.** The combination of the initial probability distribution with the likelihood function, to obtain the final probability distribution, is achieved through the **Bayes' theorem.** We shall introduce this theorem by using our example, wherein the end-point is the walking distance indicated with X and the unknown parameter is the difference between two means, $\delta_\mu = \mu_A - \mu_P$. If we use the symbols reported in Table 5.8, the theorem of Bayes can be expressed with the following formula:

$$p_{posteriori}(\delta_\mu) = const \times p_{priori}(\delta_\mu) \times L(\delta_\mu) \tag{5.8}$$

where "*const*", once again, stands for constant, i.e. a value which does not depend on the unknown parameter (it stays the same whatever the value of the parameter).

Table 5.8. Symbols used in this section and their meanings

Symbol	Meaning
$\delta_\mu = \mu_A - \mu_P$	Difference between the (true) means of the populations treated with A and P
$p_{priori}(\delta_\mu)$	Distribution of the initial probabilities of δ_μ (*a priori* probability distribution)
$L(\delta_\mu)$	Likelihood function
$p_{posteriori}(\delta_\mu)$	Distribution of the final probabilities of δ_μ (*a posteriori* probability distribution)
$\hat{\delta}_\mu$	Estimate of δ_μ

We shall now go a bit deeper into each of the three points listed above.

Point 1: a priori probability distribution. We said that the *a priori* probability distribution of the parameter, in our example δ_μ, represents the expression of a certain level of information on the unknown parameter. When informative results on the parameter of interest from previous experiments exist, the *a priori* probability distribution will be based on them, provided that they are considered reliable by the researcher. For example, let's assume we want to plan a study to compare two treatments for intermittent claudication, with walking distance as the primary end-point. We have recently completed a study with the same treatments in which walking distance was a secondary end-point. Walking distance results gave a bell-shaped *a posteriori* distribution of the mean difference δ_μ, with mean = 40 meters and standard deviation = 50 meters. With the above information we are entitled to assume as *a priori* probability distribution for our new study a normal distribution with mean = 40 meters and SD = 50 meters.

In the absence of informative data or as a complement to these, assessments not based on previous experiments, but other sources, such as for example experience, are used to determine the *a priori* probability distribution. It is in this context that we understand why the use of the *a priori* distribution presumes the adoption of a different concept of probability, which in section 5.1 we called "subjective". When there is no information on the parameter of interest, an alternative approach to the "subjective" determination of the *a priori* probability distribution also exists: the use of a special type of probability distribution, called **non-informative distribution**, that does not alter the information coming from the observation of the sample results. The idea is to use distributions which assign the same probability to all of the possible values of the parameter. In our example, for the unknown parameter δ_μ, we could adopt the distribution

$$p_{priori}(\delta_\mu) \approx \frac{1}{const}$$ as a non-informative *a priori* distribution. If a non-informa-

tive distribution is chosen as an *a priori* distribution, the *a posteriori* distribution has the same shape as the likelihood function. This can be derived from the formula (5.8), imagining that the constant (the term "*const*" in the formula) and the value $p_{priori}(\delta_\mu)$ cancel each other out.

Point 2: likelihood function. The likelihood function, as illustrated in section 5.4.2, is built from the probability distribution of the end-point. In our example, having assumed a normal distribution as the probability law for each X of the sample, the likelihood function is given by the product of normal distributions. Here we will not assume homoscedasticity, because contrary to the frequentists, the Bayesians generally do not make this assumption. Table 5.9 gives some essentials on the calculation of this function.

Table 5.9. Laws of probability for the calculation of the likelihood function in our example

---

a. Given two independent events E_1 and E_2 (that is, knowledge of E_1 does not change the probability of E_2 and vice versa), the probability of both events occurring is given by the product of the probability of each of them occurring.

b. All of the $n_A + n_P$ observations of the sample are independent from one another. The n_A observations on the patients treated with A are determinations of a random variable with a normal probability distribution with mean μ_A and standard deviation σ_A, while the n_P observations on patients treated with P are determinations of a variable with normal probability distribution with mean μ_P and standard deviation σ_P.

c. If we put together the considerations in points a and b, we realize that, to obtain the likelihood function $L(\delta_\mu)$ of the entire sample (seen as the combination of two samples, treated with A and P respectively), we must calculate the product of $n_A + n_P$ normal probability distributions, of which n_A have mean μ_A and standard deviation σ_A and n_P have mean μ_P and standard deviation σ_P. In reality, some transformations are needed to express the likelihood as a function of δ_μ; furthermore, the likelihood function is not just a function of the parameter of interest δ_μ but also of the disturbance parameters σ_A and σ_P (*).

(*) Mathematical methods aimed at eliminating the disturbance parameters exist: one of these consists in maximizing the likelihood function with respect to the disturbance parameter

Point 3: a posteriori probability distribution. We now have all the elements we need to apply the Bayes' theorem and obtain the *a posteriori* probability distribution.

So far we have approached the problem as if there were only one parameter, δ_μ, in order to simplify the outline of the basic concepts. But, at this point, we must recognize that the standard deviations σ_A and σ_P are other unknown parameters (in our case disturbance parameters) that are still present in the likelihood function, even after the sample results have been obtained. The Bayesian approach offers various methods to address the problem of the disturbance parameters and, as mentioned above, in general it does not require the assumption of homoscedasticity. These methods are beyond the scope of this book. The reader must make another leap of faith and accept that, while the likelihood function is dependent on more than one unknown parameter, there are methods to eliminate the problem of the ones that are of no interest (disturbance parameters); nevertheless *a priori* probability distributions are needed for all of the parameters involved in the formulation of the problem.

The problem encountered when comparing two means from normally distributed end-points is known in the literature as the Behrens-Fisher problem. An *a priori* distribution of reference for this problem is based on the assumption that the parameters μ_A, μ_P, σ_A and σ_P have uniform (i.e. non-informative) distributions and are independent. The *a posteriori* probability distribution obtained with this choice, known as the Behrens-Fisher distribution, cannot be expressed in terms of tabulated functions. However, as described by Box and Tiao [18], it is possible to use the approximation proposed by Patil to obtain a probability distribution (more precisely, a probability density function) of known shape[6].

Obviously it is not possible to go into the details of the calculation here. By applying this method to the walking distance example introduced in section 5.5.1, the *a posteriori* probability distribution illustrated in Figure 5.7 is obtained.

Before moving to the *a posteriori* probability distribution, it is important we understand the role of the constant in the formula (5.8). It is needed to ensure that the result obtained from the Bayes' theorem be a probability distribution, i.e. have a total area equal to 1. For this reason, such a constant is called a normalization constant.

The *a posteriori* probability distribution represents the synthesis of all of the information, available before and after the experiment, on the unknown parameter. It is to the Bayesians what the sample distribution of the test statistics is

---

6. Given the choices made for the *a priori* probability distributions concerning the parameters, μ_A, μ_P, σ_A, and σ_P, and using the approximation of Patil, the a posteriori probability distribution is a generalized t distribution, that is to say, a t distribution with a mean different from 0 and a variance different from 1. The degrees of freedom, the mean, and the variance can be calculated from the sample data (see [18]).

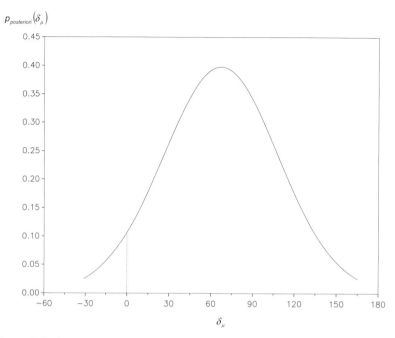

Figure 5.7. *A posteriori* probability distribution of δ_μ for the example on walking distance (it is the t distribution with mean = 67.11; variance = 1708.015; degrees of freedom = 83.96)

to the frequentists, the instrument through which all inferential processes are carried out: hypothesis testing, point estimation and estimation by interval. It is clear that, in order to carry out any form of inference, we must know the *a posteriori* distribution, which means that either we know the mathematical expression or have access to the relevant probability tables. When this is not possible, we must rely on an approximate evaluation, based on simulation techniques.

While the sample distribution of the test statistic varies with the variation of the possible sample results in the hypothetical succession of identical experiments, the *a posteriori* distribution varies with the variation of the possible values of the parameter. This difference is not trivial. It enables the *a posteriori* probability distribution to directly answer questions such as: "What is the probability that the value of the parameter is greater than a given value, or that it is included between two values v_1 and v_2?". The sample distribution of the test statistic cannot directly answer this type of questions because the areas of the sections under its curve do not express the probabilities of the different values of the parameter. They express instead the probability of the various sample results.

It is evident from (5.8) that the *a posteriori* probability distribution depends not only on the experimental result, but also on the *a priori* probability distribution chosen (in the case of more than one parameter, it depends on each of the respective *a priori* distributions).

- If there is no *a priori* information on the effect of the new treatment, a non-informative *a priori* distribution is chosen; therefore, the *a posteriori* distribution will have the same shape as the likelihood function, that is to say, it will be determined by the experimental results. This is what was done in the example illustrated in Figure 5.7.

- If *a priori* the new treatment is considered "probably inefficacious", the *a priori* distribution will be concentrated around a value of δ_μ close to zero. If the information is scarce, the *a priori* distribution will be poorly informative, i.e. very dispersed around the zero value. In this case, only very positive experimental results in favor of the new treatment will generate an *a posteriori* distribution supporting the hypothesis favoring efficacy, i.e. will be able to make us change our minds.

- If, on the contrary, *a priori* the new treatment is considered "probably efficacious", the *a priori* distribution will concentrate around a value of δ_μ close to the value of clinical relevance for the difference between treatments. If the evidence in favor of the treatment is strong, it will be very concentrated around this value. In this case a reasoning opposite to the previous one will apply, because only experimental results highly unfavorable to the new treatment will generate an *a posteriori* distribution supporting the hypothesis favoring lack of efficacy.

Conduction of the Bayesian test. From the discussion so far, it should be clear that the *a posteriori* distribution is already, to a large extent, the answer to the hypothesis being studied. However, formal tests can also be conducted in the context of the Bayesian approach. To mirror section 5.5.1, we shall submit to statistical testing the unidirectional hypothesis (5.2) for our walking distance example (illustrated in Figure 5.7). We will show how the *a posteriori* probability distribution can be used to this end.

We must calculate the *a posteriori* probabilities of the two sets of values included in the null hypothesis and in the alternative hypothesis, respectively: in the first case it is a matter of calculating the area under the curve corresponding to values of δ_μ less than or equal to 0; in the second case it is a matter of calculating the area (under the same distribution) corresponding to values of δ_μ greater than 0. For the final step of the formal hypothesis testing, the Bayesians use the so-called **loss function**, which expresses the losses associated with the decision of accepting H_0 or of accepting H_1 when one or the other hypothesis is true.[7]

Generally, the correct decisions are those that are associated with small or no losses. The concept of loss can be interpreted in monetary terms or more gen-

---

7. The loss function, which must be pre-specified in the planning phase of the experiment, is also used by the Bayesians in problems of estimation: in fact, it is used to define the "optimal" estimate.

erally as a loss of usefulness (based on subjective considerations). Losses with a negative sign are interpreted as gains.

This function plays a role somewhat similar to that of α and β for the frequentists. However, whereas the frequentists make implicit reference to considerations related to losses and subjective beliefs in choosing α and β, the Bayesians make such considerations explicitly by using the loss function.

To carry out the test, the Bayesian calculate the mean expected losses linked to the decision to accept H_0 or H_1 (this is done by calculating the weighted means of the losses linked to the choice of H_0 and H_1 multiplied by the rispective a $posteriori$ probabilities of H_0 and H_1) and choose the hypothesis corresponding to the smallest mean loss.

The discussion of this theory is definitely beyond our goals. We refer the reader to the book by Wonnacott and Wonnacott [105] for an introduction to the topic and to the previously cited work by Berry [12] and by Spiegelhalter, Abrams and Myles [97] for a complete discussion. Here we will only point out that, assuming a constant loss function, the experiment leads us to choose the hypothesis associated with the highest a $posteriori$ probability. In our example on walking distance, we obtain the following: area under the curve corresponding to the values $\delta_\mu \leq 0$ equal to 0.054; area under the curve corresponding to the values of $\delta_\mu > 0$ equal to 0.946.

The a $posteriori$ distribution of δ_μ allows us to directly calculate the probability of the alternative hypothesis, corresponding to the smallest difference considered clinically relevant. Therefore, it helps us to directly answer the question concerning the clinical relevance of the results. Let us suppose we have decided that $\delta_\mu = 50$ meters is the smallest difference in mean walking distance between the two treatment groups that still is of clinical relevance. Using the a $posteriori$ distribution, we can calculate the probability of $\delta_\mu \geq 50$. In Figure 5.7 this probability is represented by the area under the curve to the right of $\delta_\mu = 50$ meters. If this area is sufficiently large (for example 0.9, i.e. 90% of the entire probability distribution), we can accept the hypothesis that δ_μ is at least 50 meters, therefore that the difference between treatments is clinically relevant. In our example, the probability of $\delta_\mu \geq 50$ is approximately 66%, thus it is not "sufficiently" large to accept the alternative hypothesis.

In concluding this section we should point out that the assumption of homoscedasticity would have simplified the calculations. However, as we said, generally Bayesians prefer not to make this type of assumption.

5.6.2. Estimation of the Effect: the Bayesian Solution

What is the best point estimate of the parameter δ_μ? Most would agree intuitively that a "good" estimate of δ_μ is given by the mean of the a $posteriori$ probability distribution (or another statistic capable of summarizing its position or "central tendency", such as the mode or the median). In our example, the mean of the a $posteriori$ distribution is 67.1 meters.

With the Bayesian approach, as with the frequentist one, numerous types of estimation methods exist and the validity of the estimates is assessed based on a series of desirable properties, generally different from those used by the frequentists (see [76]).

In our example, the Bayesian point estimate of δ_μ coincides with the frequentist one, i.e. it is the difference between the two treatment sample means, if non-informative *a priori* probability distributions are used, as we have done. This concurrence of results does not always occur, even when non-informative *a priori* distributions are used. When *a priori* distributions other than the non-informative ones are used, the frequentist and Bayesian estimates always differ.

Moving to the interval estimate of δ_μ, the Bayesians build the **credibility** or **credible interval** (the term confidence interval belongs to the frequentist approach). This is defined as the smallest set of values of δ_μ having an *a posteriori* probability greater than or equal to a certain desired value. For example, if we wish to build a bidirectional 95% credibility interval, we must find the smallest interval of values of δ_μ which has a total *a posteriori* probability of 95%. To obtain this interval, we could take the set of values of δ_μ for which $p_{posteriori}(\delta_\mu) > h$ and then choose h so that this set has a total area of 95%. With reference to Figure 5.8, we need to choose the value h so that the set of values included between $\hat{\delta}_{Inf}$ and $\hat{\delta}_{Sup}$, identified by the two vertical lines passing through the two intersections between the horizontal line crossing h and the $p_{posteriori}(\delta_\mu)$ curve, is equal to 0.95.

The width of the credibility interval depends on the variability of the *a posteriori* distribution: the less variable (i.e. more narrow) the distribution, the more precise (i.e. smaller) the credibility interval and vice versa.

In our example comparing two walking distances, the bilateral 95% credibility interval for δ_μ, based on the *a posteriori* distribution illustrated in Figure 5.7, is (-14.7; 148.9) meters in favor of treatment A. With an analogous procedure,

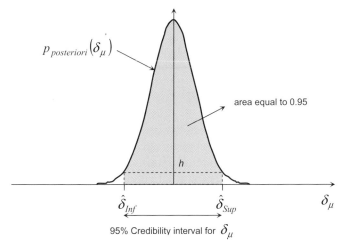

Figure 5.8. How to use the *a posteriori* probability distribution of δ_μ to estimate and build a bidirectional 95% credibility interval

the unilateral credibility interval can be calculated.

In conclusion, in our example the 95% confidence interval and the 95% credibility interval give approximately the same result (but it should be considered that with the Bayesian approach, we made no assumption of homoscedasticity). Again, this does not always occur. In any case, whether the results coincide or not, the interpretation of the two types of interval is different.

For the comparison of two means:

- The frequentists' 95% confidence interval is the smallest set of values of the statistic d_μ which includes 95% of its sample distribution, i.e. it is the smallest set of values which includes 95% of the sample estimates of the parameter that we would obtain in hypothetical future studies, all similar to the one actually performed.
- The Bayesians' 95% credibility interval is the smallest set of values of δ_μ which has an overall probability of 95%, i.e. it is the smallest set of values which includes the true value of the parameter with a probability of 95%.

Only by somewhat forcing the concept, we can say that the frequentists' interval includes the true value of the parameter with a probability of 95%.

5.7. Some Additional Considerations on the Frequentist and Bayesian Approaches

At this point, no matter which approach is chosen, the role of statistics should be clearer to the reader. It is a set of techniques for the evaluation of the degree of uncertainty, which:

- In the planning phase of the experiment, allows evaluation of the risks associated with a number of necessary choices, such as, for example, the choice of the sample size (in turn linked to many other factors – see chapter 6).
- In the assessment phase of the experiment, it allows the appropriate analysis and interpretation of results.

Also, the reader should remember that the clear-cut separation between the frequentist and Bayesian approach we maintained throughout this chapter was an intentional exaggeration, with the goal of simplifying the presentation. In fact, intermediate approaches exist and there are many statisticians who are open to adopting either approach, depending on the nature of the specific problem.

We can now attempt a comparison between the two approaches. There are two main criticisms of the Bayesian approach: the first is that it is a subjective method where results depend on the arbitrary choice of the *a priori* probability distribution; the second is that it often requires very complex calculations that are difficult to verify. The most common criticism of the frequentist approach is that it follows a twisted logic.

Concerning subjectivity, we must recognize that this is present in both approaches. It plays a big role in the frequentist approach as well, although it is, so to speak, more hidden. For example, as already mentioned, the choice of the 5% threshold of statistical significance is totally arbitrary and exclusively codified by use and by convention. The same can be said of the choice of the acceptable level for the type II error. Likewise, the choice of the threshold of clinical relevance is almost always highly subjective (see chapter 6). Nevertheless, the frequentist approach profiles itself as an objective method in which elements of subjectivity are perceived as "undesirable".

On the contrary, in the Bayesian approach, subjectivity, intended as a broader concept of probability than the one based on frequencies derived from long series of tests, is the very essence of the method. In this approach, the acquisition of knowledge is considered an interlocutory process that, by its own nature, includes elements that are openly subjective, especially in the initial phases. It is true that subjectivity should not be intended as a license to use non-sensical *a priori* distributions; on the contrary, the initial probabilities must have an acceptable basis. It is true that this choice becomes progressively less subjective, as more knowledge on the unknown parameter is acquired. It is also true that the impact of the choice of the *a priori* probability can be verified, within limits, by studying the variation of the estimate of the parameter with the variation of the *a priori* distributions. Finally, it is true that some kind of "reference threshold" can be built from non-informative *a priori* distributions, when calculating the *a posteriori* probability distribution. However, the fact remains that the subjective elements can never be completely eliminated. The acceptance of subjectivity, as matter of fact inseparable from the cognitive process, is what characterizes the Bayesian approach. From this point of view, the solution of limiting subjectivity by restricting the use of Bayesian methods to non-informative *a priori* distributions, seems to betray the foundation of the approach.

The complexity of calculations is definitely greater in the Bayesian approach. This limitation was practically impossible to overcome before the computer became a widely accessible commodity. Later, an almost equally insurmountable limitation was the lack of software allowing scientists without advanced expertise in computer programming to use the Bayesian methods. Today the situation has changed dramatically, so much so that the complexity of calculations is almost no longer an obstacle. If anything, the one thing that remains difficult is the verification of results by others, since the *a posteriori* distributions often cannot be treated with analytical methods. Therefore, simulation methods ("Monte Carlo", "bootstrap", "jackknife" and others) must be used to estimate empirically or approximately these distributions and to calculate the relevant areas, intervals, etcetera.

Let us now move to the criticism of the frequentist approach. In our view, it is difficult to deny that the reasoning behind it is not very straightforward. For example, when we perform a statistical test, what we really would want to know is whether the observed difference is due to chance or not. With the Bayesian approach we can answer this question directly. Instead, with the frequentist approach we can only manage to get this information indirectly.

If the test is statistically significant, the probability of getting a result equal to the one obtained in the study or one more extreme, under the hypothesis H_0 of absence of differences (i.e. by chance), is lower than the threshold of statistical significance (almost always 5%). This probability is considered sufficiently small to conclude that the observed difference did not result from chance. If the test is not statistically significant, then through analogous reasoning, the frequentists conclude that the observed difference is due to chance. The reader must pay attention to the roundabout way one gets to the final verdict, due to the fact that the p-value does not directly express the probability that the observed difference is due to chance.

The same consideration can be made for the confidence interval. In section 5.5.2 we saw that with the frequentist approach it is difficult to answer the question: "does the confidence interval include the true value of δ_μ?", which is what the researcher is really interested in. When we obtain a 95% confidence interval in a study, this interval either includes the true value of δ_μ or does not include it, and there is no way to know which situation we are in. What we can say is that we are applying a procedure that works (that is to say, includes the true value of δ_μ) with a probability of 95%. This is the relative frequency of the intervals including the true value of the parameter in a long sequence of intervals, stemming from a long sequence of hypothetical identical experiments. This property of the procedure is then extended to the single interval somewhat stretching the logical argument.

In our opinion, the main reason why the Bayesian approach is less common than the frequentist one in the field of clinical research is that it does not easily lend itself to a rigid decision making system. We do not mean to say that the frequentists necessarily use rigid decision making schemes, only that the frequentist approach is more suited to a final judgment of the "true/false" type. The Bayesian approach seems to us to be intrinsically contrary to this type of oversimplification: it represents well the cognitive process, the way it develops in time, that is, a gradual process of getting closer to the "truth", through various shades of gray. This explains why this approach is rarely accepted by the regulatory authorities (especially as a method of analysis of phase III pivotal trials), who must necessarily draw black or white conclusions and, consequently, why it is not used much by researchers nor appears much in applied scientific publications. Another reason is that the frequentist approach became widely used long before the computer did, at a time when the Bayesian approach was really difficult to apply. To gain back lost ground the Bayesian approach must prove itself against a widely used and accepted method.

Before bringing this section to an end, we need to stress another difference between the two approaches: the different attitude toward the multiple tests, which we discussed in section 4.7. The issue is very important and warrants a closer examination, since it influences many experimental situations, spanning from the use of more than one primary end-point to the comparison of more than two groups, to the interim analyses and so on. The conceptual model behind the frequentist approach, that of repeated sampling, entails the problem of statistical multiplicity, while this is not a problem in the conceptual model used by the Bayesians.

The frequentists define as statistically significant those differences between the sample means that are so extreme that they would occur in less than 5% of the tests, if the two groups were selected from populations having identical means (we saw that, in general, the scientific community considers that the risk of making this error is sufficiently small if less than 5%). When we perform many statistical tests, the probability of making at least one type I error increases compared to when we perform only one test. We remind the reader that for a comparison between two means, a type I error is the erroneous conclusion that μ_A and μ_P are different. This occurs when the results of the study give by chance an extremely high or low difference $\bar{X}_A - \bar{X}_P$. This observed difference leads to the wrong conclusion that there is a difference between the two population means μ_A and μ_P, when in reality there is none. When many statistical tests are performed, the probability of obtaining by chance at least one such extreme result rapidly increases with the number of tests performed.

These problems are not encountered with the Bayesian approach, since the logical process occurs in the context of the data obtained from the one experiment truly conducted, not in the prospective of an infinite repetition of the experiment. The probabilities that are calculated from the *a posteriori* probability distribution directly express the probability of the unknown parameter being equal to or greater than a certain value of interest. Therefore, no adjustments for multiplicity are required. However, what we just stated must be interpreted with caution. It does not mean that for the Bayesians it is acceptable to perform studies with many end-points of the same importance (i.e. many primary objectives), planned as if there were only a single end-point. First of all, the rule of not performing studies addressing too many questions at the same time is a principle of good clinical practice valid for everyone, including the Bayesians. The biggest problem of these studies remains that of interpreting conflicting results from different end-points. Second, if one wants to have multiple end-points of equal importance in the same study, in order to use correctly the Bayesian approach, one must face the problem of reconstructing the complex links among the end-points, and consequently among the respective probability distributions.

5.8. Parametric and Non-Parametric Inference

In this section we introduce the distinction between parametric and non-parametric inference, terms that are very often encountered in applied clinical research. This is not an easy task because in this book we have not touched upon all of the concepts required to explain this distinction. As a consequence, we can only provide rough definitions.

Parametric methods are those in which both of the following requirements are met:
- The researcher is interested in submitting hypotheses on one or more parameters of the population to statistical testing, or in estimating such parameters.

- The researcher knows the distribution of the end-point of interest in the population on which the inference will be made.

Methods for which both of these requirements are not met are called **non-parametric**.

Let us consider again the example that we have used all along in this chapter. We said that the end-point of interest, the walking distance, has a distribution of known shape, which we have assumed is normal. This distribution is completely characterized by two parameters, the mean μ and the standard deviation σ, as illustrated in Figure 1.1. For the probability theory (see Table 5.7), the difference between the walking distances of two independent populations A and P also has a normal distribution, with mean $(\mu_A - \mu_P)$ and standard deviation $\sqrt{2\sigma^2}$ (assuming $\sigma_A^2 = \sigma_P^2 = \sigma^2$).

At this point it is clear that the example falls in the parametric inference because both of the requirements stated above are satisfied.

It is important to stress that the results of the parametric analysis, both in the frequentist and Bayesian approaches, depend on the assumptions made on the distribution of the primary end-point. If these assumptions change, for example the distribution is assumed of a different shape, the results also change. For this reason it is of paramount importance to always perform a statistical verification of the assumptions whenever a parametric analysis is carried out.

Let us now imagine that the end-point walking distance has a distribution the shape of which is unknown. As usual, we are interested in testing the efficacy of a new treatment (A) and wish to perform a clinical study in which this treatment is compared to placebo (P). We extract a sample of subjects (units) from the population of patients with intermittent claudication; then we randomly assign the subjects to the two treatments under comparison so as to form two independent groups; finally, having treated the patients for an appropriate period of time, we observe the results in each group. At this point, we summarize the results appropriately, for example using the mean, median, or another estimator of central tendency. The object of the inference remains the same, that is, the extension of information obtained on the samples to the underlying populations, but there is no link between the distribution of the population and the sample distribution of the estimator. In this context we would perform a non-parametric inference.

5.9. Statistical Decision Making in the Medical Field

In **statistical decision making,** a statistical-probabilistic model for decision making is formally linked to one or more experimental models. In this context, the data collected in the experiment (or experiments) are analyzed with the explicit objective of making an optimal choice.

In the medical field, a typical decision making problem is when the doctor has to decide how to treat his/her next patient, on the basis of the knowledge of the results of clinical trials available up to that moment. This problem belongs to the category of the so-called **predictive problems**: we have a past experiment (the clinical trial) giving information pertinent to the outcome of a future experiment (the treatment of future patients), both experiments having the same inferential structure. For example, let us suppose we have performed an experiment in which the end-point walking distance is measured in n_A patients treated with compound A and n_B patients with compound B. The doctor having to choose whether to treat his/her next patient with A or B (assuming A and B are both active) would find it very useful to be able to predict the walking distance of that individual patient after A and after B.

Both the frequentist and Bayesian approaches offer statistical methods to allow such a prediction. We have no intention in this book to discuss these methods, not even superficially, because of their complexity. We refer the reader interested in the topic to the books by Piccinato [76] and by Berry [12], which however require good knowledge of mathematical analysis and probability calculus.

Our objective is to show the reader that the true essence of clinical practice is making decisions under conditions of uncertainty. When the doctor sees a patient for the first time, he/she needs to adopt a strategy to guide the plan of investigations. To begin with, the doctor must move towards a specific diagnosis (or a restricted group of options), based on a multiplicity of information obtained from different sources: the medical history of the patient, the symptoms and the signs detected during the visit, epidemiological, etio-pathogenicity and clinical knowledge of the disease, etc. To reach a sufficient degree of diagnostic certainty and to exclude alternative diagnoses (the so-called differential diagnosis), the doctor can add to the history and physical examination of the patient a set of laboratory and/or instrumental investigations. To do so, the doctor must have information, as up to date as possible, on the validity of the available diagnostic tests. Once the diagnosis is established, the attention of the doctor turns to treatment and prognosis. The question that the doctor asks him/herself is: what is the evidence supporting the different available treatments? In choosing, the doctor must also consider the potential side effects and cost implications of the different options. If a new treatment is started, the doctor must also decide what tests the patient will need to perform to monitor progress and how frequently. Depending on how the clinical picture evolves, the doctor will need to make other decisions. If the patient's problem is not solved, is it worth continuing the treatment? If the problem is solved, is it reasonable to perform further tests and/or visits? At each phase of the diagnosis and treatment process, the doctor must make decisions in a context of uncertainty.

We must admit that the decision process followed by the doctor in the practice of medicine is close to the Bayesian approach, in the sense that the *a priori* probabilities of a given diagnosis are constantly updated by new observations, new results of laboratory and instrumental investigations, etcetera. Obviously, the doctor does not formally apply the Bayes' theorem, but uses the same logic and would be helped if he/she were aware of the principles behind it. It is a fact that, whereas in the inferential field the frequentist methods are applied much more commonly, in the field of decision making problems, it is the Bayesian approach to be more frequently used .

5.10. Evidence-Based Medicine

In this last part of the chapter we will give an introduction on the so-called **Evidence-Based Medicine** (EBM), which has the primary objective of helping the doctor to make the best possible choices in the treatment of individual patients. As we will see, this approach gives an explicit recognition to statistics as a fundamental tool for drawing conclusions in clinical as well as in epidemiological studies, and for helping doctors to make appropriate decisions in the treatment of patients.

EBM is a discipline both relatively young and, so to say, fashionable. It is one of the many disciplines born from clinical epidemiology. However, more and more emphasis has been put on clinical research, intended as the group of disciplines assessing the effect of treatments, and on diagnostic research, intended as the group of disciplines assessing the accuracy and precision (i.e. the validity) of tests to diagnose and evaluate progression of diseases.

One must admit that the expression EBM is somewhat weird, in that it seems to imply that there is an alternative medical practice based on non-evidence! Unfortunately this is indeed the case, even though few physicians would be willing to admit it. Clinical practice is full of decisions based on an "ideological" approach, on sympathy, fascination, personal interest, etcetera, all of which are foreign to evidence.

EBM as a discipline was born from an idea originated by Professor Sackett and some of his colleagues at the McMaster University in Canada [89, 90]. EBM is defined as the "conscientious, explicit and judicious use of current best evidence in making decisions about the care of individual patients". This definition integrates two components of equal dignity: the personal clinical experience of the physician and the ability to critically evaluate the results of medical research, both epidemiological and clinical. It is important to stress again that the two components have equally important roles.

The success of EBM had various positive effects.
- The first and most important one is that of helping doctors to care better for their patients.
- Another important contribution is that EBM has drawn attention on the importance of scrutinizing quality of the medical information available to the public from databases, scientific journals, the web and other sources. The admonition that quality of medical literature is often poor is not new and certainly pre-dates EBM: on this issue see, for example, the articles by Altman [2], Brown [19] and Pocock, et al [78]. However, EBM made a strong contribution to this awareness. First, by highlighting the shortcomings of many high

profile studies and relative publications. Second, by giving impetus to the creation of groups aimed at performing systematic reviews of the literature and at defining and divulging criteria to discriminate reliable from unreliable research. Among these groups, the Cochran Collaboration Center [11] is particularly active. It is an international organization, established in 1992, which has the primary aim of facilitating informed decision making on medical and health care matters, by preparing, updating and divulging the so-called systematic reviews or meta-analyses (see chapter 12) of clinical and epidemiological studies, in practically all areas of medicine. This organization is well known for its database (Cochran Database of Systematic Reviews in the Cochran Library), regularly updated by the member groups.

- Furthermore, EBM has contributed to the definitive affirmation of the fundamental role of methodology and statistics in medical research, both experimental and epidemiological. In reality, for many years it has been clear that an understanding of methodological and statistical principles is indispensable for critically evaluating the results of both clinical and epidemiological research (see for example the two guidelines ICH [60] and [61]). However, such awareness has traditionally been limited to a relatively restricted number of "insiders". The broad public of "beneficiaries" of biomedical research, doctors, biologists, pharmacologists who read scientific magazines, without being directly involved in research, for a long time have been typically unaware of the methodological bases of research, which prevented them from critically evaluating it. Unfortunately, many still are. However, EBM had the great merit of bringing a broader public closer to the debate on what represents methodological rigor and statistical evidence. At the same time, EBM solicited the recognition that knowledge of methodological and statistical principles is indispensable also to doctor day to day care of individual patients.

As a rule, any experimental result should be considered as affected by accidental variability, and the statistical analysis has the aim of evaluating the disturbance resulting from it. To fully understand the contribution that statistics can give, one must be aware of the value and limitations of any statistical procedure. The measurement of evidence and the techniques to evaluate it proposed by frequentist and Bayesian statistics are different, as we attempted to explain in this chapter. The debate on the role of these approaches in the medical field, which appeared to be definitely closed in favor of the frequentists, has recently gained new impetus, and the Bayesian approach is today often seen as a more natural and conceptually easier approach to measure the statistical evidence. An interesting dissertation on the statistical concept of evidence, with applied comparisons between the two approaches, can be found in a paper by Piccinato [77], while a more practical discussion on the concept of evidence of efficacy and safety required for the regulatory approval of a pharmacological treatment can be found in a paper by Gould [52].

Many articles have been written, both in the statistical and medical literature, on the issue of statistical training of doctors: a very useful reference is an entire volume (volume 21) of Statistics in Medicine, published in 2002. As we said, EBM explicitly recognizes the need for all doctors, including those not involved in research, to understand the basic concepts of epidemiological and experimental methodology and of statistics. The doctor needs this knowledge to interpret and assess the information coming from clinical and epidemiological studies published in the literature, and to apply this information to the diagnosis and treatment of the individual patient. It is interesting to note that the UK General Medical Council has included the following requirements for all general practitioners (see again [4]):

- Ability to formulate the problems in a clear way, to implement an appropriate strategy to solve them and to critically evaluate the data collected to establish the efficacy of this strategy.
- Ability to understand the contribution of the different research methods, and to apply and interpret correctly the results of studies performed in the specific area of competence.

Summary

What characterizes the questions of inference and decision making, which are the foundations of clinical research, is that the answers are given under conditions of uncertainty. If the level of uncertainty is low, the conclusions are strong; if the level of uncertainty is high, the conclusions are weak. The probability theory provides the tools and methods to perform this kind of assessments. Several approaches to defining probability exist. In the "frequentist" approach, probability is the relative frequency of an event, calculated in an infinite sequence of experiments all performed under the same conditions. In the "subjective" approach, probability can be defined as the price that one is willing to pay to get 1 if the event occurs and 0 if the event does not occur.

A variable is called random when its value is uncertain and for this reason it is given a probability distribution. A probability distribution can be seen as the ordering (from the smallest to the greatest) of all the values or groups of values that the variable X can hypothetically assume, each quantified by the probability of it occurring (a point on the ordinate axis for a discrete variable, or an area under a specific section of the curve for a continuous variable). Each probability distribution, to be usable operationally, must be described by a mathematical expression, linking each value x of the variable X to its probability.

Statistical inference is the set of procedures through which conclusions obtained on the sample are extended to the underlying population. The need for statistical inference stems from the recognition that the result of a single experiment (a sample result) does not coincide with the true effect of the treatment, since each result is affected by accidental factors (chance), to an extent that is different with every repetition of the experiment and unpredictable.

In statistics there are several inference methods, each based on a different probabilistic approach. The best known are the frequentist approach (by far the most commonly used in the clinical field), based on the frequentist definition of probability, and the Bayesian approach, based on the subjective definition of probability. Both approaches can be used to test hypotheses and to estimate parameters, i.e. the effects or signals of interest.

In the frequentist approach, the inspiring principle is that of repeated sampling, which assumes that the experiment is performed an infinite number of times under identical conditions. The statistical procedures (both for estimation and for hypothesis testing) are evaluated with reference to this hypothetical series of repetitions of each experiment, throughout which it is assumed that all experimental conditions, including the effect of the treatment(s) under investigation, remain unchanged. The treatment effect is the unknown parameter to be estimated. It is considered to be a fixed quantity, while the statistic summarizing the experimental results is considered variable during the hypothetical repetition of the experiments. When the statistical analysis carried out with this approach shows that the result is statistically significant, the conclusion is formulated as follows: "It is very unlikely (typically with probability equal to or lower than 5%) that a difference equal to or more extreme than the one observed is due to chance". The meaning of "extreme" must be interpreted differently, depending on whether the alternative hypothesis is unidirectional or bidirectional.

In the Bayesian approach, for every experiment two phases are considered: the pre-experimental one, where the results have yet to be obtained, and the post-experimental one, where the results are available. In the pre-experimental phase both the unknown parameter (that is, the real effect of the treatment) and the set of results which are possible before performing the experiment (*a priori*) are treated as random variables, each having its own probability distribution. In the post-experimental phase, the result of the experiment is no longer a random variable, because there is no more uncertainty about it, while the parameter is still treated as a random variable. The conclusion we draw through the statistical analysis performed with this approach is summarized in the *a posteriori* distribution of the parameter, from which we can directly obtain the probability that the unknown parameter has of being equal to or greater than any value of interest.

The inference methods are divided into parametric and non-parametric. Methods satisfying both the following requirements are called parametric:
1. The researcher is interested in submitting to statistical testing hypotheses on one or more parameters of the population, or in estimating such parameters.
2. The researcher knows the distribution of the end-point of interest in the population on which the inference will be made.

The methods not satisfying both these requirements are called non-parametric.

In recent years, a new discipline, called Evidence-Based Medicine (EBM), has acquired growing standing within the medical community. This discipline has been defined by Armitage and Colton as the "conscientious, explicit and judicious use of current best evidence in making decisions about the care of individual patients". EBM facilitates the integration of two components of equal dignity in the medical decision making process: the personal clinical experience and the ability to critically evaluate results obtained from epidemiological and clinical research. To reach the latter objective it is crucial for the medical community to understand and embrace the basic principles of methodology. EBM played a very important role in elevating methodological and statistical knowledge to the prominence of a basic discipline for any doctor, even if not directly involved in research.

6
The Choice of the Sample

The sample is the group of subjects on which the study is performed. Two aspects, one qualitative and the other quantitative, must be considered when choosing the sample.

6.1. Which Subjects Should Form the Sample?

The qualitative aspect of the sample selection consists of:
- Defining the key characteristics of the subjects to be enrolled.
- Defining the mechanism for selecting the subjects from the population, which must be such that a sample representative of the underlying population is obtained.

6.1.1. Characteristics of the Patients to be Enrolled in the Study

Some characteristics will be considered indispensable for the subject to be included in the study (inclusion criteria), while others will be considered incompatible with the study (exclusion criteria).

First of all, depending on the type of clinical study, the sample can be of healthy volunteers or of patients affected by a given condition. **Healthy volunteers** are generally involved in the initial phases of the clinical drug development process (phase I, see chapter 12). The criteria qualifying a person as "healthy" are far from obvious. At one end of the spectrum, we can consider healthy any person who does not have clinically overt diseases at the time of entering the study. Most would consider such an approach problematic, because it does not account for undiagnosed diseases, nor for diseases at a subclinical stage (because mild or initial), nor for risk factors. At the other end of the spectrum, we could decide to consider healthy only the subjects showing "normal" values in a very large set of instrumental and laboratory tests. The latter approach is just as problematic as the former, if not more so, because there is practically no limit to the number of tests one can undergo and because, when many tests are performed, it is practically certain that some results will be outside the normal range, even in the absence of disease and risk factors. If such a diagnostic "furor" is used, any volunteer would violate at least one criterion for perfect health and be classified as diseased.

Clearly, the status of healthy volunteer presumes the absence of clinically relevant diseases. Routine investigations of the cardiovascular function (e.g. standard electrocardiogram), liver function (e.g. transaminases, bilirubin), renal function (e.g. creatinine clearance, electrolytes), and of the hematological profile must be assessed as normal in the context of a thorough clinical examination. This should be a true integration of information from different sources, not a mechanical screening of the test results against the respective "normal ranges". Once major organ and system impairment has been ruled out, a subject must fulfill additional criteria to qualify as "healthy", depending on the type of treatment and disease under study. Furthermore, the cultural context in which a study is performed plays a key role in defining "good health". Is a subject with a common cold healthy or not? What if he/she is anxious? If a subject is paraplegic, because of a car accident, but otherwise perfectly healthy (perhaps an elite athlete), is he/she healthy or diseased? Is an over-weight, but not obese, person healthy or diseased? Obviously, there are no absolute answers. It should be noted that the inclusion of female healthy volunteers into an early study implies that the drug being studied has already passed fertility and teratogenicity tests in animals (these tests evaluate the influence of exposure to the drug during conception and pregnancy on malformations and survival of the offspring). Sometimes these studies are not yet completed when clinical development begins; therefore, phase I studies must be restricted to male volunteers.

Except for phase I studies on healthy volunteers, clinical research is performed on patients affected by a specific disease or condition. In fact, in many therapeutic areas, including oncology, even phase I studies are increasingly conducted on patients instead of healthy volunteers. When patients are the object of a study, the first step in the sample selection must be an accurate definition of the diagnostic criteria. For many diseases diagnostic guidelines exist, published by national and international specialist bodies (such as the American Heart Association, the European Respiratory Society, etc.). In planning a study, it is generally advisable to use recognized guidelines, resisting the temptation (often very strong) of modifying them for the purpose of the study. The adoption of modified guidelines generally enhances the credibility of the study only in the eyes of the researcher who made the modifications, but diminishes it in the eyes of the rest of the scientific community.

Another very important selection criterion concerns the severity of the disease: the most severe forms of many diseases are somewhat independent entities, characterized by a special pathogenesis and clinical picture. The researcher must decide whether or not to include in the study the patients at the extreme end of the severity spectrum. In fact, sometimes it is appropriate to focus exclusively on this group of extreme patients, because that is where the therapeutic need and most of the human and financial costs are. Going back to the example used in chapter 4, asthma is generally a disease manageable with relatively simple treatments and compatible with an almost normal life. However, steroid-resistant asthma, affecting 5 to 10% of asthma patients, is very difficult to treat, causes a dramatic reduction in the quality of life (to which the side effects of the available drugs contribute), has a quite high mortality and is responsible for a disproportionate fraction of the direct and indirect costs caused by this disease.

Once the diagnostic criteria of the disease are defined and the range of severity to be included in the study is decided, the researcher must face the complex problem of the other selection criteria. The nature of the problem is similar to the one described above for the choice of healthy volunteers. Around the central criterion, the condition under study, a virtually endless constellation of factors exists, which could affect the efficacy of the treatment, its safety, or both. These criteria certainly deserve to be considered, starting with the demographic characteristics. Elderly subjects could be more prone to potential side effects than younger ones. Women in their fertile years are at risk of becoming pregnant during the course of the study (see below). And then there is the issue of children: is it ethically acceptable to experiment the new drug in children (see below)? A second group of criteria concerns the concomitant diseases: which ones will we accept in the study? And what will we do about the patients with abnormal laboratory values? A third group of criteria concerns the behavioral, occupational and life style factors, some of which carry legal implications. Should we enroll cigarette smokers? If yes, must we set a limit to the number of cigarettes smoked per day? And what about subjects taking drugs or who have done so in the past? Should we exclude some professions, for example train or bus conductors? Is it necessary to impose the HIV test? The list of categories and examples could go on for the rest of this book.

The dilemma faced by the researcher is the following: the stricter the inclusion and exclusion criteria for the study, the smaller the background noise of biological variability. Therefore, it will be easier to detect a response to the treatment. Furthermore, the risk of unexpected adverse events will be lower. On the other hand, the stricter the inclusion and exclusion criteria, the more abstract and far from the clinical reality the sample will be. The risk is to end up with an enrollment plan restricted to subjects affected by the disease under study, but otherwise super-human for physical health, psychological balance and absence of risk factors. In our career as protocol reviewers, we have seen this frequently. Apart from the practical difficulty of finding such subjects, who may only exist in the researcher's mind, what is at risk is the legitimacy of generalizing the results. The results of our study may only apply to a theoretical population that, at best, represents a minute fraction of the real population of patients.

As a general rule, it is acceptable to be more restrictive in the early phases of the clinical development (phase IIa- see chapter 12), where the principal aim of the study is to prove the biological hypothesis behind the treatment (the so-called "proof of concept studies"). When it comes to the dose-response studies (phase IIb) aimed at selecting the dose (or doses) for phase III pivotal studies, it is necessary that the selected sample be representative of the majority of the patients to whom the treatment is targeted. Since experience with a new treatment is generally still very limited in phase II, more selective inclusion and exclusion criteria in phase II dose-response studies compared to those of phase III pivotal studies, can still be accepted. However, a mistake to avoid at all costs is that of having drastically different patient selection criteria between the dose-finding studies and the pivotal phase III studies, as the dose(s) chosen for phase III could be painfully wrong.

Special groups of patients. Patients with kidney or liver impairment are generally studied separately (when such patients are relevant for the disease under investigation), under strictly controlled conditions. An alternative approach, which is relatively new and used more and more, is that of studying sub-groups of patients in large integrated databases of multiple studies. At the end of phase III, an integrated database generally includes thousands of patients. This number is even higher if, after drug approval, the database is updated with post-registration studies (phase IV - see chapter 12). Let us suppose we are interested in knowing the tolerability profile of a corticosteroid in patients with myopia, i.e. shortsightedness (corticosteroids can cause or worsen various ocular conditions including glaucoma and cataracts). Rather than performing a dedicated study in such patients, one can extract from the integrated database all of the patients for whom myopia has been reported in the physical examination performed at the beginning of the study (naturally, this implies that myopia was not an exclusion criterion in the main studies). Some of the myopic patients extracted from the database will have been treated with the experimental treatment, others with the placebo, still others with active controls. Adverse events and laboratory data can then be summarized and compared between the treatment groups. The great advantage of this approach is that it makes good use of the great amount of data generated during clinical development, and is far more rapid and cost-effective than an ad hoc study on a special population.

On the other hand, the reader should keep in mind that results of analyses of subgroups from integrated databases should be interpreted with caution. This is for several reasons, above all the imbalance, with respect to known and unknown prognostic factors, that can potentially be introduced in the comparison between treatments in a subgroup (when one extracts subgroups from a larger group, some experimental units are excluded from the statistical comparison, and consequently, the balancing effects of randomization may be jeopardized). Other reasons that suggest caution in interpreting these analyses are:

- The problem of multiple comparisons (see below).
- The problem of a post-hoc selection of subgroups, i.e. after having examined the data, which allows the "fine tuning" of selection criteria so that the results will confirm the desired hypothesis ("data driven selection"). Going back to the example of myopia, the careful examination of the integrated database could suggest that there is no difference between corticosteroid and placebo in the frequency of glaucoma and cataract when considering the subjects with more than 2 diopters (a measure of the degree of myopia), while there appears to be a higher frequency of such events in the corticosteroid group when considering subjects with 1 to 2 diopters. This knowledge could induce the researcher interested in demonstrating that corticosteroids are safe to define the subgroup of myopic subjects as "subjects with more than 2 diopters".

Some of these problems are mitigated by the fact that the special populations we are talking about are often standardized, i.e. predefined quite precisely (in which case they do not lend themselves easily to "data driven selection"). In addition, statistical methodologies exist for the subgroup analyses (interaction tests) which reduce some of the above mentioned problems [64]. Finally, the alternative of performing dedicated studies in the special populations of interest has its own share of problems, which are equally complex or even more so. Such studies are extremely difficult to conduct, long and expensive and, because of the complexity of finding patients, major issues related to the representativeness of the sample may arise.

We will conclude this section on the qualitative characteristics of sample selection by dealing briefly with three special aspects: studies on pregnant women, studies on children and informed consent.

Studies on pregnant women. Generally, before entering a clinical study, women in their fertile years must perform a pregnancy test and, once enrolled, must agree to use birth control methods for the entire duration of the study (to note that pharmacological methods such as oral contraceptives may be forbidden, because of the risk of interaction with the treatments under study). This is because a pregnancy starting during a study is generally a dreaded event to be avoided, even if doing so involves complex ethical and practical issues, for example when dealing with a teenager accompanied by her parents, and with cultural contexts where contraception can be very problematic. The reason for this extreme caution is obvious, especially in the presence of a completely new pharmacological entity. However, the consequence is that information on the efficacy and tolerability of a new treatment on pregnant women (and on the unborn) is almost never available when the treatment is approved and made available to doctors and patients. Unavoidably, the package insert will carry a warning against the use of the drug in pregnancy. Clearly, it would be very important to fill this big gap as soon as possible. After a few years on the market, when there is more confidence in the efficacy and tolerability profile of the treatment, formal studies would need to be performed in pregnant women. But this almost never happens, at least not in the structured and highly regulated form that must be followed to obtain the initial approval of the drug. In practice, in this very delicate area, the scientific community (health authority, pharmaceutical industry and academia) tends to completely shirk responsibility: initially, it relies on the uncontrolled and accidental use of the drug in pregnancy to gain experience. Later, only exceptionally will it formalize this experience with appropriate clinical studies. Naturally, there are some exceptions, but these are rare and generally occur too late.

Studies on children. It is a commonly held opinion, both in the general public and in the scientific community, that, for ethical reasons, clinical experimentation on children should be performed only much later than that on adults. Unfortunately, in general, experimentation on children either starts many years after studies on adults have concluded, or it is not performed at all. Thus, the pediatrician is left with the difficult task of empirically adapting to their little patients drugs and other treatments that really were only tested on adults. In our opinion, and in agreement with many experts in the field, this approach is neither scientifically nor ethically justified. From the scientific point of view, children are not "little adults": the efficacy of a drug can be higher or lower in a pediatric population compared to an adult one. Furthermore, children are neither necessarily more prone to side effects, nor do they necessarily require lower doses compared to adults. From the ethical point of view, it is the lack or the excessive delay of experimentation on children that is unacceptable. The pharmaceutical companies and the scientific community must be encouraged to start appropriate clinical studies in children as soon as possible, often very early in the clinical development program, for example, immediately after completing phase I or phases I and IIa (see chapter 12) in the adults. In this regard, it is interesting to recognize that for drugs of pediatric interest that were not voluntarily tested in children, the US Food and Drug Administration (FDA) often formally requests that the sponsor perform an appropriate clinical development program in pediatric populations, offering, as an incentive, an extension of the duration of the patent protection for that drug.

Informed consent. The **informed consent** to participate in a clinical study (as a healthy subject or patient), to be given by the subject him/herself, if capable of giving it, by a legal guardian when the subject is not, or by both when the subject is less then eighteen years old, is now a cornerstone of clinical research. The right of the patient to an informed consent is stipulated in the Declaration of Helsinki, already included in its original version of June 1964 by the World Medical Association and later amended several times (for the latest version see [106]). The problems related to the informed consent will not be discussed in this book. However, we do want to stress the importance and the complexity of the problem. Subjects who are asked to consent to enter a study, the "experimental units" to clinical researchers and statisticians, are real people who are generally suffering physically and psychologically, often caught at the peak of very dramatic situations. They may not be highly educated and may feel intimidated by the medical personnel asking them to give their consent. It is hard to tell what is informed consent under such conditions. What does the parent who just took his/her child to the emergency room, or the patient who has just been diagnosed with cancer, truly give consent to? How "informed" can the consent be of a semi-literate farmer intimidated by the white coats in an academic medical center? The problem is very difficult and there are no solutions that are valid for all situations. However, it is essential that researchers, who are not in direct contact with patients, keep in mind the procedures and risks for which consent is asked, and ponder whether they themselves would enroll in such a study or would enroll a loved one.

6.1.2. Mechanism of Subject Selection

As previously discussed (see chapters 2 and 5), to be able to extend results from the **sample** to the population it comes from, the former must be **representative** of the latter, i.e. all types of subjects (experimental units) included in the population must be proportionally represented in the sample.

The method generally used for selecting a representative sample is that of choosing the experimental units randomly from the population. This method insures that the units included in the sample differ only by chance from those not included. This makes it likely that the group of subjects included in the sample will not differ in any systematic and relevant way from the group of subjects not included in the sample with respect to known and unknown prognostic factors (including demographic and baseline characteristics).

The further we move from random selection, the more problematic it is to generalize the result obtained on the sample to the underlying population.

In real life clinical research, however, we do not achieve truly random samples of patients; rather, we select the sample from the cohort of patients who seek treatment at the center(s) where the study is performed. Such patients may be more or less representative of the population.

The drawback of not having truly random samples from the population is compensated by randomly assigning the patients to the treatments, a process called randomization. In reality, this solves only part of the problem. In this way the groups are not systematically different from each other, therefore, the study has internal validity, according to the definition given in chapter 4 (ability to draw comparatively valid conclusions). However, randomization cannot compensate for a distorted selection of the whole sample as far as generalization of the result is concerned. If, for example, our sample includes predominantly patients from one particular social status, because the majority of the subjects who refer to the study center belong to that social status, it will be difficult to extend results to patients of all social levels of the population. We will return to this topic in chapter 9. For the moment let us be satisfied with the internal validity of the study and suffice it to say that randomly assigning the subjects to treatments, through the process of randomization, puts us practically in the same condition as randomly extracting samples from the population.

6.2. How Many Subjects Should Form the Sample?

One cannot expect to get from the sample the exact same result that one would get if it were possible to evaluate all units of the population. We need to consider this element of variability when deciding on the size of the sample.

The number of subjects to be included in a study (the so-called sample size) is generally the result of statistical, medical and practical considerations.

6.2.1. Statistical Considerations

In this section, we will briefly discuss the statistical criteria that contribute to determining the sample size of a study and explain some of the mechanisms used in the frequentist approach. This section applies only to studies aiming at demonstrating the superiority of a treatment over another. Other methods, which will not be considered in this book, are used to determine the sample size for equivalence and non-inferiority studies.

It will be useful for the reader to refer to Figure 6.1, similar to Figure 5.5. Both refer to a unidirectional test for the comparison between means, assuming an end-point with normal distribution and homoschedasticity. However, instead of illustrating the sample distribution of the test statistic d^*_μ, Figure 6.1 illustrates the sample distribution of the statistic d_μ, both under the null hypothesis ($H_0{:}\delta_\mu{=}0$) and under the alternative unidirectional hypothesis ($H_1{:}\delta_\mu{>}0$). We remind the reader that, under the conditions considered, the sample distribution of d_μ is normal, has mean $\delta_\mu{=}0$ under the null hypothesis, and $\delta_\mu{>}0$ under the alternative hypothesis and has variance $\left(\dfrac{\sigma^2}{n_A}+\dfrac{\sigma^2}{n_P}\right)$ under both hypotheses. In this figure the areas corresponding to α, β, and $1\text{-}\beta$ (= power) for the unidirectional test of interest are shown. Furthermore, the standard deviation of the two sample distributions is reported, equal to the square root of the variance (i.e. $\sqrt{\left(\dfrac{\sigma^2}{n_A}+\dfrac{\sigma^2}{n_P}\right)}$), which we know from Figure 1.1 determines the width of the normal distributions. Before carrying on, the reader should make sure these concepts are clear, in light of what was presented in chapter 5.

In evaluating a statistical test, the concept of power is essential. The power of a test is the probability that the test will draw the correct conclusions when the treatment has a real effect. Remember that the power is calculated by subtracting the probability of obtaining a false-negative (i.e. of concluding that there is no difference between treatments when a difference does exist) from the number 1 (which indicates absolute certainty of detecting a difference when it really exists). Generally, the power is expressed as a percentage, therefore, if the probability of a false-negative is 20%, the power of the test is 80%; if the former is 10%, the latter is 90%, and so on.

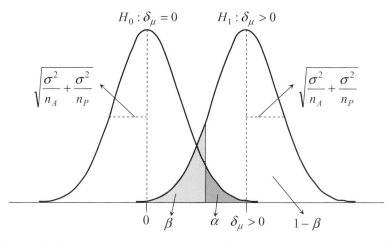

Figure 6.1. Elements for establishing the sample size of a superiority study based on a comparison between means, assuming an end-point with normal distribution and homoschedasticity

A power of less than 80% is generally considered unacceptable in the context of clinical trials.

As we will see later, all of the components of the statistical test are linked. As a starting point, let us consider the relationship between power and sample size. This is a relationship of direct proportionality, that is, as the sample size increases, so does the power, and vice versa. The concept that, if we increase the number of patients we study, we also increase the probability of reaching the right conclusion is intuitive at a common sense level, but not obvious from a mathematical perspective. We will illustrate this concept by making reference to Figure 6.1. The sizes of the two groups under comparison, n_A and n_P, can be found in the denominator of the formula for the standard deviation of the two sample distributions, therefore, whenever they get bigger, the standard deviation gets smaller. If the standard deviation gets smaller, the two curves become narrower (see also Figure 1.1). For these curves to stay centered respectively on the value 0 and on the value of δ_μ considered in the hypothesis H_1, the overlapping area between the two curves must necessarily shrink. This causes, for a given value of α, a reduction of β and an increase in the power (= $1-\beta$). Since the power and the sample size increase or decrease in a directly proportional way, if we change any of the other elements involved in the test in a way that reduces its power, we must increase the size of the sample to bring the power back to the desired level.

We will now briefly touch upon the individual components contributing to the calculation of the sample size. It is important to stress that the statements made below for each component of the test are valid under the assumption that all other remain unchanged.

1. ***Threshold of clinical relevance of the signal.*** The smaller the clinically relevant difference between treatments, the bigger the number of subjects required to detect it, that is, to separate it from the background noise and, therefore, declare it statistically significant. Figure 6.1 should help to better understand the reason for this. If we maintain unchanged all other conditions, but choose a threshold of clinical relevance smaller than the one illustrated in the figure, the distribution under the alternative hypothesis (H_1) must move to the left (because it is centered on a smaller value of δ_μ). Thus, assuming that α is kept unchanged, β will increase and therefore the power of the test will decrease. To leave the power unchanged, the sample size must be increased.

2. ***Variability of the primary end-point.*** The greater the variability of the end-point (intrinsic or induced by the measurement process), the more subjects are required to detect a given threshold of clinical relevance. Returning to Figure 6.1, if we consider a greater variance σ than the one shown in the figure, the two distributions will be larger and flatter. For the two curves to remain centered on 0 and on the value of δ_μ respectively, the area of overlap between the curves must necessarily get bigger. This in turn creates an effect similar to the previous one, i.e. it eventually leads to a reduction in power, that can only be balanced by increasing the sample size.

3. ***Acceptable risk of obtaining a false-positive result (α).*** As discussed in chapter 5, the highest probability of a false-positive result (i.e. the erroneous conclusion that there is a difference between the groups, type I error) that one is willing to accept is the threshold of statistical significance, indicated with α. The smaller the value of α we adopt for the study, the bigger the size of the sample. Returning to Figure 6.1, if we decrease α (for example, from 0.05 to 0.01), because we want to be more conservative, β will increase, therefore, once again, the power of the test decreases, unless we increase the sample size.

4. ***Acceptable risk of obtaining a false-negative result (β).*** As discussed in chapter 5, the highest probability of a false-negative result (i.e. the erroneous conclusion that there is no difference between the groups, type II error) that one is willing to accept, indicated with β, determines the power of the study ($1-\beta$). The smaller the value of β we adopt for the study, the bigger the sample size must be. In this case, the statement is obvious, considering that the power is equal to $1-\beta$.

5. ***Unidirectional or bidirectional alternative hypotheses (one- or two-tailed test).*** In the previous chapter we stated that the two-tailed test is more conservative than the one-tailed test, that is, if all other conditions are the same, the two-tailed test requires more subjects. Again, Figure 6.1 is helpful. If we perform a two-tailed test, we will have to consider another sam-

ple distribution of d_μ, to the left of the null hypothesis, as in Figure 5.6. Under these circumstances, Figure 6.1 represents only one part of the test (the one to be considered when $\delta_\mu > 0$) and the tail of area α must be reduced to $\alpha/2$. This automatically determines an increase of β and therefore a reduction in power, to be balanced with an increase in sample size (the same reasoning applies when $\delta_\mu < 0$, clearly focusing on the other distribution of d_μ).

6. **The type of test statistic.** If we change the type of test statistic we have used so far in our example, the size of the study will change: in fact, Figure 6.1 will no longer be valid. However, the intricate net of relationships existing among the various elements of the test remains the same. In general, parametric tests require less patients (i.e. have more power) than the corresponding non-parametric tests. Choosing one type of test over another depends on the nature of the end-point (for a definition of parametric and non-parametric analyses see section 5.8).

7. **Design of the study.** The way in which the subjects are assigned to the treatments and are evaluated (see chapters 10 and 11) influence the sample size in that they can modify the variability of the end-point (see point 2 above) and also the type of statistic required to conduct the statistical test (see point 6 above). For example, provided that all other conditions remain unchanged, a parallel group design requires more patients than the corresponding cross-over design, because in the former, but not in the latter, the total number of patients is obtained by multiplying the number of patients needed for one treatment group by the number of treatments and also because in the cross-over design the variability term used in the statistical test is usually smaller (see chapter 10). The stratified design or the randomized block design, both of which control some of the sub-experimental factors, generally require less subjects compared to completely randomized designs (see chapter 10). With some designs, increasing the number of measurements on each subject (repetition of measurements) has an effect similar to increasing the sample size (see section 11.4). In a particular case of experimental design, called N of 1 (described in chapter 10), the sample is only one subject. Above and beyond the design per se (intended as the mechanism of assignment of the subjects to the treatments and the plan on when to measure the end-points), many other aspects of the research protocol, such as the way patients are selected, measurements are performed, end-points and signals are defined, etc., influence the variability of the response and therefore the sample size.

8. **Frequency of premature discontinuations (drop-outs).** In any clinical experiment it is unavoidable that some subjects leave the study before it is finished. This can occur for a variety of reasons, including dissatisfaction with the treatment, occurrence of an undesired event, loss of interest in the study, change of address, etcetera. These subjects are called **drop-outs**. In general, all subjects contributing to the primary end-point, even if only to a mini-

mal extent (i.e., all subjects who have at least one evaluation for the primary end-point after the beginning of the treatment), are inserted into the statistical analysis. This approach is called "intention-to-treat" (see chapter 9). However, the true contribution of a patient to the detection of the signal generally diminishes as the actual duration of treatment, compared to the intended duration, decreases. Therefore, if the number of drop-outs is high, the variability of the response will increase and the effect of the treatment will be, on average, attenuated. Furthermore, some patients will end the study before they can give any information about the primary end-point. These patients will not contribute at all to the statistical test. It is necessary to consider all of these elements at the time of planning the number of subjects to enroll in the study. The higher the probability that patients will leave the study prematurely, especially before contributing to the primary end-point(s), the higher the number of patients to be enrolled.

9. ***Number of primary end-points and corresponding statistical tests.***
When there is more than one primary end-point, the calculation of the sample size must be repeated for every one of them. If, in order to declare a treatment efficacious, we require that statistical significance be reached for all the comparisons (tests) performed, the size of the sample will have to be the largest among the ones calculated for the individual end-points. If, instead, we are ready to declare a treatment efficacious when only some of the comparisons reach statistical significance, this rule is not sufficient because, as mentioned in section 4.7, the implications of multiple comparisons must be taken into consideration. One of the solutions to this problem is the use of an α value that is smaller than that which would be used if only one test were performed. As a consequence of this choice (see again Figure 6.1), β increases and therefore the power decreases: to keep the power at the desired level, the size of the sample must increase.

In this section we have only considered one aspect of inference, the hypothesis testing. In particular, we have described how the power of the test changes with the change of any of the other elements contributing to the statistical test. However, it should not be forgotten that the size of the sample has a similar impact on the other aspect of inference, the estimation. The precision of an estimate, i.e. its reproducibility in other experiments conducted under similar conditions, increases as the sample size increases (see section 1.3.2). If the sample size is maintained constant, the precision of the estimate and the power of the test mirror each other in the way they change with changes of the other elements described in this section. Precision, in turn, determines the width of the interval estimate (the confidence interval for the frequentists), which will therefore become progressively narrower as the sample size increases.

As anticipated in section 5.7, the role of statistics in the process of determining the sample size is that of performing an evaluation of the risks (of false-positive or false-negative results) associated with different choices. Therefore, the outcome of a sample size assessment generally is not one single number, but a range of numbers, each representing the outcome of a different scenario. This information is important in deciding whether or not to perform the study as planned, both from an ethical and a financial point of view. Performing an under-sized or an over-sized study is unethical, apart from special cases in rare diseases. From a financial perspective, the risks of performing type I and II errors translate into risks for the investment made. For example, if the researcher decides on a β of 0.3, instead of the standard value of 0.2, the money needed to conduct the study will be lower because the study will be smaller, but the financial risk for the investment will be higher, because of the increased probability of concluding the study with a false-negative result.

6.2.2. Medical and Practical Aspects

The first medical contribution to the definition of the sample size of a study is to clearly define, together with the statistician, the objective of the study and the threshold of clinical relevance of the signal(s) of interest.

Once these key aspects of the protocol are defined, the most correct approach to determining the sample size is to perform a preliminary statistical calculation to get an idea of the order of magnitude of the number of subjects required to detect the selected signal or signals. At this point the task of estab- lishing the practical feasibility of the study should start. To this end, the fol- lowing points must be considered.

1. **Expected enrollment rate.** The researchers responsible for planning a study must try hard to estimate the number of eligible patients that each study center will provide each month of recruitment (or year or other appro- priate time unit). One should keep in mind that the estimates given by the centers in the planning stage are almost always too optimistic. Pocock [79] suggests halving the initial estimates obtained from the centers, to have a more realistic idea of the enrolment rate that will actually occur when the study is underway. Our experience suggests that in many cases even Pocock's approach is too optimistic.

2. **Time required for enrolment.** The total number of patients required for the study must be divided by the projected enrolment rate, considering all of the centers involved in the study. The resulting enrolment time will have to be compared with the acceptable duration of the study.

3. **Acceptable duration of the study.** The acceptable duration of a study varies dramatically depending on the disease under investigation and the cir- cumstances of the study. However, some simple rules are always valid.
- The investigators are more motivated in the initial stages. If the study lasts too long, the motivation tends to decrease and the quality of the study tends to worsen.

- The pharmaceutical company (if any) sponsoring the study generally needs it to be completed within a given time, in order to be able to meet the timelines of the clinical development program.

If the estimated sample size of the study is at least roughly compatible with the acceptable duration of recruitment, the researchers can move on to a more comprehensive statistical assessment, which should provide sample sizes for a range of different scenarios. For example, the choices of α and β are in many ways arbitrary; therefore the consequences on the sample size of more or less conservative choices of α and β can be considered. With regard to variability, sometimes it is possible to adopt experimental designs which "control" variability in a more efficient way (see chapter 10) than others. This, of course, will impact the sample size. Sometimes, different sample size options can be proposed based on different thresholds of clinical relevance. Alternatively, if the treatment under study is considered very promising, e.g. because in previous studies it demonstrated far better effects than the threshold of clinical relevance, the size of the study can be based on the expected effect, rather than on a threshold of clinical relevance. This would obviously result in a smaller sample size. However, at the same time, the researcher must accept the danger of declaring the treatment inefficacious even if it shows a clinically relevant effect (in other words, must accept a higher than necessary risk of a false-negative conclusions).

If the estimated sample size is completely incompatible with the acceptable duration of the study, one could attempt to increase the overall recruitment rate, for example, by increasing the number of participating centers, or by changing the patient selection criteria of the protocol. Another approach could theoretically be that of modifying the specifications used for the statistical calculations, in a manner similar to that described above. However, if this is done with the sole purpose of justifying, on financial or practical grounds, a sample size much smaller than the one originally considered necessary, such an exercise can easily become ridiculous. It is indeed ridiculous when the specifications for the statistical calculations are changed over and over again, until the "acceptable" sample size decided in advance finally pops up and is considered "justified".

It is clear that costs play a crucial role in determining the size of a study. The cost per patient changes from study to study, depending on its duration, location, number of visits and on the complexity of the required medical investigations. Sometimes, when the projected costs exceed the available budget, it is reasonable to consider a simpler and cheaper experimental design. However, this may not be possible without sacrificing the main objectives of the study. Pocock [79] supports the idea that, if it is not possible to conduct the study in such a way that a clinically meaningful difference can be detected with a "reasonable" degree of certainty, it is better to forgo the study. Many other researchers, including the authors of this book, share this opinion, unless the disease under study is rare. The opinion of the supporters of the so-called meta-analyses may be different (see chapter 12). Some of them recommend that studies should be performed even if under-powered, as long as well designed and properly performed, in light of the possibility of combining the individual studies through meta-analyses.

Finally, it should be noted that the sample size of pilot studies, which have the purpose of estimating the order of magnitude of the parameters of the phenomenon of interest, is generally determined empirically i.e. without the support of formal statistical procedures.

Summary

The sample is the group of subjects on which the study is performed. The choice of the sample requires qualitative and quantitative considerations. Among the qualitative aspects of the sample selection, crucial is the need to ensure that the sample is representative of the population to which one wants to extend the conclusions of the study. Among the quantitative ones, crucial is the need to quantify the concept of "sufficiently large sample", i.e. of a sample large enough to allow the detection of the treatment effect, separating it from the variability of the phenomenon, with an acceptable degree of certainty. This is achieved through statistical methods. The size of the sample required for a given study depends on the magnitude of the signal, the risks we are willing to accept of making type I and type II errors, the type and variability of the end-point(s), the design of the study, and the number of treatments and primary end-points. Once the information on the size of the sample required for a given study is obtained, it is essential to evaluate the feasibility of the study, based on practical considerations, such as the number of patients we are likely to obtain from the participating centers, the study duration considered acceptable and the projected costs. If the study is not feasible, sometimes changes in the design will allow the researcher to conform to the limits set by the above-mentioned practical considerations. However, in other cases, it is best to give up. This is much less frustrating than proceeding with a study which is bound to fail.

7
The Choice of Treatments

aIn line with the terminology introduced in section 2.4, in this chapter we shall use the term "experimental treatment" when referring to the main object of a clinical trial (often a novel treatment), and the term "study treatments" when referring to both experimental and control treatments.

In a clinical study, in addition to the study treatments, there may also be concomitant treatments. Both categories of treatments must be described in detail in the research protocol.

7.1. Study Treatments

Experimental treatments are the intervention of interest that one wants to study in a given disease or condition. As discussed previously, they are evaluated in comparison to other treatments, called control treatments. The experimental and control treatments constitute the study treatments, to be distinguished from the concomitant treatments. The latter can be taken during the study, but are not the object of the experimentation.

As mentioned in chapter 1, the experimental treatment can be of different types, as summarized below.

- Pharmacological, for example, a novel inhibitor of cyclo-oxygenase isoenzyme-2 (COX2 inhibitor) against arthritis pain.
- Surgical, for example, a new form of partial gastrectomy (that is, partial removal of the stomach) against multiple or recurrent gastric ulcers.
- Psychotherapeutic/behavioral, for example, a specific form of psychotherapy against anxiety.

- Logistical/organizational, for example, normal hospital wards instead of intensive care units for selected patients with myocardial infarction.

The general principles of clinical research methodology are identical, whatever the nature of the experimental treatment, even if some procedural, logistical and ethical aspects may differ. Unfortunately, the experience of the authors of this book is limited to pharmacological treatments. Therefore this book is inevitably unbalanced towards such treatments. However, we want to stress that in non-pharmacological therapeutic areas the need for rigorously performed clinical experimentation is equally great, but there are relatively few researchers capable of applying the general principles of research methodology to their respective disciplines.

Control treatments should represent the state of the art therapy for the condition under study at the time the trial is performed. If no treatment of proven efficacy and/or acceptable safety/tolerability exists, the control treatment should be a **placebo**. A placebo can be defined as an inactive treatment, identical to the experimental treatment in every aspect, except for the presumed active ingredient(s) or intervention. The placebo is used as a control treatment with the aim of separating the intrinsic effect of the experimental treatment from other effects, often more powerful, linked not to the treatment itself, but to the process of treating the patient, including the expectations, psychological influences, nursing support, duration of hospitalization, etc. To this end, it is very useful that the study **treatments** be administered in a **blinded** (or **masked**) fashion, that is, such that neither the patient nor the research staff know which study treatment is administered to which patient. The methodological reasons and practical implications of the use of placebo and of the blinding of study treatments will be discussed in depth in chapter 9.

If the experimental treatment is a capsule, the matching blinded placebo will also be a capsule, as close as possible to the former in shape, size, color, appearance, flavor and smell. If the experimental treatment is a partial gastrectomy for multiple and recurrent ulcer, the corresponding blinded placebo (at least in theory) would be a surgical intervention with the same anesthetic procedures, skin incision, duration, suture and post-surgical procedures, but without the actual gastrectomy (it is obvious that there are ethical problems here - see below). In a study evaluating the efficacy of a given form of psychotherapy for treating anxiety, the blinded placebo would be a set of "mock" psychotherapy sessions identical in context and duration to the "real" ones, but in which the psychologist administers to the patients a generic form of support instead of the specific psychotherapy under study. Finally, when logistical measures are evaluated, the blinded placebo can be obtained by standardizing the logistical context in which the study is conducted. In the above mentioned example, comparing the efficacy of intensive care to that of traditional hospital stay, the patients assigned to the latter may be placed in the intensive care ward, but receive a normal level of care (i.e. with all of the bedside monitors turned on but not used), so that neither the patients nor their relatives realize that the care level administered is really that of a "normal" hospital ward.

As with many other topics in this book, it is not possible to cover the topic of placebo to the extent it would deserve. All we will do here is to briefly address some of the issues resulting from the use of this methodological artifice.

The use of a placebo in a clinical study causes many ethical problems. First of all, the basic question arises as to whether the use of placebo is in itself ever ethical: is it ethically acceptable to administer a treatment we know to be inactive? Furthermore, even admitting that the practice as such is acceptable, is it ethical to use a placebo that involves invasive procedures, such as the sham gastrectomy operation mentioned above? Many articles have been written on this topic, in support of very diverse positions. In our opinion, in the great majority of cases, the use of a placebo as a control treatment is more than acceptable ethically, it is an ethical imperative, whenever the available treatments (which may be used as controls in the study) have not been conclusively proven as safe and effective in methodologically sound confirmatory studies. The only exception may be that of advanced stages of serious diseases, characterized by very poor quality of life, almost no chance of remission, and/or very short life expectancy (in other words, situations unlikely to be worsened by the hypothetical toxicity of a non-effective treatment). Many forms of terminal cancers belong to this category. The patient may unfortunately have little to lose, but it must be the patient him/herself, or his/her guardian, to decide this, not the researcher! In such cases, the most ethical behavior is probably to accept the risks of the experimental treatment and administer it to the whole study sample in the hope that it will show some efficacy. However, we want to emphasize that the conditions belonging to this category are few. Even for diseases with fatal outcome, if the quality of life is reasonably good (for example because not in an advanced stage), the use of the placebo is recommended in the absence of an active control of proven efficacy. From these short comments, it is evident that in extreme situations the choice concerning the use of a placebo is very subjective and may be quite dramatic (as are many other medical choices in such situations) and there are no easy rules. In any case, the will of the patient (or guardian if the patient is incapable of understanding the situation and expressing his/her will) is paramount: it must be actively solicited through an appropriate explanation of the problem, and must be respected.

The ethical implications of the use of a placebo reach well beyond the basic principle. Even those who consider ethically acceptable the use of placebo, as we do, justify its use only in the absence of an active treatment of documented and adequate efficacy and safety. The problem is that there is no consensus on the clinical value of many treatments commonly used in clinical practice. For example, inhaled corticosteroids in the treatment of chronic obstructive pulmonary disease (COPD) are considered efficacious by many specialists and largely used in clinical practice. However, various studies and authoritative experts consider the continuous use of these drugs in COPD ineffective, if not harmful. Is the use of placebo as the control treatment justified in a study evaluating a new drug in COPD? To complicate matters further, many regulatory authorities including the FDA in the United States, typically impose the use of a placebo in confirmatory clinical trials, even in diseases for which the majority of experts in the scientific community agree that an active treatment of adequate efficacy and safety does exist.

The issues concerning the use of placebo are not only ethical, but also methodological and practical.

- There are situations where a placebo matching the experimental treatment to ensure blinding is either impossible to make or not compatible with the objectives of the study. For example, if one wants to evaluate the impact on quality of life of a given therapeutic regimen (as opposed to the efficacy of the pharmacological principle), one needs to compare the experimental treatment regimen (e.g. once a day) to a control treatment regimen (e.g. twice a day), which is not compatible with the use of a placebo.
- The manufacturing of a placebo requires considerable technical and economical resources. Underestimating the complexity of this process is a dangerous mistake that can delay the start of the study by many months.

Returning to the choice of the study treatments, numerous are the decisions the researcher must make and describe in detail in the protocol before starting the study. The most important ones are summarized in sections from 7.1.1 to 7.1.4.

7.1.1. How Many Treatments

It is intuitive that the more study treatments one wants to compare in the same clinical trial, the more complex the trial will be. As the number of study treatments increases, so do the many other aspects of the study: the number of patients, the methodological and statistical complexity of multiple comparisons, the logistical complexity of the production, blinding, packaging and distribution of the treatments, the amount of data generated and the consequent complexity of data management (see section 2.2. for a discussion of the consequences of an excessive complexity of the study). Among the many ways in which a study can become excessively complex, the ambition of evaluating many treatments in the same study is one of the most common. There is no general rule concerning the acceptable number of experimental and control treatments in the same trial. In dose-response studies, where the study drug is administered as single dose or for short periods of time and the end-points are instrumental measurements, a relatively high number of treatments can be feasible. The statistical analysis of these trials may benefit from numerous treatment arms, if based on regression techniques, comparing the trends of the dose-response curves (see [86]). Conversely, for studies with treatments of long duration, end-points based on clinical outcomes or measurements (which typically require large sample sizes), and objectives of confirmatory nature, that is aimed at deciding on the best treatment among those being compared, it is generally dangerous in our experience to go beyond three, maximum four, treatments per study, whatever the experimental design (see also [85]).

7.1.2.   What Treatments

In addition to choosing how many treatments one wishes to study, it is also necessary to choose which ones to study (it is obvious that in practice, these two aspects are not sequential, but concurrent). One or more experimental treatments will naturally be among the study treatments. The choice of dose(s) and frequency of administration of an experimental treatment is all but easy, especially in the early stages of the clinical development process. Clearly, in dose-response studies more than one dose will be chosen. But which ones? What should the lowest dose be? What should the highest one be? How many intermediate doses? Based on what criteria should the doses be chosen? Sometimes, even in phase III, more than one dose of the experimental treatment is tested (this occurs, for example, when phase II studies were not able to fully define the profile of two adjacent doses). The frequency of administration often determines the success of a drug on the market. Among the leukotriene antagonists, a relatively new class of drugs used in the treatment of asthma, the once daily montelukast has been more successful than other drugs of the same class that reached the market earlier, such as pranlukast, as the latter must be administered three or four times a day. Unfortunately, pharmacokinetic data alone are not always sufficient to predict the optimal frequency of administration of a drug; therefore, it can be very useful to test more than one dosing regimen before starting large phase III studies.

If the choices concerning the experimental treatment are not easy, those concerning the comparator treatment or treatments are often even more complex. We have already discussed the placebo. When it comes to **active controls** (or comparators), it is a matter of choosing a treatment of proven efficacy (and adequate safety) that is considered the "standard of care". The problem is that often many different treatments are used in clinical practice, with numerous national and even regional differences in preference. For example, the therapeutic armamentarium for hypertension offers many classes of widely used drugs (beta-blockers, diuretics, ACE inhibitors, angiotensin II inhibitors, etc.), each class including many drugs of common use. Antihistamines are frequently used in the treatment of bronchial asthma in Japan, but are hardly used in this condition in Europe and the United States. To make things even more complex, fixed combinations of drugs, often very commonly used in clinical practice, add to the list of available options (e.g. the fixed association of diuretic and ACE inhibitors in hypertension, or of β2-agonist and corticosteroid in asthma). And this is not all: in many therapeutic areas, including the above mentioned hypertension and bronchial asthma, the pharmacological treatments can be integrated with (or substituted by) dietetic treatments and physical therapies, not to mention the so-called complementary treatments, such as massage, homeopathic agents, etc. What should a researcher wishing to test a novel antihypertensive or antiasthmatics treatment compare it to, given the methodological and practical limitations described above? As always, the final choice will be a mixture of considerations of scientific, regulatory, practical and commercial nature, combined with personal preference.

From a methodological point of view, it is important to decide from the very beginning if the objective of the trial is to establish the superiority or non-inferiority of the experimental treatment compared to the active control. For non-inferiority studies, the choice of the control drug (including its dose and dosing regimen) is even more critical than for superiority studies (see ICH guideline [61]). In fact, in a superiority study, a statistically and clinically significant result favoring the experimental treatment can be taken as evidence of efficacy, even if the active control has an uncertain efficacy or is not used at its optimal dosage. It is obvious, however, that for the purpose of concluding "real superiority" of the experimental treatment over the active control, it is essential that the latter be administered with the optimal dose and dosing regimen (see ICH guideline [62]). On the other hand, in a non-inferiority study, a positive result leads to the conclusion that the experimental treatment and the active control are both efficacious. This conclusion will be all together wrong if the control is not truly active, because intrinsically ineffective or because it has been given at the wrong dose and/or with the wrong regimen. Even though it is a common belief that experiments with active controls have less ethical problems than those with placebo (because all patients receive an "active" treatment), this is not always true. It should not be forgotten that patients receiving the experimental treatment do not receive the standard therapy of proven efficacy (at least in the parallel group designs - see chapter 10).

Regulatory and practical concerns may well be the ones that prevail in the end. For example, if a study is conducted for registration, that is, its goal is to provide confirmatory evidence for the regulatory authorities to approve a new treatment, it will often be necessary (or highly advisable) to follow specific guidelines providing essential information on how to design such studies [62]. As mentioned above, placebo very often appears in registration studies for this very reason. Sometimes the regulatory guidelines also indicate what treatment is to be used as active control. From a practical point of view, if one intends to blind the study treatments (see below), it is useful to choose an active comparator that is easy to manufacture (if not protected by a patent) or to modify into a "blinded" galenical form (see below).

Finally, sometimes commercial considerations have great importance, since the pharmaceutical company sponsoring the study can, depending on the study, "strongly recommend" or "strongly discourage" the selection of specific treatments as active comparisons. For example, remaining in the field of hypertension, an article in the Journal of the American Medical Association (JAMA) has recently been published on results of a clinical trial comparing a diuretic, a calcium channel blocker, and an angiotensin converting enzyme (ACE) inhibitor [1]. The conclusion of this study was that diuretics have an effect very similar to that of the other two treatments in reducing the incidence of coronary heart disease and of other cardiovascular diseases. Considering these data, and in light of the fact that diuretics are very cheap and generally well tolerated, one would think that a company developing a new treatment for hypertension should plan at least one clinical study with a diuretic as the active control.

In fact, most likely, if such a study were to succeed in demonstrating the superiority of the new treatment over diuretics, its results would be "valuable" in supporting a premium price of the new treatment once it reaches the market. Sometimes commercial rationales like the one mentioned are legitimate, but at other times they are not. The researcher must be able to make his/her own mind up and must have the strength to refuse to collaborate with companies that force (or deny) the choice of active controls (as well as of other key aspects of the experimental design), based on reasons that in his/her opinion are not legitimate.

To conclude this section, the so-called **"add-on" studies** deserve mention. The classic design of this type of study has two treatment groups: the experimental treatment group receives the new treatment in combination with the standard treatment (which can itself be a combination of several treatments), while the control group receives only the standard treatment. Therefore, the experimental treatment is "added-on" to the standard treatment. In this particular case, the experimental treatment is the combination of the new treatment and the standard therapy, since in this experiment one can only verify the efficacy and safety of the combination. To establish the efficacy of the new treatment alone it is necessary to administer it in mono-therapy to patients in a third treatment group.

7.1.3. Blinding of the Study Treatments

Having chosen the number and nature of the study treatments, we are only half way done. At this point we need to decide whether or not we want to "blind" them and, if so, the level of blinding desired. Blinding is a very important aspect of the methodology of clinical research, both conceptually, as an instrument for avoiding some very frequent forms of bias, and practically, for the challenge of pharmaceutical development and manufacturing of blinded treatments. Section 9.3 is dedicated to a more detailed discussion of these issues, while here we will only remind the reader that the manufacturing of blinded placebos and active controls can require many months and, if underestimated, can delay the start of the study. It is not rare that the company responsible for the production of blinded placebos and active controls requires more than one year of advance notice before delivery.

7.1.4. Packaging and Logistics

Once the study treatments are obtained, they must be properly packaged. Each package will contain the study treatment for a single patient. Sometimes it will also contain one or more concomitant treatments, such as rescue medications (see below) or drugs used as background therapy in add-on studies (see section 7.1.2).

In some cases, it is possible to include the entire treatment destined to a single patient in one "patient pack" and prepare all of the patient packs from the same production batch. However, in many other cases this is not possible. The reason for this is that all pharmacological and dietary treatments (including placebos) have expiration dates, after which they cannot be used. Therefore, in studies with long enrolment and/or long treatment duration, one or more study or concomitant treatments may expire before the projected end of the trial. This implies a very complex process of staggered packaging, which must take into account the expiration date of each of the study treatments, as well as that of the concomitant treatments, if packaged together with the study treatments, the duration of enrolment of the study subjects, and the length of the treatment.

Furthermore, an "adequate" label must be attached to each patient pack. The labeling of the patient pack, far from being a simple administrative act, is an important, complicated and treacherous process, for several reasons, not least because it is full of legal implications. The label must contain many types of information. First, it must be identified by a unique identification code (numerical or alphanumerical). In randomized clinical trials, this code is the only link between the treatment contained in the pack and the randomization list. Consequently, mistakes in coding the labels generate confusion over the assignment of treatments. A mistake of this type (or even the suspicion that one has occurred) can destroy the credibility of a study, to the point of preventing its use for registration purposes. The process of randomization was introduced in chapter 2 and will be discussed in depth in chapter 9. In non randomized studies, the code in the label will coincide with the treatment number assigned sequentially to each treated patient (note that the treatment number may be different from the enrolment number since some patients who enter the screening process may never receive the study treatment for a variety of reasons).

In addition to the randomization code (or the treatment number for non-randomized studies), the labels must contain a considerable amount of information, including the medication batch number, the country of production, the expiration date, a warning that the content of the pack is (or may be) an experimental treatment. Some of this information is required by law in the country in which the study is performed, and must be in the local language. When multicenter studies are performed in multiple countries, another level of logistical complexity is added: an accurate estimate of the number of patients to be enrolled in each participating country is needed, since, once the patient packs have been delivered, it will not be easy to transfer them from one country to another. Multilingual labels sometimes represent a partial solution to this problem.

Finally, the patient packs, properly labeled, must be shipped to the study centers. Once again, this process conceals numerous risks. Many drugs require special couriers to avoid breakage and/or to ensure proper transport conditions (for example, refrigeration). In some countries, there are long waits at customs (sometimes for "quarantines" imposed by local laws, other times for inefficiency and slowness). More than once we have had treatments become unusable due to problems occurring in this final stage.

In clinical studies, there are many other issues related to the production and logistics of the study treatments, so many, in fact, that we cannot even begin to mention them here. However, we hope that through this short overview we managed to give an idea of the complexity of the process, which requires highly qualified specialists who are an integral part of the research staff. The experienced clinical researcher will always have a special regard for the advice from colleagues in charge of treatment logistics, because often they will be the first to realize the excessive complexity of the study. For trials conducted as collaborations between a pharmaceutical company and the clinical centers, it is generally the industry that is responsible for treatment logistics (entire departments are dedicated to these tasks). For trials performed independently from industry, we recommend that the issue of treatment logistics be addressed in the very beginning of the planning process. If the study is carried out in one or few centers, sometimes an experienced pharmacy of one of the participating centers can take responsibility for this task. However, in most cases, we strongly recommend that treatment logistics be delegated to a company specializing in this area.

7.2. Concomitant Treatments

Concomitant treatments are all the treatments allowed during the study without being the object of the experimentation. For example, if in a study aiming to evaluate the pain killing effect of a novel COX2 inhibitor in rheumatoid arthritis, the patient takes an aspirin for a headache (adverse event), aspirin represents a concomitant treatment. Concomitant treatments are not necessarily pharmacological. For example, physiotherapy for headache caused by cervical spine problems, if allowed during a study, would be a non-pharmacological concomitant treatment.

It is not possible to exclude with certainty the possibility of a concomitant treatment interfering with the desired and/or undesired effects of one or more of the study treatments. In some cases, these interferences are completely unpredictable; in other cases they can be predicted or at least suspected on the basis of the mechanisms of action of the concomitant and study treatments. In the above example, we know that aspirin can influence both the efficacy and the safety/tolerability profile of COX2 inhibitors. Aspirin will positively affect efficacy, as it is proven to be efficacious against pain in rheumatoid arthritis, in addition to being active against headache. Vice versa, safety and tolerability will be negatively influenced, since aspirin damages the gastric mucosa, with consequences ranging from gastritis to ulcer to hemorrhage. Such a negative effect is especially damaging in the context of our example, since the class of COX2 inhibitors has been specifically developed to reduce the gastric side-effects of the other non-steroidal anti-inflammatory drugs (including aspirin).

Therefore, it is clear that the use of concomitant treatments must be carefully regulated by the protocol of a clinical study. This does not mean the solution is simplistically that of prohibiting all concomitant treatments. This approach (which unfortunately we see with some frequency) is almost never useful. Even in the early studies on healthy volunteers (phase I), the complete elimination of all concomitant treatments dramatically reduces the number of subjects that can be enrolled in a study and the number of subjects completing the study without violating the protocol.

Generalizing, the earlier the phase of the clinical development of an experimental treatment, the more restrictive one must be concerning concomitant treatments, since it is necessary to assess the "intrinsic" efficacy (or activity) and tolerability of the new treatment at an early stage. However, in our view, even in these early phases it is appropriate to make concessions for some commonly used concomitant treatments, unless there are obvious reasons to suspect interactions with the study treatments. Pain killers, oral contraceptives and vaccines can be included in the category of concomitant treatments for which a concession should be considered even in the early phases of clinical development.

When one reaches the stage of large, phase III pivotal studies, in our opinion, it is very important to be as liberal as possible with concomitant treatments. If we are evaluating a corticosteroid in COPD, as in one of the previous examples, we know that the population under study will have a large proportion of subjects who are elderly and suffering from cardiovascular diseases (cigarette smoking predisposes to both COPD and cardiovascular conditions). What value would there be in evaluating the efficacy and safety/tolerability of the experimental treatment when all of the drugs used in the therapy of angina, heart failure, arrhythmias, etc. are excluded? Naturally, if there is a reason to believe that specific concomitant treatments may worsen the side effects of the experimental treatment or reduce its benefits, these must be excluded also from phase III studies. However, the researcher must be aware of the consequences of such an exclusion, which will necessarily translate into a contraindication or warning in the "package insert" once the experimental treatment eventually reaches the market. If the excluded concomitant treatment is truly important, special studies aimed at investigating potential interactions at the pharmacokinetic, pharmacodynamic and therapeutic level will need to be planned.

In practice, some level of restriction on concomitant treatments must also be applied in phase III studies. In the post-registration phase (the so-called phase IV), these restrictions can be eliminated for the most part.

Finally, it should be noted that concomitant treatments can be used as markers of the efficacy and/or tolerability of the study treatments. For example, the efficacy of a new COX2 inhibitor in the treatment of pain from tooth extraction can be evaluated by measuring the time between the extraction and the first "rescue" intake of a pain killer or by counting the number of rescue doses taken in the first six or twelve hours after the operation. Likewise, the efficacy of an inhaled corticosteroid in the COPD can be evaluated by calculating the mean number of daily inhalations of rescue albuterol (also known as salbutamol, a reliever of shortness of breath with fast onset and short duration of action) over a sufficiently long period of time (1-3 months). The intake of concomitant treatments functions well as an end-point in many therapeutic areas, since it is clearly linked to the level of control of the disease under study and is generally easy to quantify.

Summary

In a clinical trial one should carefully define both the study treatments, i.e. the experimental and control treatments, and the concomitant treatments. The experimental treatments are the main objects of the experimentation and are evaluated in comparison with the control treatments. The experimental and control treatments, which include the placebo (an inactive treatment, identical to the experimental treatment in every aspect except for the presumed active substance), as a whole, constitute the study treatments. The concomitant treatments are drugs or other forms of treatment that are allowed during the study, but are not the object of experimentation. For each type of treatment, the researcher must make many choices, from the selection of the treatments, to their mode of administration, to the method of blinding the experimental and control treatments. These choices must be described in detail in the study protocol, as most of them directly influence both the conduct and analysis of the study.

8

Experimental Design: Fallacy of "Before-After" Comparisons in Uncontrolled Studies

The design of an experiment is defined as the method by which subjects (experimental units) are assigned to treatments. The chosen method of assignment in turn determines the way in which the data collected in the study are analyzed.

It is important for the reader to keep in mind that, although we use this technically rigorous definition [24, 27], often the expression "experimental design" is used with a broader meaning, to indicate all the methods and procedures used in a study: these include, in addition to the method of assignment of subjects to treatments, the criteria for the choice of control group(s), masking of treatments, study subjects and sample size, as well as the number and sequence of visits, the measurement modalities, the statistical analysis plan, etcetera. These aspects will be covered in other chapters of the book.

8.1. Experimental Design: Introductory Concepts

In this field, even at the most basic level, there are differences in terminology between physicians and statisticians. One is, in our opinion, revealing: whereas the physician refers to the assignment of treatments to patients, the statistician refers to the assignment of patients to treatments. This distinction may appear pedantic, and in practice it is, but conceptually it alludes to the different way of "seeing the world" that permeates so many aspects of the collaboration between the two professions and contributes to the difficulties in communication: the physician has an anthropocentric perspective (treatments are things, patients are persons and it is obvious that things are assigned to persons); the statistician has a methodological perspective (treatments, once decided, are fixed, whereas patients are variable, i.e. individual patients are not known *a priori*; thus patients, as they enter the study, are assigned to the predefined treatments). On this aspect we will adopt the statistician's vision and will talk of assignment of patients to treatments.

By controlling the assignment of patients to treatments, the researcher controls the experimental factors and some of the most important sub-experimental factors (see chapter 2), with two main objectives:

- Minimize the bias between the groups being compared, thus allowing accurate comparisons.
- Minimize the "unexplainable" variability of observations, i.e. the component which cannot be attributed to known factors. The expression "explain the variability" has a technical meaning, which will be clarified in chapter 10. Also, see chapter 5 for an introduction to the measurement of variability. As discussed, variability impacts the precision of the estimate and the power of the statistical test: the greater the former, the smaller the latter two (see paragraph 6.2.1). Therefore, for a given sample size, if one minimizes the variability of observations, one also maximizes the precision of the estimates and the power of the statistical tests.

Furthermore, in choosing the experimental design, the researcher must always keep in mind the need for reasonably simple study procedures which must be feasible in real life situations. The importance of not complicating things too much has already been emphasized several times in previous chapters. This need must be prominent in the design selection, to some extent even at the expense of the accuracy and precision of comparisons (estimates and tests).

The theory of experimental design is dedicated to reaching these objectives.

An important preliminary remark is that the experimental design must be appropriate for the characteristics of the disease, end-points and treatments and not vice versa. Unfortunately the "vice versa" is often chosen: the experimental design is decided a priori, based on tradition in a given therapeutic area, on the experience of a given research team or, more often, on a preconceived idea that a standard of perfection exists in a single design (e.g. the randomized, double-blind, parallel group design, see paragraph 10.2). We want to warn the reader against this simplistic approach, which can be the source of many mistakes and complications.

We shall start our coverage of experimental designs with the simplest one: the before-after comparison in a single group of subjects. The illustration of this design will be followed by the description of its many limitations, the majority of which can be solved through the use of an adequate control group (see chapter 9). The most common experimental designs will be presented in chapter 10.

8.2. Before-After Comparison in a Single Group of Subjects

Let us go back to the example of the analgesic (pain killer) effect of a new COX2 inhibitor (COX is an acronym for the enzyme cyclo-oxygenase type 2) in rheumatoid arthritis patients with chronic pain. Why not treat all patients in our sample with the experimental medication and compare the intensity of pain before treatment with the intensity of pain after treatment? This design is called **before-after comparison** or within-patient comparison in a single group of subjects. In this experimental design the comparative nature of the experiment is respected: the group receiving the control treatment is represented by the whole sample before the start of treatment with the COX2 inhibitor, whereas the group receiving the experimental treatment is represented by the same group during and/or after treatment with the COX2 inhibitor.

The before-after comparison has several features that make it attractive. First of all, this approach is frequently used in real life situations ranging from advertisement campaigns for washing powders and slimming products to the assessment of a patient's evolution by his/her family doctor; as a consequence it is easy to explain, for example, to patients when seeking their informed consent to a study. Second, since the group undergoing the control treatment and that undergoing the experimental treatment are identical (or almost, if we concede that some subjects will discontinue the study prematurely), one would intuitively assume that the biological variability is minimized and thus the likelihood of showing a response to treatment (if it exists) is maximized. As a consequence, all other conditions being equal, the sample size will be smaller compared to alternative experimental designs, i.e. we will need fewer patients to reach the same objective. In reality, as anticipated in section 4.4, this is not always true, because the convenience of within-patient compared to between-patients comparisons is dependent on the degree of correlation between pre- and post-treatment measurements on each patient: if high, within-patient comparisons are convenient, otherwise they are not.

Unfortunately, in addition to these advantages, the before-after comparison suffers from the huge disadvantage of not offering any protection against the main enemy of an experiment: bias. As repeatedly mentioned in previous chapters, in clinical research a **bias** or **distortion** is an error that systematically favours one treatment over another. The fact that the error always goes in the same direction is what distinguishes bias from random error and what makes bias so dangerous in the context of clinical trials. An error that favours at random sometimes one treatment and other times the other treatment increases the variability of the response and thus makes it more difficult to separate the signal from the background noise (see chapter 5); however, this variability is manageable (within limits) through an adequate sizing of the sample (see chapter 6). Instead, a systematic error is a very serious one because it cannot be managed in any definitive way, neither by increasing the sample size, nor by changing the statistical analysis. There are techniques of statistical analysis which may suggest the existence of bias and give "adjusted" estimates of the treatment effect, somewhat "purifying" results from the influence of bias. However, such analyses are of exploratory nature and their outcomes cannot confirm or reject in any definitive way the study hypothesis (see also section 9.1).

The only way to convincingly "manage" bias is to prevent it in the planning stage of the experiment by choosing an appropriate experimental design.

There are many potential sources of bias in a before-after comparison, five of which are of special importance:

1. The temporal variations of the disease.
2. The temporal variations of staff, equipment and environment.
3. The "regression toward the mean" phenomenon.
4. The learning effect.
5. The psychological effect.

Because minimization of bias is the main objective of the methodology of experimental designs, its main causes deserve to be discussed in some detail: these will be covered in sections 8.3 to 8.7. The last paragraph takes into consideration a special situation, namely the oncology therapeutic area, where before-after designs are heavily used.

From now on, for the sake of brevity, we will use the terms "before" and "after" to indicate all evaluations conducted before and after treatment, respectively. Although items # 1, 2, 4 and 5 can favour both "before" and "after", almost always in a before-after comparison in a single group of subjects, it is the "after" that is favoured. As a consequence, the vast majority of experimental treatments assessed in this way tend to appear effective, only to fail later on, when tested in other experimental designs offering greater protection against bias. In our view, the high proportion of "positive" outcomes is the main reason for the continuing popularity of the before-after design among researchers.

8.3. Temporal Variations of the Disease

Let's assume we are responsible for a new antihistamine compound targeted against allergic rhinitis. In a typical before-after comparison, we start a group of 30 children with overt symptoms on the new treatment. Our patient sample is recruited over a two-week period during the second half of April in the region of Umea, in the northern part of Sweden. Let's assume that the treatment lasts for two months and that patients undergo a visit at baseline and after two, four and eight weeks of treatment. At the final visit we notice with joy that 28 children out of 30 show a dramatic improvement compared to the baseline visit. We conclude that the new antihistaminic agent is very promising, potentially superior to those currently available on the market. In our final report we make a recommendation to the management of our institute to proceed as soon as possible with a full clinical development aimed toward registration and commercialization of the drug. In the meanwhile, we are busy preparing a quality manuscript for submission to a prestigious medical journal.

Unfortunately, the conclusions we reached are not supported by the experiment we conducted. In attributing the whole merit of the improvement observed in the young patients to the new treatment we forgot, first and foremost, the temporal evolution of the condition being studied. Allergic rhinitis has typical seasonal recrudescence which coincides with an increased concentration in the air of specific pollens and other allergens. In our case it is likely that the majority of patients were allergic to the pollen of birch, a very common tree in Sweden, which reaches its blossoming peak in April-May. At the start of our study, in April, birch was in full bloom and all patients were highly symptomatic, whereas at the end of the study, in August, the pollen season is generally coming to an end. In other words, patients allergic to birch pollen would have improved anyway, with or without our treatment. The question that must be asked in a clinical trial is not "how are patients doing after treatment compared to before treatment", but "how are patients doing after treatment compared to a situation identical under all respects, except for the treatment itself." Our new antihistaminic agent may well be truly effective, i.e. reduce symptoms and accelerate their disappearance; on the other hand, it may be totally ineffective or even detrimental for patients, by making their symptoms worse and delaying their disappearance. Unfortunately, our before-after design in a single group of patients does not help in any way to clarify the situation.

Many diseases have a well-known temporal evolution toward improvement (e.g. healing of a bone fracture or of a wound, common cold, influenza) or toward deterioration (e.g. most cancers, amyotrophic lateral sclerosis, chronic obstructive pulmonary disease, Alzheimer's disease) or in the form of **seasonal cycles** (e.g. many allergic conditions, Raynaud syndrome). A special form of cyclic variation is the so-called **circadian rhythm**, where the duration of each cycle is roughly 24 hours. Numerous symptoms, signs, and laboratory measurements fluctuate with a circadian rhythm. For example, it is well known that asthmatics tend to be at their worse during the early hours of the morning ("morning dip"): a before-after comparison in which "before" is the evening and "after" is the following morning almost inevitably will suggest a negative effect of treatment, whereas the opposite sequence will suggest a positive effect.

Only in very rare cases in which a treatment is associated with a massive departure from a well-known temporal evolution of a disease, will a before-after comparison in a single experimental group provide useful information. But these are exceptions. Instead, in the vast majority of cases a well-crafted before-after comparison lends itself perfectly to confirming what we want to believe, i.e. the efficacy of a new treatment. To complicate matters further, temporal fluctuations of a disease often do not follow a known pattern, as in the examples mentioned above, but are totally unpredictable (see chapter 1). Unpredictable fluctuations may overlap with the "normal" evolution of the disease being studied, thus making impossible any rationalization of results of a before-after study (which may be at least attempted if the temporal evolution is predictable). A pollen season with very low counts in a region typically characterized by very high counts; food poisoning due to a highly virulent strain of salmonella; a cancer with rapidly fatal evolution which "miraculously" disappears; a measles epidemics which causes high mortality in an aboriginal population. Temporal variations that are unexpected and different from the known pattern are not the exception but the rule. The researcher must expect them and address them by means of an adequate experimental design rather than be taken by surprise.

8.4.   Temporal Variations of Staff, Equipment and Environment

The disease or condition being studied is not the only factor capable of influencing the results of a clinical trial because of temporal variations. Any change of personnel, directly or indirectly involved in the study, can have exactly the same effect. Let's assume that during a study requiring endoscopic evaluation of the gastric mucosa, a young colleague who is involved for the first time in a clinical trial replaces the senior endoscopist. It is very likely that the two researchers will reach different, even very different, conclusions, because of an unavoidable difference in approach, experience and enthusiasm. Clearly, differences in their technical ability in the execution of measurements can cause the after-treatment assessment to be radically different from the before-treatment one, even in the absence of any effect of the treatment itself. But this is not the only factor. The quality of the relationship between the medical and nursing staff and patients is of paramount importance, as it often influences not only the symptoms or even the natural history of the disease (see below), but also numerous other aspects, just as important in determining the outcome of a clinical study. For example, as time goes by, especially in a long-term study, a relationship of mutual liking may grow between patients and study personnel. If this happens, patients will tend to miss fewer visits, fill-in their daily diaries (used in many studies to collect various types of information) more accurately, cooperate better in diagnostic procedures, etcetera. The overall outcome will be that the data collected at the end of the study will be better than those collected at the beginning. Obviously, the opposite will happen if a deterioration of the relationship develops over time. Changes over time in the administrative setting of a study are also key: if a study, initially characterized by an efficient scheduling of patient visits and management of case report forms and by a pleasant assistance to patients, with time becomes sub-optimal in such areas, either for lack of funds or for "drying up" of enthusiasm, changes in results over time are to be expected, independently of any effect of the experimental treatment.

Furthermore, it is intuitive that changes in hardware and software used to measure the end-points of a study can radically influence results.

Changes in personnel, equipment and environment, capable of influencing the results of a study, are by no means limited to the study centre: the same considerations apply to groups responsible for data collection and data management and monitoring of the study.

In conclusion, temporal variations of disease, personnel, equipment and the environment of a study are important sources of bias, i.e. of systematic error. Although in theory the bias caused by these factors can be in favor or against the experimental treatment, in a before-after design in a single group of subjects, it generally tends to favor the "after", i.e. the experimental treatment, compared to the "before", i.e. the "non-treatment", used as control. The reason is that the treatment is known (there is no blinding of treatment, see chapter 9), thus all the hopes and interests for a "positive" result can exercise, unchallenged, their powerful influence.

8.5. Statistical Regression Toward the Mean

8.5.1   The Basic Principle

Hypercholesterolemia (elevated levels of cholesterol in plasma) is an important risk factor for cardiovascular diseases. For this reason numerous drugs capable of reducing the levels of plasma cholesterol (cholesterol lowering agents) have been developed and introduced onto the market in recent years.

In a large prospective study conducted in the United Kingdom and known with the acronym of UKPDS, a group of approximately 2000 patients with diabetes mellitus was followed for five years and submitted to yearly measurements of plasma cholesterol, among many other tests [107]. Over the five-year duration of the study no temporal trend was observed for cholesterol levels. A subgroup was extracted from the total study sample based on high cholesterol levels, namely greater than 6.5 millimoles per liter (mmol/L). Approximately 200 patients were eligible for this subgroup, with a mean cholesterol at screening of 7.2 mmol/L. One year into the study, whereas the whole patient sample did not show any reduction in mean cholesterol, the subgroup showed a decrease from 7.2 to 6.6 mmol/L, equal to a non-trivial reduction of mean cholesterol of about 9% ((7.2-6.6)/6.6=0.09). The interesting aspect of this story is that, in this study, no cholesterol-lowering drug (proven or putative) was being tested. The reduction of 0.6 mmol/L in mean cholesterol observed in the subgroup between the initial measurement at screening and that taken one year later is due not to a biological phenomenon, but to a statistical one, known as statistical regression toward the mean.

The expression statistical regression toward the mean (from now on for brevity referred to as **regression toward the mean**) refers to a phenomenon by which, when a variable takes on an extreme value in the first measurement (i.e. much greater or much smaller than the mean of its distribution in the population), in successive measurements it will tend to take on values closer to the mean of its distribution, i.e. less extreme values. This phenomenon will occur every time a group of subjects is selected based on "extreme" (high or low) values of a variable, when that same variable is measured again in the same subjects. Again, the mean of the values obtained in the second measurement will tend to be less extreme compared to the mean of the values obtained in the first measurement (lower if the initial mean was high and higher if it was low), thus it will be closer to the population mean. This explains the term "regression", i.e "turning back" to the mean. This phenomenon will occur in the absence of any treatment effect. Of course, as it is always the case with probabilistic phenomena, there will always be exceptions, but these are rare: regression toward the mean is increasingly likely when increasingly extreme threshold values are chosen for the initial selection of subjects (and consequently the mean value of the first measurements becomes more extreme compared to the population mean).

If the variable used for the selection of patients is also used as an end-point in the study (in our case cholesterolemia was used as the end-point in patients selected based on high cholesterol levels), in a simple before-after comparison, the effect of treatment (wanted, but uncertain) will be confounded by the effect of regression toward the mean (unwanted, but almost certain); thus it will be very difficult, if not impossible, to separate one from the other. Methods exist to reduce or estimate regression toward the mean (see paragraph 8.5.3), however such methods are approximate, relatively complex and at times impossible to put into practice.

In real life, the researcher who observes the improvement he/she hoped for will tend to ignore (or forget) the effect of regression toward the mean and to attribute the improvement to the treatment. Attributing an effect due to regression toward the mean to the experimental treatment is one of the main reasons why studies based on a before-after comparison in a single group of subjects frequently give "positive" results.

We will now go back to the study on high cholesterol in order to explain on an intuitive level why the regression toward the mean phenomenon occurs. Each patient has a "true" value of plasma cholesterol level, which could be approximated by the mean value of the daily measurements taken at the same time of the day for one year. The intent of researchers is to select patients with "true" values above the threshold of normality of 6.5 mmol/L. In reality, however, the "true" value of cholesterolemia of any individual patient is unknown; thus a surrogate will have to be used, generally represented by a single value of plasma cholesterol measured before entry into the study (screening or baseline value). However, such measurement is subject to spontaneous fluctuations both real (e.g. due to diet) and due to measurement errors (e.g. mistakes in blood drawing, blood handling, use of reagents, functioning of analytical equipment, identity exchanges, transcription errors, etc.). As a consequence, the value of the single measurement will almost inevitably be higher or lower than the "true" value. Two situations are of interest to explain regression toward the mean: the first is when patients with "true" values below or equal to 6.5 mmol/L show by chance a screening value above that threshold; the second situation is the opposite of the first: when patients with "true" values above 6.5 mmol/L get by chance a screening value equal to or below the threshold. When a second measurement is taken, it is unlikely that the same combination of accidental circumstances that caused the initial departure of screening values from "true" values will occur again. Therefore, when a second measurement is taken, a patient in the first category will likely show a lower value of plasma cholesterol, whereas a patient in the second category will show a higher value. Since the fluctuations occur at random in both directions, the mean cholesterol level of the whole population will not be impacted much. However, because of the selection criterion used in the study, only patients of the first kind will have been entered into the study. Patients of the second kind will have been excluded. Therefore, downward changes will be much more frequent than upwards changes and consequently the mean value of plasma cholesterol in the group of patients with high screening values will tend to decrease at the second measurement.

Regression toward the mean can be demonstrated mathematically. For a clear illustration of this phenomenon in numerical terms we refer to a paper by Bland and Altman [16], which is part of a simple and exhaustive pair of papers on this topic published by the British Medical Journal in 1994 [15, 16]. We recommend these papers, together with the above mentioned paper by Yudkin and Stratton [107].

8.5.2. *Areas of Biomedical Experiments Affected by Regression Toward the Mean*

Once the basic concept is understood, one realizes that regression toward the mean is present in many areas of biomedical research. Referring once more to Bland and Altman [16], we will briefly describe three of the most important areas affected by this phenomenon.

*1. **Study of a treatment aimed at reducing high values (or at increasing low values) of an outcome variable.*** This is the case we have considered so far, the most common and important one. There are many examples where subjects with a given disease or risk factor are selected for enrolment in a clinical trial based on a threshold baseline value of a variable linked to the condition being studied, that same variable being the actual end-point of the study: diastolic blood pressure in the study of hypertension and hypotension; body weight in obesity and chachexia (pathologically low body weight); body height in gigantism and dwarfism; blood glucose in diabetes mellitus; forced expiratory volume in the first second of forced expiration (FEV1) in asthma and COPD; walking distance in intermittent claudication, etcetera. As discussed above, every time a group of subjects is selected from the population based on a measurement value above or below a given threshold, regression toward the mean will occur to simulate or amplify a treatment effect.

*2. **Study of the relationship between the initial value of a measurement and the magnitude of its change over time.*** We are often interested in finding out if the change of an outcome variable is related to its initial value. For instance, with a bronchodilator drug it is reasonable to assume that the greater the degree of airway obstruction (i.e. the lower the pre-treatment baseline FEV1 value), the greater the efficacy. Although the underlying biologic hypothesis is absolutely plausible, to verify it one cannot simply group patients in several classes based on baseline FEV1 values and then compare the magnitude of post-treatment improvement between these classes. The reason why this approach is erroneous is that regression toward the mean will not be the same for all groups. Indeed it will be proportional to the degree of baseline anomaly: it will be greatest in the group with most extreme baseline FEV1 values and will grow smaller and smaller in the groups with baseline values closer to the "norm": thus the greatest improvement in the average FEV1 value is to be expected in the group with worse (i.e. lowest) screening values, even in the absence of any beneficial effect of the treatment.

3. Comparison between two methods of measurement. This section may be somewhat obscure to the reader who is not familiar with regression analysis. For an introduction to regression analysis the reader may consult (among others) Wonnacott and Wonnacott [105].

The degree of agreement between two methods used to measure the same quantity is often assessed by means of linear regression analysis between two series of measurements, each generated by one of the two methods. The underlying assumption is that, if the two methods are in perfect agreement, the regression line coincides with the bisector line, (i.e. has equation $y=x$, where y and x indicate the measurements generated by the two methods – see Figure 8.1). The slope or regression coefficient of this line will therefore be equal to 1.

Such an approach is problematic because regression toward the mean will always make the slope smaller than 1 even in presence of a perfect agreement between the two measurement methods, independently of which measurement method corresponds to variable X and which to Y. In subjects with an extreme first measurement, repeated measurements will tend to be less extreme and vice versa, in subjects with an extreme second measurement the first measurement will tend to have less extreme values: this will simulate or amplify a "disagreement" between the two methods. Let's assume we wish to establish if body weight as reported by the patient ("referred weight") accurately reflects body weight as measured by the doctor with a well calibrated scale ("measured weight"). We ask each subject of our sample to declare his/her weight and then measure it on the scale. Let's assume we carry out a linear regression analysis using the measured weight as the predictive variable (X) and the referred weight as the outcome variable (Y). The regression coefficient will be smaller than 1: from this result we conclude that body weight as referred by the patient does not accurately reflect the weight as measured with the scale, namely, fat subjects declare a weight which is lower than the corresponding measured weight, whereas thin subjects declare a weight which is greater than the corresponding measured weight. This result is perfectly acceptable and consistent

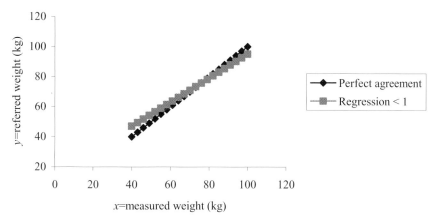

Figure 8.1. Regression between "measured weight" and "referred weight"

with common sense. Unfortunately, however, it is not supported by the data because a regression coefficient <1 is to be expected in any case due to the effect of regression toward the mean, even if the two measurement methods were in perfect agreement. Indeed, if we carry out the regression analysis again, but this time using the referred weight as the predictive variable (X) and the measured weight as the outcome variable (Y), we will once again obtain a regression coefficient which is smaller than 1. Thus the same data would suggest the opposite conclusion, namely that fat subjects tend to overestimate their weight and thin subjects to underestimate it. Bland and Altman, from whose paper the above-mentioned example was taken, propose adequate methods to evaluate the degree of agreement between two measurement methods [15].

8.5.3. How to Minimize the Effect of Regression Toward the Mean

What can we do against such a potent confounding element? In the context of clinical trials, the best way to remove the effect of regression toward the mean is to include a control treatment in the study, with randomized assignment of subjects to the treatments, as will be discussed in chapter 9. In this way, the effect of regression toward the mean is likely to be equally distributed between treatment groups and will therefore disappear when the responses of the treatment groups are compared by subtraction. Of course, regression toward the mean will still affect the response in each treatment group, thus the absolute value of the response to each treatment will remain unknown. Methods exist to minimize the problem of regression toward the mean in a simple before-after comparison (see, for example [107]). These approaches are also useful in a randomized study to estimate more accurately the absolute value of the effects of individual treatments.

1. *Estimate the magnitude of the effect of regression toward the mean and subtract it from the overall effect.* It is possible to estimate the magnitude of regression toward the mean using mathematical formulas and the following information: the distribution of the outcome variable in the population, the mean, the standard deviation and the correlation among repeated measures (known or approximated, e.g. from the literature or from screening measurements on the whole study sample), as well as the threshold value used for the selection of subjects. As an alternative to formulas, the magnitude of the regression toward the mean can be estimated through simulation. This requires a software capable of generating series of random extractions from two normal distributions (one for pre- and one for post-treatment measurements), each with a known distribution, mean and standard deviation and linked to each other by a known correlation coefficient. These methods are outside the boundaries of this book; however a simple introduction can be found in the above mentioned paper by Yudkin and Stratton. The effect of the regression toward the mean, once estimated, can be subtracted from the overall effect (obtained as a difference between pre- and post-treatment measurements), to get a more realistic idea of the true treatment effect. Clearly, all the other problems of the before-after comparison in a single group of subjects, as discussed in this section, will remain unchanged.

2. *Conduct two or more screening measurements and use their mean as baseline value.* The more accurate (i.e. less erratic) the baseline measurement is compared to the "true" value, the smaller the regression toward the mean will be. The baseline value can be "stabilized" by using the mean of multiple screening measurements instead of a single measurement. For example, going back to the UKPDS study, Ludkin and Stratton have demonstrated that, whereas the reduction in plasma cholesterol at year 2 was 9% compared to the initial screening value, the reduction of plasma cholesterol at year 5 was about 3% compared to the mean of the previous four years, indicating that regression toward the mean decreased by approximately three fold when the mean of four measurements was used as the baseline value instead of a single measurement. It should be noted that increasing the number of baseline measurements above 4 would not be of much use to further reduce the effect of regression toward the mean, therefore it can be reduced but not eliminated in this way.

3. *Conduct two screening measurements and use the first to select patients and the second as baseline value to assess the response to treatment.* The idea, proposed by Ederer [32], is that regression toward the mean can be greatly reduced if two baseline measurements are taken before treatment is started: the first is used as criterion for inclusion of patients into the study, the second as baseline value, i.e. as reference value to evaluate the treatment effect. Regression toward the mean will have occurred between the first and the second measurement; therefore, any further change between the second baseline measurement and a third measurement conducted during or after treatment can be attributed to the treatment itself and not to regression toward the mean. Such a simple approach is very appealing. However, the effect of regression toward the mean will be eliminated only if the correlation between the first and the second measurement is identical to that between the second and third measurement, which is not necessarily true, and in any case is impossible to demonstrate in the presence of treatment.

8.6. Learning Effect

Let's assume we wish to assess the effect of a new statin (a class of cholesterol lowering medications) in improving the walking ability of patients with peripheral arterial disease. We chose as primary end-point the distance covered by the patient on a treadmill under standardized conditions. The treadmill test is conducted before the start of treatment and thereafter every two months for the six-month duration of treatment. Let's assume we allocate all patients in our sample to the study treatment in a typical before-after comparison. Patient number 058, a 65 year old farmer, enters the cardiovascular physiology center for his first test: machines everywhere, cables, electrodes, monitors, an intense smell of disinfectant, white coats dashing in all directions. The patient listens to the instructions from the study nurse but is somewhat intimidated. The test starts: our patient is above all afraid of falling and the nurse's instructions are all but forgotten; the only thing on his mind is to get back home as soon as possible.

Approximately six months later the fourth and last test is reached. Our patient by now has gotten to know the nurses and technicians and finds that they are good kids. Even the doctor is not too bad after all. A friendly relationship has developed with several fellow patients and jokes are made on the distance covered during the treadmill test. The machines and the treadmill are no longer intimidating to our patient and the test day represents a pleasant diversion from the routine work at the farm.

When do you believe the patient has performed best, at the first or the fourth test? Naturally at the fourth, and this result will be totally independent of, and confounded with, any effect of the statin on peripheral arterial disease. The patient has learned how to conduct the test, how to use the machines and how to interact with the environment.

This is the so-called learning effect (in fact, in the example there may be a mixture of learning effect and placebo effect described in the next paragraph: the two are often concomitant and interdependent). The learning effect does not affect only patients, but all involved in the study: investigators, nurses, lab technicians, clinical research associates, data managers, etcetera.

The learning effect, i.e. the effect linked to the progressive familiarization with the procedures and context of a study, merges with the treatment effect: in a before-after comparison in a single group of patients it will be impossible to distinguish one from the other.

8.7. Psychological Effect

The last of the factors capable of confounding (amplifying or reducing) the effect of an experimental treatment is the **psychological effect**. A psychological component is certainly embedded in the learning effect, as shown in the previous section. However, the psychological effect is much further reaching and is one of the most potent contributors to the magnitude of the treatment effect. It can both augment and diminish the magnitude of the response to treatment, depending on the circumstances.

The psychological effect affects everyone involved in a study, from patients to researchers to support staff. It has two main components: the influence of the investigator (or other health care provider) and the placebo effect.

Influence of the investigator. A patient who recently suffered a myocardial infarction receives a phone call. To her great surprise on the line is the head of the cardiology department in person, who is very well known in town for his scientific as well as philanthropic merits. The professor congratulates the patient, as she is among the lucky few selected for an important multinational study, which has the goal of discovering the effect of a new medication on survival after a myocardial infarction. "This study -explains the professor - is the culmination of 10 years of research and, although obviously the outcome cannot be guaranteed, we are very optimistic as to the chances of the new drug to revolutionize the prognosis of myocardial infarction". "With your consent - concludes the professor - we will use the data we already have on you as the starting point (baseline) in order to evaluate the effect of the treatment on you. All you need to do is to come tomorrow to our clinic to receive the medication, take it without fail once a day for one month and report back at the end of the treatment period for a final evaluation". Our patient cannot believe her luck and of course accepts. She is enrolled in the study after signing the informed consent. At the end of treatment, she declares she feels wonderful and indeed she looks like a different person: she has gained weight, is in a good mood, energetic and optimistic on what life holds for her in the future. The truth is that our patient had already improved at the end of the phone conversation with the professor, before the start of treatment. It is clear that the circumstances have influenced her psychologically in a positive way and this, in turn, had a beneficial influence on her overall clinical condition. Obviously the doctor (or other health care provider) can have a negative influence as well when the patient does not trust him/her. The only way to dramatically reduce this cause of bias is to conduct the experiment in a blinded fashion (see chapter 9).

Placebo effect. The act of taking a treatment contributes to the psychological effect independently of and in addition to the influence of health care providers: it has been repeatedly proven that an inactive treatment which resembles an active one, namely a placebo, can have the same effect as the active treatment. This results from a combination of behavioural factors, including changes in life style due to the consciousness of being treated, and from self-suggestion.

The power of the **placebo effect** is considerable and well documented, not only on subjective end-points, such as mood or motivation, but also on objective end-points such as remission time or mortality [9, 66]. Naturally the placebo effect can also be negative, when there is a general distrust in drugs, lack of motivation, etcetera. However, it is well documented that, much more often, it has a positive influence, i.e. tends to favor the effect of a new treatment. The only way to minimize the bias caused by the placebo effect is to introduce a control group and blind the treatments being compared; if no active comparator is available, the control group should receive a treatment that is identical to the one under study, but lacking the substance presumed active, indeed a placebo.

8.8. The Before-After Design Without Control Group in Oncology

In oncology, despite all the limits described in this chapter, the before-after design in a single group of patients is frequently used in the early development stage of new compounds: the two-phase design described by Simon [95] and that described by Gehan [47] are two of several examples.

In oncology, the use of placebo (see chapter 9) poses major ethical problems: given the seriousness of the disease, how can some patients be denied standard treatment (which, although far from solving the problem, does show some efficacy) and be assigned instead to an experimental treatment, the efficacy of which still remains to be verified? Clearly, for the same reasons, it would be even less acceptable to deny all patients the standard treatment and to treat them all with the experimental one. In order to overcome this ethical obstacle, oncology compounds in general are initially tested in patients who did not respond to available standard treatments, the so-called non-responders, or patients for whom disease progression is no longer controllable. For these patients there is no remaining therapeutic option. One could consider a randomized, controlled comparison between experimental treatment and placebo in a non-responder population. But, once more, the problem is ethical in nature: since the prognosis for these patients is almost invariably unfavourable and the experimental treatment may offer some benefit, is it acceptable to deny patients this last chance? For this reason, in the early stages of development, new oncology compounds are tested on non-responder populations by means of before-after designs without a control group. In addition, again for ethical reasons, these designs include multiple steps, most frequently two (two-stage designs): the objective of the first stage is to reduce as much as possible the exposure to the experimental treatment if this does not show any sign of activity.

Clearly, as for all before-after designs in one group of subjects, the observed results could be due not to the treatment, but to one (or more) of the phenomena described in this chapter. The influence of these phenomena is however mitigated by the nature of the experimental conditions, as briefly described below.

The temporal variations of the disease are predictable within acceptable limits (although exceptions are always possible). For instance, if the response to treatment is defined as a "reduction of at least 50% of the tumor mass", the percentage of patients with tumors poorly responsive to available treatment expected to achieve a response is basically nil. If in a clinical trial conducted with a before-after design in this kind of patients, the percentage of subjects with positive response is different from 0, the study is considered a success. Obviously, depending on the type of tumor being studied, the expected result without treatment could be that 10 or 20% of patients respond; in this case it would be necessary to observe responses in at least 20 or 30% of patients to hypothesize the success of the new compound. The basic point is that the expected outcome is known with reasonable certainty. Temporal variations in personnel, equipment and the context of early phase II oncology studies can be kept under control, because typically these studies are small in sample size and short in duration. Regression toward the mean has a negligible effect compared to the natural progression of the disease. Psychological effects, including the placebo effect, certainly play a role, but this is limited by "objective" end-points.

Notwithstanding what we just said, we want to stress that, in oncology, before-after studies in a single group are used only as a screening instrument for new compounds: if an experimental treatment gives good results in these early studies, then the development plan is continued. In oncology, as in any other therapeutic area, the before-after studies without a control group cannot replace, in any way, controlled studies, which are absolutely necessary to confirm efficacy and safety of new treatments.

The before-after designs most commonly used in oncology are illustrated in greater detail in section 10.9. The use of these designs could apply to other diseases that, just like some cancers, have an "inexorable" evolution that is well known in terms of time and dynamics.

Summary

By means of the experimental design the researcher controls the experimental factors and some of the most important sub-experimental factors, with two principal objectives:

1. Minimize the bias between the groups being compared.
2. Minimize variability.

In choosing the study design, the researcher must always keep simplicity in mind (studies which are too complex are not feasible).

The most elementary experimental design is based on the before-after comparison in a single group of subjects, i.e. without a separate control group ("before" and "after" refer to the beginning and the end of treatment, respectively). There are numerous sources of bias in this design:

- Temporal variations of the disease.
- Temporal variations of personnel, equipment and the context of a study.
- Statistical regression toward the mean, a phenomenon by which a variable having an extreme value (very high or very low) in the first measurement will tend to be closer to the population mean in subsequent measurements.
- Learning effect.
- Psychological effect, basically caused by the physician and/or by the awareness of being treated.

Despite these limitations, before-after comparisons without a control group are used extensively in oncology in the early stages of the development of new compounds, mainly for ethical reasons.

9
Experimental Design: the Randomized Blinded Study as an Instrument to Reduce Bias

9.1. Introduction

From the previous chapter it should be clear that in most cases the before-after comparison in a single group of patients is an inadequate experimental design, as it fails to achieve comparisons free from bias. "Before" is not a good control for "after", since the effects of many factors are mixed with the effect of the treatment, introducing all kinds of systematic errors. Generally, in this type of experimental design, bias has the effect of simulating or exaggerating the effect of the treatment.

At first glance, the so-called **historical control** seems an attractive and cost-effective alternative. In this kind of study, the control group is a group of patients with the disease of interest and documented selection criteria and endpoints, who were however diagnosed and treated in the past, i.e. before the beginning of the study (hence the term "historical"). Unfortunately, many of the sources of bias discussed for the before-after comparisons also apply to comparisons with a historical control. In particular, it is likely that the temporal, learning and psychological effects influence the two groups in a quite different way. Often, the historical control does not come from a clinical trial and this enhances the differences from the experimental group. Furthermore, the quality and quantity of health care available to the historical group (nursing support, organization of the hospital, psychological support, etcetera) can be very different from that available to the group prospectively followed in the study. As for the before-after comparison, the historical control design also tends to exaggerate the effect of the treatment.

In order to reduce the probability of bias distorting the results of a study, it is therefore necessary to divide the sample into two or more groups to be treated and followed prospectively and simultaneously: the so-called **concomitant** or **concurrent controls**. A treatment or a sequence of treatments is assigned to each group. The former case is referred to as a parallel group design, the latter as a cross-over design. Let us suppose we have three study treatments (A, B, C), each lasting one week. In the parallel group design the sample is divided in three groups, each receiving one of the study treatment: the first group is assigned to A, the second to B, and the third to C. The three groups, sometimes called arms of the study, are treated and followed up in parallel (hence the name of this design) for the duration of the treatment (one week in our example). Since each group corresponds to one treatment, conclusions are drawn by comparing the groups. In the cross-over design, each group receives a different sequence of treatments, instead of a different treatment. With three treatments six sequences are possible (A-B-C, B-A-C, C-B-A, B-C-A, A-C-B, C-A-B). Therefore, in the simplest form of cross-over design with three treatments, the sample is divided into six groups: the first group receives a week of treatment A, followed by a week of B and finally a week of C; the second group receives a week of B followed by A, followed by C; the third group receives C, followed by B, followed by A, and so on (the term cross-over refers to crossing over from one treatment to another, within the same group). Since each group receives a sequence of treatments, conclusions on individual treatments are made by comparing treatments within subjects even though, as we will see in chapter 10, the concept of comparing groups (i.e. sequences) is maintained. We will come back to these two fundamental types of experimental design in chapter 10.

At the end of the study we summarize the results obtained for each treatment using a measure of central tendency (for example the mean) and a measure of variability (for example the standard deviation). Unavoidably, there will be differences between the treatments. For simplicity, let us consider only two treatments: A (experimental treatment) and B (control treatment). Let us suppose that A and B are two treatments against obesity and that the primary end-point is the weight of the patient, measured at the end of one month of treatment. To further simplify matters, we shall ignore the standard deviation (assuming that it is similar in the two groups). At the end of the study, results are as follows: the post-treatment mean weight is 104 kg after A and 114 kg after B. We are naturally tempted to attribute the 10 kg mean difference entirely to the treatments, concluding that A is more efficacious than B in reducing weight in obese patients. Unfortunately, things are not this easy. Various causes, of which treatment is only one, can contribute to the observed 10 kg mean difference. As discussed in section 2.4, one possible cause is chance, the combined effect of non-systematic, unpredictable and unknown phenomena, escaping every control. This effect is not reproducible by definition (see section 1.3.2). The influence of chance is evaluated through the statistical analysis, as discussed in chapter 5. All other possible causes, other than the treatment itself, are sources of bias. Sackett [88] described many types of bias, which can be summarized in three main categories:

1. **Selection bias**, defined as a non-random imbalance among treatment groups of the distribution of factors capable of influencing the end-points, that is, of sub-experimental factors (including prognostic factors) discussed in sections 2.3 and 2.4 [26].

2. **Assessment bias**, defined as a non-random imbalance among treatment groups in the way subjects are followed and assessed during the course of the study [26]. This category includes all forms of bias discussed in chapter 8.

3. **Analysis bias**, defined as a distortion in favor of one of the treatments, intervening during the data analysis.

For the observed difference to reflect a true difference between treatments, it is necessary that the design and procedures of the study remove (or render negligible) the three categories of bias mentioned above.

An appropriate statistical analysis allows the exclusion of chance (in probabilistic terms), but does not allow one to definitively establish if the observed difference is due to the treatments or to one or more types of bias. Statistical methods for the detection of selection and assessment bias do exist but, because of their intrinsic weaknesses (see below), are to be considered exploratory.

As far as selection bias is concerned, the statistical analysis can detect the presence of imbalances between treatment groups occurring at baseline (i.e. before the start of study treatment administration) for a limited number of known sub-experimental/prognostic factors. When these imbalances are detected it is possible to "adjust" the results. "Adjustment" in this context means that, on the basis of an appropriate statistical model (suitable for the data being analyzed), the result is "enhanced" in the group with a baseline disadvantage and "reduced" in the group with a baseline advantage. The magnitude of the adjustment is established by the statistical model and by the magnitude of the baseline imbalance. Unfortunately, such adjustments are questionable for three reasons:

- They can only be applied to known sub-experimental/prognostic factors, whereas the majority of such factors, causing bias, are unknown.
- They are performed "*post hoc*", that is, are decided upon and applied with the full knowledge of the results for each treatment.
- They dependent heavily on the selected statistical model and, because of this, are partially arbitrary.

For all of these reasons, the results of such adjusted analyses have an exploratory value and are in general not usable for confirmatory purposes.

With regard to assessment bias, some statistical techniques, mostly descriptive, can either confirm or alleviate doubts on the bias-free conduct of the assessments. For example, consistency in the correlations among study endpoints can be verified by comparing different centers or different evaluators, or even different studies. These techniques are also exploratory and do not offer solutions if the suspicion of assessment bias is confirmed.

In conclusion, the statistical methods cannot definitively confirm or rule out selection bias or assessment bias. It is crucial for researchers to understand this concept. The only way to avoid the risk of attributing to a treatment what is in fact the effect of bias is to perform bias-free comparisons (see section 2.1). The only way to ensure that the comparisons are bias-free is to design and execute the study properly. In reality, the risk of bias can never be totally eliminated; therefore, the expression "bias-free" refers to situations in which the probability of bias is sufficiently remote to allow us to ignore it in drawing our conclusions.

The logical sequence in the reasoning is as follows:

- The study is planned and executed so that comparisons are likely to be bias-free; therefore a difference between groups, if any, can be attributed either to the treatment or to chance.
- The statistical test is performed to exclude the effect of chance.
- If the test is statistically significant one concludes that the effect is not due to chance, i.e. it is due to the treatment.

In this chapter, we will deal with two fundamental procedures typical of experimental studies that are used to minimize selection and assessment bias: randomization (against selection bias) and blinding of study treatments (against assessment bias). The next two sections (9.2 and 9.3) are dedicated to these procedures. Furthermore, as mentioned above, the statistical analysis can itself be the cause of various types of bias, collectively indicated as analysis bias. Section 9.4 is dedicated to this topic. The chapter ends with a comparison between observational and experimental studies, mainly concerning the reliability and generalizability of the conclusions (section 9.5).

9.2. Randomization as Antidote Against Selection Bias

9.2.1. Definition and Conceptual Framework

Randomization is the assignment of subjects to treatments (or sequences of treatments, in the case of cross-over designs) with a predefined probability and by chance. This implies that each individual assignment cannot be predicted based on the previous assignments. In this chapter we refer to treatments, but what we state is also applicable to sequences of treatments in cross-over designs.

The word randomization is derived from "random", meaning **chance assignment**. In its simplest form, at each assignment, each subject has the same probability of being assigned to each treatment: this probability is 50% in a study with two treatments, 33.3% in a study with three treatments, 25% in one with four treatments, and so on. However, as we will see, there are forms of randomization, so-called unequal or unbalanced, in which the probabilities of assignment to each treatment are not equal. Therefore, once the randomization is completed, the sample is unevenly divided between treatments, generally with more subjects assigned to the experimental treatment than to the control (or controls). Whatever the probability of a subject being assigned to a given treatment, the essence of randomization is the chance nature of the assignment, so that the outcome of an assignment cannot be predicted on the basis of the previous ones. There are some partial exceptions to this fundamental rule (see for example the randomization in blocks in section 9.2.2). However, for the process of assigning the subjects to the treatments to be called randomization, it is imperative that the fundamental characteristic of chance assignment be maintained in essence.

It is important to distinguish between random assignment, i.e. randomization, and haphazard assignment. Random assignment follows the precise rules just described, while haphazard assignment does not really follow any rule. Therefore, in the latter assignment the preferences, conscious or unconscious, of the person in charge of the assignment may influence the outcome.

Alternatives to randomization have been sought. To this end various forms of so-called **systematic assignment** have been proposed. One could assign patients seen on odd numbered days to one study treatment and patients seen on even numbered days to the comparator treatment, or patients hospitalized in rooms on the left side of the ward to one treatment and patients in rooms on the right to the other, or patients with last names from A to L to one treatment and the remaining to the other treatment, and so on. These procedures are to be avoided, because they are susceptible to both conscious manipulation and unconscious mistakes, and in any case lend themselves to suspicion and accusations of manipulation when results are critically assessed and interpreted. For example, the above mentioned criterion based on last names easily creates a racial bias between the groups under comparison, because each ethnic group tends to have a small number of very common last names. Furthermore, such procedures are often more complicated than the true randomization. However, there are "hybrid" forms of assignment, with a systematic and a random component, that are acceptable in special situations. These will be introduced in section 9.2.3.

Randomization has two main justifications.

The first justification of randomization is that it eliminates selection bias for both known and unknown sub-experimental factors capable of influencing the response to treatments (see section 2.4). Let us consider a study with the objective of comparing the effect of a new thrombolytic agent to that of tPA (tissue Plasminogen Activator) on the survival of patients with myocardial infarction. We shall assume that 90% of the patients assigned to tPA were more than 70 years old, against 30% of the patients assigned to the experimental treatment. It is easy to realize that age influences the mean survival time: older patients generally have less time ahead of them compared to younger ones, irrespective of myocardial infarction; furthermore, older patients tend to respond less to many drugs and have an overall worse prognosis following angioplastic procedures, which sometimes follow treatment with thrombolytics. An imbalance in mean age between treatment groups is a classic example of selection bias that, in our case, will almost unavoidably determine a longer survival time in the group assigned to the new thrombolytic agent compared to that assigned to tPA, independently of the efficacy of the two drugs. If a treatment effect does exist, it will be contaminated by the effect of the selection bias. Age is a known prognostic factor. In fact, the imbalance of known sub-experimental and prognostic factors is only the most obvious and least problematic aspect of the selection bias problem. If it were the only problem, "matching" techniques, that control the distribution of these factors in the groups under comparison, would contribute to creating comparable groups even better than randomization, although the practical feasibility of matching decreases with increasing numbers of factors to be matched, becoming unrealistic if there are too many of them. Furthermore, imbalances of known sub-experimental factors can be compensated (within limits) through appropriate statistical procedures, as mentioned earlier in this chapter. The true problem lies with the unknown sub-experimental factors, which may not even be recorded or measured, for the very reason they are unknown, and for which balancing through matching and statistical "adjustments" is obviously impossible.

It should be emphasized that randomization does not always create balanced (homogenous) groups for known and unknown sub-experimental factors. The outcome of a random assignment of subjects to treatments may well be that of unbalanced groups (see below). The fundamental point however is that any imbalances are by definition due to chance.

The second justification of randomization is that it legitimizes the frequentist approach to statistical inference. The foundation of the frequentist approach to statistical inference is the assumption that the sample is extracted randomly from the population. As mentioned in chapter 6, strictly speaking this does not happen in clinical studies, because the study sample is not selected in a truly random fashion from the overall population of patients affected by the disease of interest. For this reason, the sample may not be representative of the underlying population. For example, the sample may consist mostly of subjects living close to the hospital, or belonging to the same socio-economic level, or frequently needing hospitalization. Patients of different nationality, ethnic background, socio-economic level or who are treated in different centers (with unavoidable differences in the quality of patient care and of the procedures needed for the study) may not respond to the treatments in the same way. As mentioned in section 6.1, if the sample does not represent the population, the legitimacy of generalizing results from that sample to the overall underlying population is questionable. To what population can we truly extend the result obtained on the sample? Randomization cannot eliminate this problem (see section 9.5). However, it compensates for another very important implication of the lack of a random extraction of the sample from the population: without the random element, the frequentist approach cannot be applied, because the conceptual foundation of repeated sampling (repetition of the experiment under the same conditions) would be missing. Randomization, by reintroducing the random element in the assignment of the "extracted" subjects (i.e. the sample) to the different treatments, ensures the applicability of the statistical significance test. The reader interested in an illuminating example can refer to chapter 10 of Colton's textbook of medical statistics [26]. This is an important concept often underestimated, which brings into question the application of any frequentist method of statistical inference to non-randomized experiments. From the Bayesian perspective (see chapter 5), randomization is important only as an instrument to eliminate bias, while it is not seen as the basis for the application of statistical methods, since the Bayesian approach does not use the concept of repeated sampling.

We have stated above that randomization does not in itself ensure homogenous groups, which is somewhat intuitive, especially if the sample size is small. The fact that we have obtained unbalanced groups only as a result of chance is not necessarily reassuring, especially if an imbalance observed at baseline concerns a known prognostic factor and is quantitatively relevant. For example, if the imbalance between the groups concerns a quantitative selection criterion, which is also used as an end-point (for example, an imbalance between the groups in the mean cholesterol levels at baseline, in a study on a cholesterol lowering drug), there will be an uneven effect of the statistical regression toward the mean, which will be greater in the group with the more extreme mean baseline value (see chapter 8). As mentioned already, the smaller the sample size, the greater the likelihood of a relevant imbalance due to chance. For example, if a sample of 1000 patients is randomized to two study treatments, it is very unlikely that one group will have twice the number of females than the other. On the other hand, if the sample is of only 10 patients, such an outcome is not rare at all. Randomization techniques exist that are useful not only to eliminate bias, but also to reduce the probability of relevant imbalances between the groups due to chance. These techniques will be presented later in this chapter.

9.2.2. Types of Randomization

Randomization is carried out through lists of random numbers, which can be taken from published tables or generated *ad hoc* using special computer algorithms. A list of random numbers is a sequence of numbers (for example from 0 to 9, from 0 to 25, etc) which follow one another without any discernible order or trend, i.e. each number has the same probability of appearing at any position of the list. By assigning each study treatment (or sequence of treatments) to one or more numbers, the random succession of numbers is transformed into a random succession of treatments (or of treatment sequences) called randomization list. Straight from chapter 5 of the Pocock's textbook on clinical trials [79] (in our opinion one of the best introductory texts on clinical research methodology) we report the first 30 positions of a list of random numbers, which uses numbers from 0 to 9:

0-5-2-7-8-4-3-7-4-1-6-8-3-8-5-1-5-6-9-6-8-1-8-0-5-7-8-8-7-4.

Simple randomization. In the so-called **simple randomization,** each patient has the same probability of receiving each of the study treatments (or sequence of treatments). For simplicity, we will limit the examples to the parallel design, but the reasoning is identical for the cross-over design, where the patients are randomized to sequences of treatments instead of single treatments.

When there are two study treatments (A and B), a simple randomization list can be generated by assigning A to the numbers 0, 1, 2, 3, 4 and B to the numbers 5, 6, 7, 8, 9 and then by appropriately replacing the numbers with the letters A and B. The following randomization list is obtained:

A-B-A-B-B-A-A-B-A-A-B-B-A-B-B-A-B-B-B-B-A-B-A-B-B-B-B-B-A.

In a study with three treatments (A, B and C), A can be assigned to the numbers 0, 1 and 2, B to 3, 4 and 5, and C to 6, 7 and 8 (the number 9 is ignored, with no treatment assigned to it). In this way the following randomization list is obtained:

A-B-A-C-C-B-A-C-B-A-C-C-B-C-B-A-B-C-C-C-A-C-A-B-C-C-C-C-B.

In a study with four treatments (A, B, C and D), A can be assigned to the numbers 0 and 1, B to 2 and 3, C to 4 and 5, and D to 6 and 7 (numbers 8 and 9 are ignored). The following randomization list is generated:

A-C-B-D-C-B-D-C-A-D-B-C-A-C-D-D-A-A-C-D-D-C.

In the simple randomization, a single list prepared in this way is used. Taking for example the four treatment list, the first patient entering the study will be assigned to A, the second to C, the third to B the fourth to D and so on, until the total number of patients required by the protocol has been randomized.

When the treatments are blinded (see section 9.3), it is necessary to transform the sequence of treatments of the randomization list (A-B-A-B-B, etc.) into a sequence of unique codes, each corresponding to a patient pack (for example, CX2224, CX2225, CX2226, CX2227, etc.). The researcher will know only which patient pack he/she must give to each subject, and will have no knowledge as to which treatment each code corresponds to. The list linking patient pack codes to treatments will be kept by personnel not involved in the study in a sealed envelope under lock and key or in an electronically protected file.

It must be possible to trace, justify and document any access to the randomization list, from the moment it is generated, to the moment it is formally "opened" at the end of the study. If the randomization process is managed through a computerized system, the randomization list must be located in a protected area throughout the study and subject to "**audit trail**", i.e. every access must result in the automatic registration of user, date, time and reason for access.

Once the randomization list and the corresponding list of unique patient pack codes have been generated, the actual randomization, that is the assignment of individual patients to the study treatments, can be directly executed by the researcher, by following a list specific to his/her center containing the order of assignment of the patient pack codes. The list is to be followed rigorously: the first pack code must be assigned to the first eligible patient, the second pack code to the second patient, and so on.

Alternatively, randomization can occur through a centralized service, to which investigators can request patient pack codes by phone, e-mail or fax. Each investigator receives a certain number of patient packs of each study treatment. The link between the randomization list and the patient pack codes is not pre-fixed but determined by the centralized allocation system, using the sequential order as the matching criterion: this means that each new request is given the first patient pack code available at the center corresponding to the first available treatment of the centralized randomization list. This method is called **centralized randomization** and it is especially useful in large, multi-center studies, to reduce logistical complexity and avoid waste of study medication.

Randomization in random permuted blocks. When the sample of a study is large (say, more than 100 subjects per treatment or sequence of treatments), simple randomization will most likely achieve a similar number of subjects in each treatment group, through the effect of chance alone, just as when one tosses a coin hundreds or thousands of times, the heads and tails tend to occur with a similar frequency. The number of subjects assigned to each treatment or sequence will obviously almost never be identical, but the differences will be small, and will not affect the statistical analysis or the interpretation of the results.

However, the picture can be completely different in small studies. A coin tossed only 10 times could easily give eight heads and two tails or even nine heads and only one tail, even though head and tail have the same probability of occurring. The same is true for a sequence of random numbers: if a short list is used, it is not rare that, by chance, it will generate an imbalance in the size of the groups under study. The shorter the list, i.e. the smaller the sample size, the more marked the imbalance can be. For example, if we were to use the last 14 positions of the sequence of random numbers reported above to generate a randomization list with two treatments (0-1-2-3-4=A, 5-6-7-8-9=B), we would end up with 11 subjects assigned to B and 3 assigned to A; if we were to use the last 10 positions, the split would be 8 units assigned to B and 2 to A. To avoid extreme inequalities in the size of the groups under comparison, when dealing with small samples, a special form of randomization, called **randomization in random permuted blocks** or simply **randomization in blocks,** is used.

Let us suppose we have two treatments, A and B, to be assigned to 32 patients. With simple randomization, the 32 patients are assigned to the study treatments based on a random sequence of 32 extractions of one of the two treatments, without any other condition.

With the randomization in blocks, the assignment occurs in subgroups, called

blocks. Each block must have a number of units equal to the number of treatments under study or to a multiple of this number. Furthermore, within each block, each treatment must appear the same number of times. The randomization in blocks serves two purposes:
- To obtain numerically balanced groups (i.e. of equal or approximately equal size).
- To obtain a constantly balanced recruitment, that is, a similar size of the treatment groups throughout the enrolment process, from beginning to end.

We shall illustrate a method for creating a randomization list in blocks, assuming two study treatments (A and B) and a block of four units. This method uses the so-called **permutations**, defined as groups that include all of the elements under study and differ from each other only in the order in which the elements appear. In our example we must consider permutations of four elements, two of which are repeated twice (permutations with repetition). There are six possible permutations: AABB, BBAA, ABBA, BAAB, ABAB and BABA. The succession of the permutations is dictated by a list of random numbers. Considering the random list of numbers from 0 to 9 described above, we could assign each of the six permutations to a number from 1 to 6, in the order they appear above, and ignore the numbers 0, 7, 8 and 9. The list of randomization in blocks of four will be as follows:

[A-B-A-B]-[B-B-A-A]-[B-A-A-B]-[A-B-B-A]-[B-A-A-B]-[A-A-B-B]-[B-A-B-A]-[A-B-B-A]-[A-B-A-B]
   5   2   4   3   4   1   6   3   5

It is easy to verify that randomization in blocks results in a balance between the two treatment groups, both during enrolment (in the example, with every four randomized subjects there will be exact parity), and at the end of enrollment (if exactly 32 subjects are randomized, 16 will receive A and 16 B; if more or less than 32 subjects are randomized, the difference in the number of subjects assigned to each treatment will never be more than two units).

Groups of equal size often facilitate the statistical analysis. A balance maintained throughout recruitment (the smaller the block, the more constant the balance) can be useful for balancing sub-experimental factors linked to time (including seasonality). The use of randomization in blocks for this purpose will be clarified in chapter 10.

Strictly speaking, randomization in blocks is not true randomization, because it is not always true that a single assignment cannot be predicted based on the previous ones. Going back to our example, if we know the size of the block and we know the first three assignments of the block, we can predict the fourth. If we know that the first two assignments are to the same treatment, we also know the remaining two. However, the blinding of study treatments described in the next section generally makes the "decoding" of the blocks very unlikely, and therefore makes the process of assignment in blocks close to a true randomization. If relatively large blocks are used and their size is not revealed to the researchers conducting the experiment, the probability of decoding the blocks is so low it can be ignored. Instead, the situation is problematic if the study treatments are only partially blinded, and even more if they are not blinded at all, in the so-called open label studies (see below). So far we have assumed **fixed size blocks**, in the example the size being four. If we wish to make it more difficult to decode the treatments, we may use **variable size blocks**, with the size of the blocks used in generating the list changing randomly from block to block.

Randomization in blocks, seen as a tool to obtain groups of equal size, in addition to being useful for samples of small size, can also be advantageous in three other situations.

- In **multi-center studies.** These are often very large studies, for which simple randomization would be completely appropriate. However, to enroll all patients in an acceptable amount of time, many centers are used, each enrolling a small part of the sample. Often the centers are in different countries, with very different cultures and socio-economic backgrounds. For these reasons the center itself is one of the most powerful sub-experimental factors. Therefore, to avoid selection bias and also to ensure that each center has all of the study treatments, stratified randomization in blocks is typically used, with each center treated as a stratum (see below) and given a number of blocks compatible with the number of patients it expects to enroll. It is to be noted that in a multi-center study, at the end of the study there will be many incomplete blocks (the last block of each center). Therefore, the overall balance between the treatments will never be as good as that achievable when randomization in blocks is performed for a single center study.

- In studies with a sequential design (treated in chapter 11). As we will see, such studies have variable size and are stopped as soon as the preestablished objective is achieved. Therefore, at no time during the study should there be an excessive imbalance in the number of subjects assigned to each treatment.

- Randomization in blocks is at the heart of the so-called randomized block design. In this kind of design, assuming k study treatments, randomization lists in blocks of k patients are used. Each block is a set of k patients, similar in respect of certain predefined characteristics. The patients of each block are randomly subdivided among the k study treatments. We will return to this topic in chapter 10.

Randomization in blocks does also present some disadvantages, not to be underestimated. If the blocks are small, the researcher may be able to guess the sequence, even in the presence of blinded treatments (see below), in which case all of the advantages of both blinding and randomization are lost. This can happen when the nature of the treatments under study makes the blinding incomplete. For example, let us suppose we are conducting a study comparing the β2-antagonist drug salmeterol to placebo in asthmatic patients. In addition, let's assume that the treatments are blinded, that is, salmeterol and placebo are indistinguishable to the researcher, who therefore does not know to which treatment each individual patient is assigned. Finally, let's assume that the researcher knows from the study protocol that randomization in blocks with a block size of four has been applied. The first two patients are randomized and, shortly after the administration of the treatment, they both show tremor, a typical side effect of the class of drugs to which salmeterol belongs. At this point, the investigator knows (or strongly suspects) that the following two patients will receive placebo, and may consciously or unconsciously select the two following patients based on his/her personal opinion of salmeterol. The investigator may also monitor the two following patients in a "special" way (e.g. less closely than the rest). Thus, both a selection bias and an assessment bias are introduced. We can reduce this risk by avoiding very small blocks. However, the blocks cannot be too big either, otherwise any advantage of this kind of randomization is lost (unless all we only want is a very rough balance between groups). In addition, if very large blocks are used, a numeric balance is achieved only at long intervals during the course of the study. In any case, it is appropriate never to report the size of the blocks in the protocol, nor any other detail of the randomization list.

Stratified randomization. The so-called **stratified randomization** takes into account the prognostic/sub-experimental factors considered most significant. It allows for such factors to be evenly distributed among the treatment groups. The stratified randomization requires that each pre-selected factor be subdivided into categories or classes, referred to as **levels**. The levels must be exhaustive (i.e. they must include all of the values the factor can take) and mutually exclusive (i.e. a given value can only belong to one level). We want to compare, in a parallel group study, a new antiviral with zidovudine in the treatment of HIV infection, with mortality as the primary end-point. We know that a low number of CD4+ lymphocytes ($<100/mm^3$) and opportunistic infections reported in the patient's clinical history are important negative prognostic factors. We want to make sure that these two prognostic factors are balanced in the groups under comparison. To this end, we divide each of the two factors into two levels (presence/absence of low CD4 counts, presence/absence of opportunistic infection in the patient's history). To ensure a balance between treatment groups for the two pre-selected prognostic factors, we assign the patients to one of the following four categories or **strata**:

1. Absence of low CD4 counts + absence of history of opportunistic infections.
2. Presence of low CD4 counts + absence of history of opportunistic infections.
3. Absence of low CD4 counts + presence of history of opportunistic infections.
4. Presence of low CD4 counts + presence of history of opportunistic infections.

Each stratum is made of one level for each factor, therefore the total number of strata is obtained by multiplying the number of levels of each factor (in this case 2 x 2).

To obtain a stratified randomization, an independent randomization list must be generated for each stratum. In our example, each patient entering the study is first assigned to one of the four strata on the basis of his/her CD4 count and history of opportunistic infections. Then, the patient is assigned to either the new antiviral or to zidovudine by following the randomization list of the stratum to which he/she belongs. Through this procedure, at the end of the randomization, we can be sure that no major treatment imbalance for the two selected prognostic factors will be present.

Often the study center, which is a sub-experimental factor of potentially great influence (even though not a proper prognostic factor - see section 2.4), is treated as a stratification factor. As mentioned above, in multi-center studies the randomization procedure is often not only stratified, but also in blocks (that is, for each stratum a randomization list in blocks is prepared). The reason for this is that in each individual center at least one of the strata is likely to end up with few patients. The blocks will make sure that no large imbalance between treatment groups occurs, especially in the scarcely populated strata. This approach is useful for any study with stratified randomization in which it is expected that one or more strata will have few patients.

The stratified randomization can be used with two primary objectives:

• Obtain balanced groups for important prognostic factors or other important sub-experimental factors such as the center, even though the interest is on the overall effect of the treatments on all strata combined.

• Perform subgroup analyses, especially study the interaction between the effect of the study treatments and that of the stratification factors.

Stratified randomization has the great disadvantage of complexity. Let us consider prognostic factors with two levels. For two such factors there will be four strata, as in our example. Three factors will generate eight strata, requiring eight randomization lists. If the factors have more than two levels, the number of strata increases very rapidly. Considering, for example, three factors with three levels each, 27 strata will be obtained, which is already far beyond a reasonable threshold of feasibility. More than three factors are generally not to be considered for many reasons, the most obvious being that, with many strata, some of them will certainly be scarcely populated and the final effect will be a serious treatment imbalance. Stratification is generally useful when limited to one or two sub-experimental factors (prognostic or not - see section 2.4) of documented importance, especially in studies with a small sample size.

Sometimes in multi-center studies, when the number of stratification factors is high, the centers are not treated as additional strata. This is done in order to reduce the overall number of strata and is justified when the center effect is deemed less important than the effect of the factors selected for stratification. In these circumstances, the use of a centralized randomization (see above) is mandatory. In fact, if non-centralized randomization were used, each center would be provided with sets of pre-coded patient packs, one set for each stratum, which implies that each center is treated as an additional stratum.

Unbalanced or unequal randomization. There are situations where an imbalance in the size of the groups under study is an advantage and facilitates achievement of the objective of the study. Let us suppose that we are responsible for the clinical development of a new monoclonal antibody directed against the immunoglobulin E (anti-IgE antibody), a biotechnological product, resulting from complex genetic engineering processes, belonging to a new therapeutic class. It is clear that, in such a situation, gaining experience concerning the safety and tolerability of the new product is of paramount importance. Therefore, in the clinical trials it would be an advantage to assign more patients to the anti-IgE agent than to the placebo (or active comparator). Another reason justifying the use of unequal randomization is of practical/commercial nature, mainly pertinent to phase IV studies, where it is considered important to give the chance to experience a new treatment to as many doctors and centers as possible.

Unbalanced or **unequal randomization** can be obtained through randomization lists built in such a way that not a 1:1 allocation, but an unequal allocation (3:2, 2:1, 3:1, etc.) between the groups is achieved. Let us suppose we want to build a list in blocks with a 2:1 allocation, so that each subject entering the study has twice the probability of being assigned to one study treatment than to the other. In building such a list, we could, for example, consider a block of size 3, in which two positions are assigned to A and one to B. The possible permutations are: AAB, ABA, BAA. We could assign the first block to the numbers 0, 1, 2; the second to 3, 4, 5; the third to 6, 7, 8 and not consider the number 9. If we use the sequence of random numbers presented at the beginning of this section, we will generate the following list:

$$[A\text{-}A\text{-}B]\text{-}[A\text{-}B\text{-}A]\text{-}[A\text{-}A\text{-}B]\text{-}[B\text{-}A\text{-}A]\text{-}[B\text{-}A\text{-}A]$$
$$0 \qquad 5 \qquad 2 \qquad 7 \qquad 8$$

This list assigns to A twice as many subjects than to B, balancing the 2:1 assignment every three subjects.

The advantage of unequal randomization, that of exposing more patients to the new treatment, has a price. A study with unequal randomization will have reduced power compared to a study with a 1:1 randomization of identical design and size. Consequently, if all other conditions are the same, a study with unequal randomization will need a higher total number of patients, compared to an otherwise identical study with a 1:1 randomization, in order to obtain the same power (see section 6.2). For small imbalances in the allocation ratio between the groups, the loss of power (or the increase in patient numbers required to maintain the same power) is relatively limited. However, with increasing imbalances in the allocation ratio, the power diminishes considerably (or, likewise, the sample size must increase considerably to maintain the same power). For example, if a study with two treatments and a 1:1 randomization has a 95% power for the primary end-point at a pre-fixed significant level, the same study with a 3:2 unequal randomization (that is, with 60% of the patients randomized to the experimental treatment and 40% randomized to the control) will have a power of approximately 92.5%. With a 2:1 allocation ratio (that is, with 66.7% of the patients randomized to the experimental treatment and 33.3% to the control), the study will have a power of approximately 90%. With a 4:1 allocation ratio (that is, with 80% of the patients randomized to the experimental treatment and 20% to the control), the power will be around 80% and with a 9:1 unequal randomization (that is, with 90% of the patients randomized to the experimental treatment and 10% to the control) the power will be around 60.5%. A useful graph relating the extent of the imbalance between the group sizes and the resulting power (from which we took the above example) can be found in chapter 5 of Pocock's textbook [79]. Of course, if the initial power with a 1:1 randomization is less than 95% (as often occurs), the reduction in power with increasing imbalance between the group sizes will reach values below 80% well before the 4:1 allocation ratio, as in the example above.

In spite of the above mentioned limit, unequal randomization is very useful to maximize the information on safety and tolerability of a new treatment, while keeping intact the methodological rigor of a study, and also to give as many researchers as possible the chance to work with the new treatment. It can be very useful in dose ranging studies with many groups (each assigned to one dose), where the primary objective is a comparison between a combination of doses and a single control group (for example, a placebo or the lowest dose). In this case, it is convenient (from the point of view of the statistical power of the test) to have a control group of a size greater than that of the other treatment groups.

An introduction to the logistics of randomization. The process of randomization is not only of crucial importance, but often also of considerable complexity. A proper discussion of its logistics is beyond the limits we set for this book, but a few broad strokes may help the reader to have an idea of what it implies. For example, a stratified randomization in blocks for a study with four treatments, to be conducted in 200 centers, located in 20 countries, is anything but easy to set up. The randomization lists must be kept sealed until the final database of the study is declared complete, that is, ready for the analysis and "locked" ("frozen") to any further change. On the other hand, in case of need (generally a serious adverse event) the researcher must be in a position to open the code of any patient (that is, to find out which treatment or sequence of treatments the patient has been assigned to) without jeopardizing the randomization and the blinding of the entire study. Mistakes related to the randomization process are disastrous, since they irreversibly destroy the credibility of the study. It is essential that the process be regulated by **standard operating procedures** (SOPs), be planned down to the smallest details under the guidance of experts and be documented exhaustively. It is important for regulatory purposes to show that the randomization list was truly obtained from a list of random numbers, through appropriate tables or specific software. In both cases, the documentation (to be kept in a sealed envelope or "locked" electronic file for the duration of the study) must include the so-called "**seed**", the starting point of the list, which is essential to show that it is reproducible. The procedure generating the randomization lists, if computerized, must be validated. Finally, as discussed at the beginning of this section, access to the list must be documented by an audit-trail.

9.2.3.   Other Methods for Assigning Patients to Treatments

There are methods that allow the allocation of patients to the treatments based on information collected during the study. These methods can be divided in two broad categories:

1. Methods where the assignment to the treatments is decided based on the distribution among treatment groups of preestablished prognostic factors at the time a new patient is ready for treatment allocation (the assignment that generates the least imbalance between groups is made).

2. Methods where the assignment is determined by the results for a pre-established end-point, generally the primary one, at the time a new patient is ready for treatment allocation (the patient is assigned to the group showing the best result).

The methods of the first category are sometimes referred to as "**dynamic assignment**", while those of the second category are referred to as "**adaptive assignment**". It should be noted that in this area the terminology is confusing; therefore, to identify a given method, one should pay more attention to how it works than to how it is called.

Historically, these methods were born as non-random (with deterministic or systematic assignments, i.e. based on a predetermined set of rules). Only later, because of the problems surrounding the methods of systematic assignment (described in section 9.2.1), a random component was introduced. This involves the patient being assigned to the selected group not with certainty (i.e. with probability of 1), but with a greater probability compared to that of being assigned to one of the other groups. This mechanism of assignment is generally called "**biased coin**" assignment.

The goal of the dynamic assignment methods is to obtain balanced treatment groups with respect to a set of baseline characteristics (typically prognostic factors). Such methods are therefore an alternative to stratification and blocking. They are to be preferred to stratification and blocking only when the sample size is small, but it is still necessary to consider many strata or blocks, that is, in the situation in which stratification and blocking become inefficient. A detailed overview of the dynamic assignment methods can be found in Kalish and Begg [63].

The goal of the adaptive assignment methods is ethical in nature, i.e. to minimize the exposure of patients to the less promising treatments. The most popular in the context of clinical trials is the so-called "**play-the-winner**" method (see [104] for the randomized version). Given m patients enrolled in the study, the method requires the knowledge of the results for these patients before enrolling in the study patient $(m + 1)$. Therefore, it is only applicable to very special situations.

A highly debated point is the validity of the traditional (frequentist) statistical tests when these methods of patient assignment to treatments are applied. Since the different sequences of assignment are not equally probable (as when randomization is used), the distributions of the test statistics are not the same as with randomization. Therefore, when these methods are applied, it is necessary to introduce some corrections to the traditional tests, possible in theory, but not easy to implement.

9.3. Blinding of Treatments as Antidote Against Assessment Bias

Blinding is an essential procedure for minimizing the assessment bias. This term embraces a multiplicity of situations in which the researcher systematically favors the patients belonging to one treatment group over another, when carrying out the procedures linked (directly or indirectly) to the assessment of the response to treatments. The assessment bias is very similar to the observation bias discussed in section 3.2 for the epidemiological studies. In a clinical trial, blinding of study treatments (also referred to as "masking") consists of making the treatments under comparison indistinguishable from one another. Commonly a study is defined as **double-blind** when neither the research staff, nor the patients can tell which study treatment is administered to an individual patient. When instead, only the patients are unaware of the study treatment, the study is defined as **single-blind**. A study in which there is no blinding is defined as **open-label**. Even though such a distinction into three categories is useful, in reality there is a gradient, a continuum of blinding levels ranging from a totally open label study to a study in which nobody, neither patients, nor researchers, nor support staff, can even suspect which treatment is given to an individual patient. For example, even in the context of a double-blind trial, there can be tiny differences in the appearance of the study medications that cannot be avoided for technical reasons. A typical example is that of the placebos matching aerosol inhalers that some times have a slightly different valve or a canister of slightly different diameter compared to the inhaler containing active substance. Furthermore, the administration of a treatment may reveal its nature. In such cases, in order to keep the study blinded, the study treatments must be administered by someone not involved in the measurements (see below). In some situations an experienced researcher can strongly suspect the nature of the treatment under study in the presence of a known positive or negative pharmacodynamic effect: the example of the tremor in studies with β2-agonist drugs has already been mentioned. The appropriate level of blinding for a study is the result of the interaction of many factors, including the complexity of the pharmaceutical formulation and production, the therapeutic regimens, the mode of administration, the costs, the therapeutic area and the importance of the study.

It is important to keep in mind that when we talk of blinded researchers, we refer not only to those directly in contact with the study subjects, but also to all the researchers who deal with the study treatments and with the data, including those responsible for the packaging and shipment of the study treatments, for the collection, review and correction of the case report forms, for the entry of data into the database, for resolving discrepancies and errors in the database, and for conducting the statistical analysis. In the blinding process the control of the randomization list is clearly of paramount importance. It would be ridiculous to embark on the complex process of blinding a study when, for example, the personnel who prepared the patient packs (who must have access to the randomization list) are also involved in other aspects of the study, or when the randomization list is kept in a drawer accessible to everybody.

The blinding of a study includes both the drugs (when used) and the procedures. It should be noted that the terms "drug" and "medication" imply a recognized therapeutic effect, thus, strictly speaking, would not apply to experimental compounds. However, in this section we need to distinguish pharmacological treatments from other forms of treatments, therefore, for simplicity we will use the term drug or medication when referring to a substance introduced into the body for therapeutic purposes, even when the actual therapeutic value has not been demonstrated.

Blinding of drugs. The ideal situation is when it is possible to obtain drugs differing in active component(s), but otherwise identical with regard to shape, dimension, color, taste, viscosity, excipients (substances other than the active component(s) that are used in the pharmaceutical formulation) and any other feature that would allow to distinguish the study drugs from one another. As mentioned already, an inactive drug identical to an active one (or presumed active) is called a placebo. Even in the simplest blinding situations, generally with oral drugs, the production of placebo and blinded active drugs requires a considerable pharmaceutical development effort, not to be underestimated. In addition, there are often important legal and commercial implications. The rigorous laws and regulations on the production, quality control, transportation and storage of marketed drugs also apply to the placebos, to the active controls and the experimental drugs used in clinical studies. Furthermore, a long series of additional regulations specifically targeted to experimental drugs must be adhered to. Finally, if the active substance of a study drug (used as active control) is patented, it cannot be manufactured without the permission of the patent holder, who may not necessarily be interested that the study be performed (on the contrary, often the interest is that the study not be performed). In some cases it is possible to bypass the problem by purchasing the active control on the market and "over-encapsulating" it to match the experimental drug.

For drugs with a route of administration other than the oral one, e.g. parenteral, inhalatory, transdermal, etc., the situation is often even more complicated. Firstly, the physicochemical characteristics of the compound take on decisive importance for the blinding. For example, if two drugs administered parenterally have identical appearance, but different viscosity, they will be distinguished immediately by both the patient and the investigator at the time of administration; aerosol metered dose inhalers (MDI) generating different "clouds" can be easily distinguished by spraying a dose against a sheet of paper. Secondly, local reactions become very important as they can "give away" the nature of a study treatment despite perfect visual blinding. Examples are a burning sensation after an injection, a sensation of "cold" in the back of the mouth after a puff from an aerosol MDI, local irritation at the site of application of a transdermal delivery system (patch). Thirdly, the device used for the administration of the study drugs, such as syringe, inhaler, patch, etc., deserves careful consideration. Devices are often technologically complex and difficult to manufacture. As an example, just consider the patches for transdermal administration of estrogens and progestinic hormones: fare from being simple plasters, these drug delivery devices are complex structures with multiple membranes. Furthermore, the devices themselves are usually covered by patents and so cannot be copied. Finally, it is not possible to transfer a compound from one device to another without altering (often profoundly) its pharmacodynamic and therapeutic properties, even when the two devices are very similar or even when it is the same device made by a different manufacturer. In conclusion, there are many situations in which the manufacture of perfectly blinded study drugs is practically impossible. In these cases, blinding can still be obtained through the so-called "double-dummy" technique or by having different investigators dealing with different aspects of the study (see below).

Blinding of procedures. To begin with, the frequency of dosing must be identical. When drugs with different duration of action are compared (for example, formoterol, a β2-agonist active for at least 12 hours and salbutamol, a "classic" β2-agonist active for 4-6 hours), all blinding efforts would be in vain due to the differences in administration frequency. In this case, the "double-dummy" technique can sometimes be a solution (see below). The blinding of procedures is crucial when the treatments under comparison are not drugs, but, for example surgical procedures. In the case of a study in which a surgical intervention is compared to a placebo, the procedures to be simulated include preparation of the operating theater and personnel, anesthesia (local or general), incision and sutures. In many situations there are a series of ancillary procedures that must also be simulated to ensure that the treatments are blinded, such as for example the sampling of blood for measuring drug levels.

From this brief overview on blinding, it is clear that neither the study drugs nor the related procedures can always be made identical. In these cases two approaches can come to the rescue: the "double-dummy" form of blinding and the separation of tasks between the person who administers the study treatments and the person who carries out the measurements.

Blinding through "double-dummy". Let's go back to the example of the comparison between the β2-agonists formoterol and salbutamol, and assume that the purpose of the study is to compare formoterol powder, administered by a specific inhaler twice per day (upon awakening and at dinner) with salbutamol aerosol, administered by an aerosol MDI four times per day (upon awakening, at lunch, dinner and bedtime), and with a placebo. As mentioned above, it is neither possible (for legal and commercial reasons), nor useful (for pharmacological reasons) to transfer the three drugs to the same inhaler; furthermore, the different frequencies of administration would make any effort to blind the drugs futile. What can be done instead is to manufacture one placebo identical to the formoterol dry powder inhaler and another placebo identical to the salbutamol aerosol metered dose inhaler. The result is a "**double-dummy**". Each patient will receive a dry powder inhaler, say, blue, and two aerosol inhalers of different colors, say, one green and one red. Each patient will be instructed to take the treatments four times per day, always with the scheme: blue + green upon awakening, red at lunch time, blue + green at dinner, red at bedtime. Therefore, all patients will have exactly the same therapeutic regimen. What changes in the three groups is the content of the different inhalers, as shown in table 9.1.

In this way the treatments are completely masked, even though they require different devices and frequencies of administration.

Clearly, the double-dummy technique requires the production of different placebos for the different study treatments, which is not always possible. Furthermore, the therapeutic regimens required to execute a double-dummy blinding can become very complex for the patients and, beyond a certain limit, counterproductive: the risk is that one problem is solved (potential assessment bias) at the cost of introducing another equally serious problem (mistakes in the intake of study medication and/or poor compliance to the therapeutic regimen). For example, we have used many times the above mentioned three-inhaler system in pivotal studies lasting up to six months. However, with such a regimen we believe that we are at the limit of feasibility, in terms of both duration and complexity, of the double-dummy approach.

Table 9.1.   Content of inhalers for the double-dummy blinding of three study treatments (salbutamol, formoterol and placebo)

Study treatment	**Blue inhaler (for powder)**	**Green inhaler (for aerosol)**	**Red inhaler (for aerosol)**
Salbutamol	Placebo	Salbutamol	Salbutamol
Formoterol	Formoterol	Placebo	Placebo
Placebo	Placebo	Placebo	Placebo

Blinding through assigning different tasks to different researchers. This option is feasible if the study treatment can be administered directly by the researchers, for example when the patient is hospitalized or when the treatment can be given during the study visits. In these cases, it is possible to achieve blinding by delegating the administration of the study treatments to a researcher who is otherwise not involved in the study. He/she should not have any contact with those who examine the patients and carry out the measurements. Such a procedure is relatively simple and efficient. However, it ensures a "lower level" of blindness, because it is impossible to reassure a third party (such as the reviewer of the regulatory authority or the reader of a scientific paper) that there has not been communication, direct or indirect, between the treatment administrator and the staff examining the patients and carrying out the measurements. In spite of such limits, there are situations in which this form of blinding is the best obtainable and, under well-justified circumstances, it is accepted by the regulatory authorities in pivotal studies for registration. Naturally, since this approach requires the administration of the treatment directly by the researchers, it is not feasible if it must be taken by non-hospitalized patients daily, or on days different from those of regular visits.

Advantages and disadvantages of blinding. The great advantage of blinding, especially when associated with randomization, is that it protects the study from the assessment bias. As stated above, this term embraces a multiplicity of situations in which the post-treatment measurements systematically favor one treatment group over the other(s). This can occur directly or indirectly, consciously or unconsciously. For example, if a researcher is convinced of the efficacy of a new treatment, or is financially interested in its success in reaching the market, he/she could round upwards the measurements on patients assigned to the new treatments and round downwards the measurements on patients assigned to the control treatments, or could be much less strict in searching and evaluating signals of adverse events in the patients assigned to the new treatment, or could assign these patients to the best rooms and the most skilful and pleasant staff, and so on.

As another example, if the patient knows which treatment he/she is receiving, he/she can be strongly influenced in the response to the treatment, based on previous experience, the opinion of other physicians and friends, or simply prejudice. Finally, blinding renders the use of placebo possible. Few patients would knowingly take a placebo and, anyway, the use of placebo would be meaningless in such circumstances, because the psychological component of taking a treatment would be lost.

But, as always, the advantages should always be weighed against the disadvantages. In the case of treatment blinding, there are two main issues: logistical complexity and ethical complexity.

Logistical complexity. From the previous discussion, it should be clear that the manufacturing of blinded placebos and active controls is no easy task. Even in large pharmaceutical companies, it can take many months, and be very expensive. As we saw, the logistical complexity can also apply to the patients when the double-dummy technique must be used, and to the researchers when the separation between those who administer the treatments and those who examine the patients is necessary. At this point, we feel the need to take a stand against dogmatism. A perfect blinding is worthless if it reduces the quality of the experiment for other reasons, or, even worse, makes the experiment practically impossible to execute. The level of blinding must always be assessed in the context of the specific study. Sometimes, a lower level of blinding will be the best decision to ensure the overall quality of the study. The important thing is that the researchers accurately describe the procedures they followed in the final study report and the corresponding paper, without hiding behind standard labels such as "double-blind randomized study", which are often not very informative, if not misleading, on the level of masking actually obtained in a study. When an open-label or single-blind approach is chosen, it is indispensable to "protect" the randomization process by making sure that it occurs in a blinded fashion. In small studies, this can be obtained by delegating randomization to personnel otherwise not involved in the study, for example, to one of the hospital pharmacists. In large, multi-center studies, the toll-free number for centralized randomization (which we mentioned previously) is the best approach. Each researcher calls a dedicated toll free number every time a new patient is to be assigned to a treatment. In addition, in these cases it is appropriate to avoid randomization in blocks, whenever possible. If this must be used for some reason, the blocks should be of variable sizes.

Ethical complexity. If we go out in the street and approach any group of lay people asking, without further explanation, what they think about the administration of a fake drug to a sick patient in order to perform an experiment, most will express dissent and will look at us with suspicion. If we then ask what they think about an experiment involving fake surgery including anesthesia, incision and suture, they may well consider us raving mad and call the police. The point we want to make is that the blinding of treatments, when it implies the use of placebos, has obvious ethical implications, from which it is impossible to escape. First, the researchers must themselves be convinced of what they are doing, and second, once they convince themselves, they must metaphorically go out in the street and convince their patients and the patients' families. Some of the controversies regarding the use of placebo are discussed in chapter 7.

9.4. A Priori Definition of the Statistical Methods and Populations as Antidote Against the Analysis Bias

At the end of a study, during the so-called "data cleaning" and the subsequent statistical analysis, very serious forms of bias can be introduced that favor or undermine one of the treatments. To limit these forms of bias it is necessary that all methods and populations to be used in the statistical analysis be predefined.

9.4.1. Methods of Statistical Analysis

First of all, situations in which the data are consciously manipulated must be mentioned. The range of these manipulations is very broad, going from the true fabrication of entire sets of data to a series of small "corrective" actions, such as the elimination of "inconvenient" values, the adjustment for factors apparently irrelevant but that actually favor the preferred treatment, the use of inadequate methods of statistical analysis. All have the overall effect of "creating" the desired result. The systematic use of such small "corrections" has the same moral implication and practical consequences of data fabrication.

Apart from the conscious manipulation of data and of analyses, one can unconsciously put the experimental treatment in a position of advantage (or disadvantage) over the control treatment. For example, the final decision on the assumptions for the applicability of a given method of statistical analysis always encompasses a degree of subjectivity. Thus the statistician, in deciding whether that method is applicable or not, may unknowingly influence the result.

For this reason, all of the decisions related to the statistical analysis must be made before starting the study, if the study is open-label, or before opening the randomization code, if the study is blind. These decisions concern the methods of analysis to be applied and a number of related details. In practice, in double-blind studies, all important planning decisions are generally made before the trial is started, while the more detailed, operational ones are made before the randomization code is broken. The former are included in the study protocol and, if truly necessary, may be modified through formal amendments (see section 2.2); the latter are documented in the so-called Statistical Analysis Plan (SAP), an operational document which is finalized before breaking the randomization code.

The decisions to be inserted in the protocol include:

- Methods of statistical analysis for the primary and secondary end-points.
- Verifications to be performed on the data and criteria for deciding the applicability of the proposed methods of analysis.
- Alternative statistical methods, to be used in case the data are distributed differently from what was anticipated, to the point that methods originally proposed are no longer applicable.
- Definition of the primary and secondary populations to be analyzed (see section 9.4.2).
- Definition of the threshold of statistical significance and power of the statistical tests (see chapter 5).

Examples of operational procedures to be included in the SAP are:

- Verification of the assumptions of applicability of the statistical methods.
- Options for pooling of strata (if too small to be analyzed individually in a stratified test).
- Detailed definition of the analysis populations, with detailed description of the inclusion criteria for each population, based on study protocol.

In open-label studies and in studies with low levels of treatment blinding, all the details related to the statistical analysis, even the smallest ones, must be defined before starting the study and documented in the protocol. The only partial exception may be when the statistical analyses are performed by independent groups (both from the researchers in contact with patients and from those in contact with the data), who are blinded to treatments and far removed from the study.

9.4.2. Analysis Populations

The set of patients on which a statistical analysis is performed is defined as the **analysis population.** Since it is very easy to introduce bias at this level, we have dedicated a separate section to this topic.

Generally, in a clinical trial more than one analysis population is defined, each with a different goal. Three are the most frequently used analysis populations: "safety", "intention-to-treat" and "per-protocol", the first for safety and tolerability end-points, the other two for efficacy end-points.

The **"safety" population** is generally defined as the set of all patients taking at least one dose of the study treatment. The analyses conducted on this population must answer the question: " what is the safety/tolerability of the treatment, taken under any condition and for any reason?"

The **"intention-to-treat" population** is defined as the set of all randomized patients, including those who prematurely discontinued the study (i.e. have missing evaluations and received shorter study treatment administration or even none at all) and those who were enrolled in violation of one or more selection criteria (i.e. should not have entered the study). The analysis performed on this population answers the question: "what is the effect of the treatment under condition close to real life?"

The **"per-protocol" population** generally includes only the patients who met the main selection criteria (inclusion and exclusion) and underwent the main procedures as instructed in the protocol: for example, patients who took the study treatment for the planned duration at the right dose, did not take prohibited concomitant medications, attended every visit (or at least the visit(s) crucial for the primary evaluation), etc. Clearly, the criteria for considering a patient sufficiently compliant to be included in the "per-protocol" analysis must be defined *a priori* in the protocol itself. The analysis performed on this population answers the question: "What is the effect of the treatment under the best experimental conditions?"

By definition, only the analysis based on the intention-to-treat principle does not alter the effects of randomization and therefore guarantees comparisons free from selection and assessment bias. For this reason, this analysis is considered most important in any context, including the regulatory one.

Vice versa, the analysis based on the per-protocol population does not guarantee bias-free comparisons. For example, by including in the analysis only patients who have completed the study, we could be selecting the patients responding better to the experimental treatment, thus introducing a serious bias in the comparison between groups. The result obtained on this population is the best obtainable by the experimental treatment (i.e. this result is the closest to the underlying scientific model as outlined in the protocol), but it is not attributable with certainty to the treatment.

The analysis conducted on the intention-to-treat population not only does not alter the effect of randomization, but also allows evaluation of the experimental treatment under conditions closest to those that will eventually occur in reality, when the treatment is in clinical practice. Many departures will occur in real life from the ideal situation, as described in the package insert, in terms of the type of disease and of patient suitability for the treatment, compliance to dosing instructions, treatment duration shorter or longer than prescribed (or even none at all), concomitant intake of non-recommended drugs, etc. These and many other forms of deviations from the instructions of the package insert will be the rule, not the exception, once the drug is available to the public. Therefore, the effect of the treatment observed in the intention-to-treat population will certainly be closer to the real one compared to the one observed in the per-protocol population.

Historically, the medical community has struggled to accept the intention-to-treat principle. Today, apart from few exceptions, it is universally recognized that the judgment on the efficacy of a new treatment must be based on this population. In other words, the primary population of pivotal clinical trials must always be the one based on the intention-to-treat principle.

In addition to the strict definition of intention-to-treat, which includes all randomized patients, a number of variants have been introduced in practice, such as the exclusion of patients who did not even receive a single dose of the study drug and/or those without any post-baseline evaluation. These variants may be used, as long as the patients included in the analysis represent almost all of the randomized patients (as a rule of thumb, patients excluded must not be more than 5% of patients randomized).

From a practical point of view, the biggest problem in performing an intention–to-treat analysis is how to evaluate those patients who miss the key measurement(s) at the end of the study or at the visit(s) where the primary evaluation is scheduled. The most widely used methods for this purpose are the use of the last available measurement for the primary evaluation (the so-called **"last-observation-carried-forward"** or LOCF method) and the use of preestablished rules, which link the missing outcome to the reason for the patient's premature discontinuation from the study. For example, if the endpoint is based on a score system, the worst possible score is assigned to a patient leaving the study because of unsatisfactory therapeutic effect, or a serious adverse event; the mean score of the group to which the patient belongs is assigned to a patient leaving the study for a reason unrelated to the study treatment; the best possible score is assigned to a patient leaving the study because the symptoms have disappeared. Among the many articles dedicated to this important subject, we recommend, in addition to the ICH guidelines [61], those by Gillings and Kock [48], Gould [50] and Lange [65].

9.5. Comparison Between an Observational and an Experimental Study

As discussed in chapter 2, the crucial distinction between an observational and an experimental study is that in the latter the researcher controls the assignment of the experimental units (patients or healthy volunteers) to the study treatments, while in the former the researcher is an observer and has no control over which study treatment each subject will take. It should be clear by now that control over the study treatments (experimental factors) by the researcher does not mean that he/she actually decides what treatment each subject should take. That assignment is in fact delegated to the randomization, the instrument through which the researcher controls the assignment of the experimental units to the study treatments.

At this point in the book, we hope that the reader has gained sufficient knowledge to appreciate the implications of the difference described above. It is for this reason that we have postponed the comparison between observational and experimental studies to this chapter.

This comparison will focus on the following aspects:
- The range of applicability.
- The reliability of conclusions on the cause-effect relationship.
- The generalizability of conclusions.

The fact that in experimental studies treatments are chosen by the researcher, restricts the **range of applicability** of such studies to interventions that one hopes can positively influence the evolution of the disease being studied. It is hard to imagine that a researcher would intentionally expose subjects to potentially harmful interventions. Vice versa, in observational studies, interventions (or characteristics) that are both potentially positive, such as a pharmacological treatment, or potentially negative, such as cigarette smoke or an inappropriate diet, can be studied. Therefore, experimental studies conducted in the human species can address a narrower spectrum of questions compared to observational studies.

With the expression **conclusions on the cause-effect relationship** we mean the ability to establish a causal link between the characteristic and the event in an epidemiological study and between the treatment and the response (signal) in a clinical study.

We know that experimental studies are generally more appropriate for drawing this kind of conclusion. Let us see why. When confronted with a statistically significant association between a characteristic and an event in an epidemiological study, or with a statistically significant difference in the responses to the different treatments in a clinical study, one tends to conclude that the characteristic/treatment is linked to the event/response by a cause-effect relationship. In reality, such a conclusion is not necessarily true. As we have repeatedly stated throughout this book, statistical significance can be due to a bias favoring or penalizing one of the groups under comparison. For example, an imbalance between groups can occur with respect to a prognostic factor impacting the event/signal. Thus, the cause-effect relationship between the event/signal and the characteristic/treatment is not direct, but mediated by this factor. In epidemiology, the phenomenon of "confounding" must also be considered: we know that when an association between a characteristic and an event is not due to a direct cause-effect relationship but to the presence of a third factor, associated with the characteristic and having an effect on the event independent from that of the characteristic, it is said that a confounding phenomenon has occurred (in clinical research this problem is avoided through randomization). Finally, the problem of the multiplicity of statistical tests must always be kept in mind. If hundreds of risk factors and/or hundreds of endpoints are considered and a threshold of 5% is used to discriminate the true associations/differences from the false ones, a substantial number of false associations/differences will be considered true, on the basis of their being statistically significant. If then the investigator "smartly" chooses to publish only the statistically significant associations/differences, the result will be a very interesting article (likely to carry professional and financial benefits) and a great lie.

The occurrence of bias, confounding and problems linked to statistical multiplicity can never be completely overcome, neither in an observational nor in a clinical study. However, in a clinical study the probability of running into the first two problems is reduced mainly through randomization, which cannot be applied in observational studies. Instead, the probability of running into the third type of problems is the same, being linked to the "smartness" of the researcher. On the topic of bias, confounding and "data dredging" we recommend an excellent editorial by Davey Smith and Ebrahim published in the British Medical Journal in December 2002 [31].

The above statements are generally valid, but should not be interpreted dogmatically. The conclusions of a randomized clinical trial are not always more reliable than the ones of an observational study. One must consider firstly the quality of the study, secondly its aim. It goes without saying that a badly planned and badly performed clinical trial does not allow firm conclusions, whereas a well planned and well performed observational study can give very reliable results.

The different approach of clinical and epidemiological studies has an effect also on the ***generalizability of the conclusions*.** **Generalizability** is the degree to which the conclusions made on the sample can be extended to the underlying population. On this front, the comparison between the experimental and the observational studies does not end with an obvious winner. Assuming that a clinical trial was properly planned, performed and analyzed, the conclusions made on the units constituting the sample can be extended, under the particular conditions of the study, to the units of the population having the same characteristics. However, there are at least two problems undermining generalizability in clinical trials. The first stems from the fact that the sample is not extracted from the population in true random fashion (see section 6.1.1 and 9.2.1). The second stems from the fact that, by definition, a clinical trial is performed under "controlled conditions". If these are too "artificial", i.e. too far from reality, one wonders if a population exists at all to which the conclusions of the study can be extended. The epidemiological studies, performed under real life, "not manipulated" conditions, give results which are easier to generalize, although also in these studies the sample is often not random (see chapter 3). On the other hand, the generalizability of results is not independent from their validity, which, as we said, is greater in clinical trials. This complicates the comparison between the two types of studies in terms of generalizability of conclusions.

Putting aside the complex judgment on generalizability of conclusions, and assuming a good quality of study planning, conduct and analysis, we can conclude that the experimental study has a narrower range of application (only positive interventions) but a greater likelihood of drawing valid comparative conclusions, from which valid conclusions on the causal relationship between treatment and effect derive (internal validity). Therefore, in situations in which the intervention under study has therapeutic aims, the experimental approach is usually "the best".

Summary

In a comparative study, the observed difference between treatments can be due to three possible causes (that can occur concomitantly and to a different extent):
1. Chance.
2. Bias, the various forms of which can be grouped in three categories: selection, assessment and analysis.
3. Treatment.

The influence of chance is evaluated through the statistical analysis, while the influence of bias must be prevented in the planning phase of the study. Three key procedures are used to minimize bias in experimental studies: randomization (against selection bias), blinding (against assessment bias) and *a priori* definition of the statistical analysis, i.e. before results are known (against the analysis bias).

The randomized, double-blind clinical trial, with concomitant controls is the type of study that is most likely to achieve bias-free results, minimizing the impact of errors systematically favoring or penalizing one treatment with respect to another.

Non-randomized and non-blinded designs cannot achieve a similar degree of methodological strength. However, one should not be dogmatic: a before-after comparison in a single group can be the best way to start experimentation of a new treatment on a cancer with rapid and predictable outcome; an open-label randomized design can be stronger than a double blind study, if the latter results in poor compliance to study medication by patients, because too complex. The experienced clinical researcher will try to get as close as possible to the standard of the randomized, double-blind design with high level blinding of the study treatments. However, he/she will also give due consideration to the practical, logistic, technical and economic aspects in making the final decision. Finally, he/she will make a transparent report on the methods followed and on the reasons for the choices made at the time of presenting the results.

The observational study can be more extensively applied than an experimental one, because it is not limited to favorable interventions. However, the observational study does not guarantee the same degree of reliability in establishing cause-effect relationships.

10
Experimental Designs

10.1. Introduction

A preliminary remark for those readers who master some statistics: this chapter is limited to the linear model, which anyway is a sufficiently broad platform to cover most of the clinical applications.

The choice of the experimental design has two main objectives:

- Minimize bias, with the aim of obtaining bias-free comparisons.
- Minimize the variability of observations, with the aim of obtaining powerful statistical tests and precise estimates.

We discussed extensively the various forms of bias in chapters 8 and 9. It remains to be clarified how the design can help minimize variability. To this end, we must return to the topic of the statistical test discussed in chapter 5. For simplicity, we will limit the discussion to the frequentist approach.

In general terms, we defined the statistical test as a ratio between the estimate of an effect of the treatment and the estimate of the variability of this effect, which is unexplained and therefore considered to result from accidental factors, i.e. chance (the background noise). How can this variability due to accidental factors be measured? The answer to this question depends on the design used for the study. Since we still have to introduce the different types of design, here we present only the basic concept. We will return later to this topic, with specific examples, when discussing the individual experimental designs.

A first and basic classification of experimental designs is in two large categories:

- Designs based on **between-subjects comparisons.**
- Designs based on **within-subject comparisons.**

The first category encompasses designs in which each experimental unit (subject) receives just one of the study treatments (or a combination, tested as a single study treatment). The second encompasses designs in which each experimental unit receives more than one study treatment. In the designs of the first category, the between-subjects variability is used in the test statistic, whereas in the designs of the second category, the within-subject variability, i.e. the variability of measurements repeated on the same subject, is used.

In general, for a given end-point, the variability of measurements carried out on the same subject is smaller than the variability of measurements carried out on different subjects. As a consequence, assuming that the other conditions are the same (the threshold of clinical significance, the acceptable thresholds of false-positives and false-negatives, etcetera - see chapters 5 and 6), the designs based on within-subject comparisons, generally require a smaller sample compared to those based on between-subjects comparisons.

A second major classification of designs is again in two categories: those explicitly taking into consideration (in jargon, "controlling for") only the experimental factor (i.e. the treatment) and those also controlling for one or more sub-experimental factors (which, as discussed in section 2.4, include prognostic factors). Through the statistical analysis, we can attribute part of the total variability of the end-point to the factor or factors "controlled for" in the design. This attribution, as mentioned in section 8.1, is defined in statistical terms as "explaining the variability". Let's assume we decide to use the variance as the measure of variability (see section 5.4.1). We know from chapter 5 that the standard error used as denominator of the test statistic d_μ^* is a function of the variance of the end-point in the population (see (5.3) in section 5.5.1). If the design of the study only controls for the treatment, we can break down the total variance as follows:

total variance = variance explained by the treatment +
residual (unexplained) variance (10.1)

The break down (10.1) is valid both for the population, i.e. for the true variance of the phenomenon, and for the sample, i.e. for the estimate of such variance. Since we can attribute a component of the total variance to the treatment, the unexplained variance (background noise) to be used in the statistical test is reduced to the **residual variance**, given by the difference between the total variance and the variance explained by the treatment. In other words, the residual variance is the part of variance that we cannot explain through the study design, and therefore must attribute to accidental factors, collectively referred to as chance.

If the design controls not only for the treatment, but also for one or more sub-experimental factors (typically prognostic factors, and/or non prognostic factors potentially of great impact on the result, such as the study center), we can break down the total variance as follows:

total variance = variance explained by the treatment + variance explained
by the sub-experimental factor + residual (unexplained) variance (10.2)

It should be noted that, in the break down (10.2), only one sub-experimental factor of interest is considered, with no interaction between this factor and the treatment (see section 10.3.2). If an interaction cannot be excluded, another component must be added to the break down, namely the variance explained by the interaction.

Again, the variance to be used in the test is the residual one. As shown in (10.2), in this type of design, it is given by the difference between the total variance, the variance explained by the treatment and the variance explained by the sub-experimental factor (or by the combination of sub-experimental factors, if more than one). Therefore, unless this last term is equal to zero, the residual variance in designs controlling for experimental and sub-experimental factors is smaller than that in designs controlling for the experimental factor (the treatment) only. Consequently, the background noise, which we cannot explain, and thus ascribe to chance (because we are unable to ascribe it to the treatment, or to other factors), is smaller.

In the design controlling for the treatment only, the estimate of the residual variance is obtained by "averaging" the sample variances calculated within each treatment group (see section 10.3.1). This was the approach taken for the test discussed in section 5.5.1, which implied a design of this kind (although this was not specified).

In the design controlling for other factors in addition to the treatment, the estimate of the residual variance is obtained by "averaging" the sample variances calculated within each of the groups that result from combining each treatment with each of the levels of these factors (see section 10.3.2). For example, let us assume we want to compare two treatments, A and P, and that gender is the prognostic factor we decide to "control for". Four groups will result from combining each treatment with each gender: females treated with A, females treated with P, males treated with A, and males treated with P. It is intuitive that, if gender really has an effect on the end-point, the variability of the observations within each of the four "treatment by gender" groups will be smaller compared to the variability within each of the two treatment groups (which combine the two genders), since the subjects belonging to each of the four groups are more homogeneous, that is, more similar to one another. When treatments and sub-experimental factors are included in the design, the statistical test is performed with a procedure similar (from a logical but not from a mathematical perspective) to that described in section 5.5.1, but using a smaller residual variance. Therefore, all other conditions being equal, the test has a greater power, i.e. a higher probability of being statistically significant when there is a true difference between the treatment groups (see chapters 5 and 6).

The distinction between designs controlling just for the treatment and those controlling also for the sub-experimental factors (prognostic or not), can be applied both to designs based on between-subjects comparisons and to those based on within-subject comparisons. The completely randomized parallel group design (see section 10.3.1) falls in the category of designs controlling just for the treatment, while the stratified parallel group design (see section 10.3.2) and the design with randomization in blocks (see section 10.3.3) fall into the category of designs controlling also for other factors.

We must admit to the reader that in the discussion above we have been quite simplistic. For example, in reality, the within-subject variability is not always smaller than that between subjects. Furthermore, the inclusion of a prognostic factor in the design does not always guarantee a gain in power of the statistical test. We have opted for this simplification to better illustrate a basic concept: if appropriate designs capable of explaining meaningful parts of the total variability are adopted, the resulting statistical test will have a greater power. With regard to the statistical test, it is important to stress that, in the parametric context (see section 5.8), all test statistics, including those for designs more complex than the completely randomized parallel group one, are derived through the same logical process used in section 5.5.1 to get to d_μ^*, that is, we have to compute a ratio between the estimate of an effect and the standard error of this estimate. However, the formulas appropriate for the test statistics for more complex designs cannot be easily derived from (5.3), and the resulting sample distribution is not necessarily a Student's t distribution.

A fundamental assumption which underlies this chapter is that the effects of the different factors are additive. Because of this assumption, the measurement obtained for an individual subject is given by:

(a quantity depending on the treatment) + (a quantity depending only on the subject).

If the design "controls" for other factors, sub-experimental or prognostic, beyond the treatment, for example gender, the measurement obtained for an individual subject belonging to a specific treatment-by-factor group, is given by:

(a quantity depending on the treatment) + (a quantity depending on the other factor considered) + (a quantity depending only on the subject).

In the example above we have assumed only one sub-experimental factor of interest, which does not interact with the treatment. If an interaction cannot be excluded, another component, i.e. the one relative to the effect of the interaction, must be added.

We will add no more on the assumption of additivity, other than reiterating that the components are added (instead of being for example multiplied) and that the effects of the treatment and of any other factor included in the design are considered constant. For a more in depth discussion of these topics, we refer the reader to the book by Cox [27], which does not require advanced mathematical skills.

The first and most important consequence of the law of additivity is that the differences between the effects of the factors included in the design can be estimated in terms of differences between means, proportions or other appropriate group indicators. This applies to the treatment, as well as to the other factors included in the design: for example, the effect of the factor "gender" can be expressed as the difference between the mean effect in males and the mean effect in females (or vice versa). The second consequence is that the total variance of the observations can be factorized as illustrated above.

In the discussion of the different designs, the reader should keep in mind that the control for factors other than the treatment (e.g. gender) implies the inclusion of other unknown parameters (to be estimated) in the so-called statistical model underlying the design. These parameters are the effects of the factors, taken independently and jointly (see main effects and interaction effects below) in the population, that is, the true but unknown effects. So as not to overly complicate the discussion, we will only refer to the sample estimates of these effects, without explicitly introducing the parameters representing the same effects in the population. It is obvious that, since these estimates are calculated on samples, to be fully interpreted they must be accompanied by the appropriate standard error giving a measure of the variability of their distribution in the sample. The formulas for calculating the standard errors of the estimates of these effects are not reported in this book. In order to perform statistical tests on these factors (for example, to verify if there is a difference between males and females), the estimate of each of these effects (considered in comparative terms) must be related to the estimate of the corresponding standard error: this ratio represents the test statistic for that factor (gender in our example).

Going back to the initial distinction between designs based on between-subjects comparisons and those based on within-subject comparisons, the most "representative" design of the first category is the parallel group one, while the most "representative" design of the second category is the cross-over one. There are other representatives for each category (for example, in the first, the dose escalating design - see section 10.4; in the second, the design in which two treatments are tested at the same time on two matching organs of the same patient, and the single patient design - see section 10.6). However, the parallel group and the cross-over designs are by far the most used in clinical research, to the point that, from now on, we will use the definitions "parallel group" and "between-subjects comparison" designs interchangeably and we will do the same for the definitions of "cross-over " and "within-subject comparison" designs.

We will compare the different designs for their ability to generate bias-free comparisons (accuracy), powerful tests and precise estimates (precision, sometimes referred to as efficiency in the jargon of experimental designs). We will also compare the designs for their ability to ensure simplicity of the studies in terms of planning, conduct and analysis. Finally, we will evaluate the conditions under which the various designs are applicable.

10.2. Parallel Group Design

10.2.1. Characteristics

Leukotriene antagonists are a class of anti-asthma drugs. Let us suppose we are responsible for a new drug of this class, fortelukast (the name is fictitious) and that we want to evaluate its effect on lung function during a two-week course of treatment. The optimal dose for fortelukast, an oral drug, has been established as 5 mg once a day. The primary end-point of our choice is the mean of the pre-medication morning values of expiratory flow rate (PEFR), measured daily throughout the two weeks of treatment.

We decide for a randomized, parallel group, placebo controlled design. As already discussed, in the **parallel group design** there are as many groups as study treatments under comparison (two in our example, fortelukast 5 mg and placebo) and each patient is assigned to only one of the treatment groups through randomization. All treatment groups are treated and evaluated simultaneously (hence the name of the design). Therefore, each patient receives just one treatment, that assigned to the group to which he/she is randomly assigned, for the duration dictated by the protocol (in our case, two weeks).

In section 10.3 we will examine the different types of parallel group designs, which differ from one another based on the type of randomization applied, and assess their strengths and weaknesses. For now, we will assess the advantages and disadvantages of between-subjects comparisons (parallel groups) with respect to within-subject comparisons (cross-over).

10.2.2. Advantages and Disadvantages

The parallel group design has two great advantages over the cross-over design:
- All other conditions being the same, the duration of the study is shorter and the visits fewer, which results in a study less burdensome for the patient.
- The statistical analysis requires fewer assumptions, which, if not verified, would reduce the reliability of the conclusions.

In summary, the parallel group design is to be preferred to the cross-over one because it's simpler and because it makes bias-free comparisons easier to obtain.

The weakness of the parallel group design is that, all other conditions being the same, it requires a larger sample size compared to the matching cross-over design, as we anticipated in section 10.1. Or, for the same sample size, it allows for less powerful tests and provides less accurate estimates. It must be noted that the sample size advantage of designs based on within-subject comparisons is not guaranteed, since it occurs only when the measurements repeated on the same subject are well correlated to one another. This condition, which guarantees that the within-subject variability is lower than that between subjects [39], is indeed met for the majority of the instrumental end-points. However, for other end-points, such as for example the scales for evaluating pain, it should not be taken for granted.

10.2.3. Conditions of Applicability

The parallel group design is applicable in a very broad range of experimental conditions. For this reason and for its simplicity, it represents the "gold-standard" of clinical research, especially in phase III (see chapter 12).

However, there are specific cases in which a true parallel group design cannot be applied. One example of inapplicability of a parallel group design is when the treatments under comparison are different doses of the same active compound and, for safety reasons, it is unacceptable to randomize patients to the different doses (see section 10.4). Another example is when it is necessary to ask the patient to express a preference between two or more study treatments.

Overall, the situations in which the parallel group design cannot be applied are in fact very few. However, when it comes to feasibility and convenience the matter becomes more complex, as we will see later in this chapter.

10.3. Variants of the Parallel Group Design

There are three main variants of the parallel group design:
• The one with simple randomization, called completely randomized design.
• The one with stratified randomization, called stratified design.
• The one with randomization in blocks, called randomized block design.

10.3.1. Completely Randomized Parallel Group Design

The **completely randomized parallel group design** is performed by applying the logic of the parallel group design with a simple randomization (see section 9.2.2). It is the simplest among the randomized controlled designs.

The **completely randomized design** is called **balanced** if the treatment groups have equal (in practice, approximately equal) size, otherwise it is called unbalanced. Generally, for reasons of statistical convenience (greater power of the test for the same overall sample size), the assignment of the experimental units to the treatment groups is made such that groups of approximately equal size are obtained.

In the completely randomized parallel group design, only the effect of the treatment can be studied, because no other factor is taken into account in the design.

If two treatments are compared, for example one active and one placebo, the data from a study of this design can be summarized as illustrated in Table 10.1. In the table, the numbers in parentheses represent the appropriate group indicators for the corresponding cells. For simplicity, assume that the appropriate indicator is the mean. The **treatment effect** (A-Placebo) is estimated by the difference between the two means calculated within each treatment group.

The advantage of the completely randomized parallel group design is basically the simplicity with which the study can be performed and the results analyzed.

The disadvantage is the limited power of the tests and the limited precision of the estimates. In fact, as touched upon briefly in section 10.1, in the completely randomized design, the residual variability of each treatment group, to be used in the statistical test on the treatment effect, is the highest with respect to every other experimental design. In practice, σ_A^2 (variance of the subjects treated with A) and σ_P^2 (variance of the subjects treated with P) are estimated with the formula shown in Table 5.2 (formula for $\hat{\sigma}^2$). Then, the "weighted" mean of $\hat{\sigma}_A^2$ and $\hat{\sigma}_P^2$, where the weights are the size of the groups, is calculated with the formula shown in Table 5.3. Finally, the standard error of the difference between two sample means is calculated (see again Table 5.3).

Table 10.1.   Completely randomized parallel group study with two treatments

Treatment A	Subjects assigned to treatment A
	(1)
Placebo treatment	Subjects assigned to placebo
	(2)

The difference between the group indicator for treatment A and that for placebo estimates the effect of treatment A. Using the numbers in parenthesis for the group indicators of the corresponding cells, the treatment effect (A-placebo) is estimated by [(1)-(2)]

Another potential disadvantage of the completely randomized design is that, by chance, the distribution of important baseline features may not be homogeneous across the treatment groups. The smaller the sample size, the more likely it is that a meaningful imbalance will occur. For example, in a small trial with two treatments (say with 30 patients in total), we can easily end up with one treatment group consisting of subjects on average younger than the other group. If younger patients have a different response to the treatment compared to the older ones, when the two groups are compared, the effect of the treatment will be "confounded" with the effect of age. In other words, it would be difficult to establish how much of the difference observed between the treatment groups in the chosen end-points is actually due to the treatments and how much is instead due to the difference in age between the groups.

When it is possible to identify in the planning phase of the study one or more characteristics of the experimental units that are likely to influence the response to the treatment (that is, sub-experimental/prognostic factors), it is possible to reduce the risk of obtaining non-homogenous groups, and at the same time reduce the residual variability, by explicitly accounting for these characteristics in the design of the study. Stratified designs and designs with randomization in blocks are typically used for this purpose.

10.3.2. Stratified Parallel Group Design

The **stratified design** is performed by applying the logic of the parallel group design with a stratified randomization (see section 9.2.2). The sub-experimental factors considered in this type of design (generally prognostic factors) are either categorical variables or continuous variables that are divided in classes or levels. For example, let us suppose we want to compare two treatments in HIV infection. The time elapsed between the initial diagnosis and the study start and the viral load at study start are two important prognostic factors for this condition. We decide to categorize each factor into three classes, thus obtaining nine strata, by intersecting each level of one factor with each level of the other (3x3). A separate and independent randomization list is used for each stratum for the assignment of the subjects to the treatments (see section 9.2.2). In our example, the stratified parallel group design requires the generation of nine separate randomization lists. In this way, within each stratum, the subjects are distributed in equal numbers among the treatment groups. For the analysis, we pool all strata for each treatment group. Therefore, the treatment groups will have a homogenous distribution of the two prognostic factors considered: this is, in fact, the main goal of **stratification**.

The **stratified design** is called **balanced** if all of the strata are of equal size (in practice of approximately equal size). In this section, we will base the discussion on the balanced design and briefly cover the imbalanced designs towards the end.

In a parallel group design, stratified for the levels of a given factor, the following effects can be studied:

- The main effect of the treatment.
- The main effect of the stratification factor, i.e. of the sub-experimental/prognostic factor.
- The effect of the interaction between the treatment and the stratification factor.

The **main effect of the treatment** is the treatment effect without considering the stratification factor, as it would be in a completely randomized design where the patients are assigned to the different treatments through simple randomization.

The **main effect of the stratification factor** is the effect of this factor without considering the treatment, as it would be in a completely randomized design where the patients are assigned to the different levels of the stratification factor through simple randomization. If randomization is not possible, the analogy is with a design where the patients are divided into groups corresponding to the different levels of this factor.

Let us suppose we want to compare two treatments, one active (A) and one placebo, using gender as the stratification factor. Data from this type of study can be summarized as shown in Table 10.2. We shall assume that the appropriate group indicator is the mean. In the balanced design, referring to Table 10.2, the main effect of the treatment is estimated by $\{[(1)-(3)]+[(2)-(4)]\}/2$ (because the strata have equal sizes) which is equivalent to $[(5)-(6)]$ and the main effect of the stratification factor is estimated by $\{[(1)-(2)]+[(3)-(4)]\}/2$ which is equivalent to $[(7)-(8)]$.

The **interaction effect** between the treatment and the stratification factor addresses the question: "what happens to the treatment effect at different levels of the stratification factor?" or "what happens to the effect of the stratification factor with different treatments, i.e. at different levels of the treatment factor?"

Referring to Table 10.2, there is an interaction effect between treatment and gender (also referred to as treatment by gender interaction) when the difference between the mean responses to the two treatments is not the same for the two levels of the gender factor, that is, the treatment effect is not equal in males and females. Generalizing, there is an interaction between two factors when the difference in mean response between two levels of the first factor varies for different levels of the second factor and vice versa. Referring once more to Table 10.2, the interaction effect is estimated either by [(1)-(3)]-[(2)-(4)] or by [(1)-(2)]-[(3)-(4)], which are algebraically equal. Since we have only one estimate of the interaction effect, we do not divide the result by 2, as we do when calculating the main effects.

In the absence of interaction, it is sufficient to present the main treatment effect, while in the presence of interaction, the treatment effect must also be reported separately within each stratum (the treatment effect at the stratum level is sometimes called "simple effect"). The implications of the interaction effect are further discussed in section 10.8 on factorial designs.

Naturally, when more than one stratification factor is considered, there is an increase in the number of effects that can be evaluated and their interpretation becomes more complex. For example, with one treatment factor and two stratification factors, in addition to the main effects of the three factors, we should consider the three **two-factor interaction effects**, i.e. the interactions between pairs of factors. The three effects are obtained by intersecting each treatment with each level of the first and, separately, of the second stratification factor, and finally each level of the first stratification factor with each level of the second one. Furthermore, we must consider the **three-factor interaction effect**, i.e. the interaction among all three factors considered simultaneously. This effect is obtained by simultaneously intersecting the levels of the treatment factor with the levels of the first and the second stratification factors, in all possible combinations.

If the stratification factors are gender (male/female) and age (adult (<65)/elderly (≥ 65)), an example of interaction between two factors would be a different mean effect of the treatment in males versus females, or in adults versus elderly. An example of an interaction among three factors is a different treatment by gender interaction effect between adults and elderly, i.e. the difference in the treatment effect between males and females changes when considering the adult and the elderly age groups.

In the case of imbalanced designs, the estimates of the main treatment effect and the interaction effect are more complex. In the absence of the main effect of the stratification factor and of interaction, the main treatment effect is estimated by the difference between the mean of treatment A and the mean of placebo, without taking into account the stratification factor (referring to Table 10.2: [(5)-(6)]). In the presence of a main effect of the stratification factor, but in the absence of interaction, the main treatment effect is estimated by the

Table 10.2. Parallel group study with two treatments and one stratification factor (gender) with two levels

	Level 1 of the stratification factor: females	Level 2 of the stratification factor: males	Total
Level 1 of the treatment factor: treatment A	Females treated with A (1)	Males treated with A (2)	Females and males treated with A (5) The group indicator of this cell estimates the overall effect of treatment A on males and females
Level 2 of the treatment factor: placebo	Females treated with placebo (3)	Males treated with placebo (4)	Females and males treated with placebo (6) The group indicator of this cell estimates the overall effect of placebo on males and females
Total	Females treated with any treatment (7) The group indicator of this cell estimates the overall effect of being female on patients treated with either A or placebo	Males treated with any treatment (8) The group indicator of this cell estimates the overall effect of being male on patients treated with either A or placebo	

Assuming a balanced design and using the number in parenthesis for the group indicator of the corresponding cell, the following applies:

1. The difference between the cell indicators (1) and (3) estimates the effect of the treatment (A-placebo) in females; likewise, the difference between the cell indicators (2) and (4) estimates the effect of the treatment in males.
2. The mean of the two differences [(1)-(3)] and [(2)-(4)] estimates the main effect of the treatment and the mean of the two differences [(1)-(2)] and [(3)-(4)] estimates the main effect of the stratification factor. These correspond to [(5)-(6)] and [(7)-(8)], respectively.
3. The difference between the two differences [(1)-(3)] and [(2)-(4)] (or analogously [(1)-(2)] and [(3)-(4)] estimates the effect of the interaction between the treatment and the stratification factor.

When there is interaction, to quantify the treatment effect, it is mandatory to present the estimate reported at point 1 in addition to the one reported at point 2 "weighted" mean of the treatment effects in the different strata, using the sample sizes of the strata as weights (referring to Table 10.2: {[(1)-(3)] w1+[(2)-(4)]w2}/(w1+w2), where w1 and w2 are calculated from the sample sizes of the treatment groups). In the presence of an interaction effect, the main treatment effect is estimated by the arithmetic mean of the treatment effects in the different strata (referring to Table 10.2: {[(1)-(2)]+[(3)-(4)]}/2). In addition, the estimates of the treatment effect must be provided for each stratum (referring to Table 10.2: [(1)-(3)] for females; [(2)-(4)] for males). The statistical justifications for this approach can be found in [39].

In the balanced designs all types of estimate of the main treatment effect discussed above coincide.

In the stratified parallel group design there is usually little interest in the main effect of the stratification factor (or factors): in fact, since stratification is applied to factors known (or strongly suspected) to influence the end-point of the study, a difference in response between the different levels of these factors is expected.

Vice versa, the evaluation of the interaction effect (or effects) is generally of interest, though rarely the primary objective of the trial (which is normally the treatment effect). The reason for such an interest is that the existence of an interaction effect has an impact on how the treatment effect is to be estimated (see above) and interpreted.

Usually, the stratified design is used, not because there is interest in studying the individual strata, but because, under the same conditions, it is more **efficient** than the completely randomized design, requiring fewer patients to detect a given difference between treatments (see section 10.1). Referring to Table 10.2, the residual variance, used for the statistical test, is estimated within each of the four cells, because the variability among the units belonging to the same cell cannot be explained by the factors considered in the design. The estimate of the residual variance can be seen as a weighted mean of these four estimates. Since subjects belonging to the same stratum are homogeneous with respect to the stratification factor, by design, the variability within each cell is expected to be lower than the variability we would find in treatment groups without further subdivision. However, in order to have a real gain in efficiency, we should only consider those stratification factors that have a relevant impact on the response, and that can therefore explain relevant parts of the variability.

Only rarely are the strata of primary interest in the experiment, i.e. the objective of the study is to compare the responses to the treatment in the different strata. These are called interaction studies (the interaction is between the stratification factor, i.e. the prognostic factor, and the treatment). In these studies, in determining the sample size, one must explicitly take into consideration this objective.

10.3.3. Parallel Group Randomized Block Design

Another method for reducing variability based on the grouping of subjects with common characteristics is the so-called "blocking", also known as "matching".

The design deriving from it, called parallel group design with randomization in blocks or **randomized block design**, is performed by applying the logic of the parallel group design with randomization in permuted blocks (see section 9.2.2).

This design is frequently used in agricultural and in preclinical research. In clinical experiments, it is primarily used to reduce time-related imbalances between the treatment groups. The advantage of this design is that temporal changes are balanced between the treatment groups at regular intervals, the smaller the block, the shorter the intervals. This is useful when the recruitment time is long, especially if the size of the study is small. Two cases can be distinguished:

- The first is when time is a sub-experimental factor but not a prognostic one, for example unpredictable changes in study personnel, or concomitant medications, or investigator's commitment to the study, etcetera.
- The second is when time is a prognostic factor, that is to say its effect is predictable and reproducible, which is the case of diseases with a seasonal trend, such as some forms of asthma and rhinitis, many infectious diseases, Raynaud syndrome, etc.

An example of an application in which time is a sub-experimental but not a prognostic factor is described by Fleiss in [39]. It concerns a study that is approaching completion of enrolment, but may miss the pre-planned deadline. There is growing pressure from the sponsor that the agreed deadline be met. Because of this pressure, there is the risk that the inclusion/exclusion criteria be "interpreted" more flexibly toward the end of the study than at the beginning. Consequently, patients enrolled in the first part of the study could have different characteristics, including prognosis, compared to the ones enrolled in the second part. Randomization in permuted blocks allows this problem to be overcome, because it balances such differences among the treatments under comparison.

An example of an application in which time is a prognostic factor, although not the only one, is the following. Suppose we want to compare three treatments, fortelukast (our new leukotriene antagonist), montelukast (the gold standard for this class of drugs) and placebo, on patients with seasonal asthma, i.e. asthma with seasonal recurrences. We decide to use the mean value of morning PEFR measurements carried out in the last week of treatment as the primary end-point. Clearly, the time of enrolment is a key prognostic factor (some seasons are worse than others for this type of asthma). In addition, gender and age (young/adult/elderly) also represent two important prognostic factors. If we were to take both factors into account in our study, we would have the following six combinations:

- Combination 1: male, young.
- Combination 2: male, adult.
- Combination 3: male, elderly.
- Combination 4: female, young.
- Combination 5: female, adult.
- Combination 6: female, elderly.

Since the time of enrolment is a key prognostic factor, we need to enroll blocks of three patients belonging to the same combination within a short period of time, and randomly assign one patient to each of the three study treatments. It is not important to fill every combination, but for every combination that does get filled, it is important to enroll simultaneously (or almost) a number of patients (i.e. a block) equal to the number of treatments. This will allow a balanced randomization. With k treatments, each block of k patients enrolled simultaneously (or almost) and matched with respect to the other predefined characteristics, is randomly subdivided among the k treatments. For example, three young males (combination 1) are simultaneously enrolled in the study, and randomized, one to each of the three study treatments.

If only two treatments are compared in the study, only two subjects are to be enrolled simultaneously for each combination of factors considered (block of size 2). This special case is referred to as the **matched-paired design** (this technique was mentioned in chapter 3 with reference to observational studies, clearly without randomization).

What are the differences between the randomized block design and the stratified design?

The stratified design does not control for the factor "time of enrolment", while the design with randomization in blocks does. In the previous example, had time of enrolment not been important, we could have used a stratified design: the six combinations of factors would have been six strata. We would have constructed a randomization list for each stratum, assigning patients to the treatments within each stratum. In a given stratum, a patient could easily have been assigned to a treatment many months after the other patients of the same stratum had been assigned to the other treatments. Furthermore, the randomized block design generates a completely balanced scheme of assignment to the treatments (i.e. each treatment group gets the same number of patients), while the stratified design does not. This has an effect on the statistical analysis.

The statistical analysis of the randomized block design is different from that of the completely randomized design and that of the stratified design. However, when time is a sub-experimental factor and it is the only factor for which randomization in permuted blocks has been applied (i.e. the only purpose is to achieve numerical balance of the treatment groups at close intervals throughout the study and overall), the statistical analysis does not take the block into consideration and the study is analyzed as if it were a completely randomized parallel group design. In fact, when time is a sub-experimental factor, but not a prognostic one, the estimate of the time effect is not of interest, because it cannot be interpreted from a clinical point of view and because it is difficult to predict whether "controlling" for this factor causes a decrease or an increase of the residual variability. In this case, by far the most common, the only effect that can be studied is that of the treatment. On the other hand, when time is a prognostic factor, the block has meaning in itself and it is appropriate to explicitly consider it in the statistical analysis. In this case both the main effects and the interaction effects can be studied, as in the stratified design.

Table 10.3. A balanced incomplete block design in a study with 5 doses of the same treatment and 10 incomplete blocks of size 3

Incomplete Block	Treatment				
	Dose 1	**Dose 2**	**Dose 3**	**Dose 4**	**Dose 5**
1	✓	✓	✓		
2	✓	✓		✓	
3	✓	✓			✓
4	✓		✓	✓	
5	✓		✓		✓
6	✓			✓	✓
7		✓	✓	✓	
8		✓	✓		✓
9		✓		✓	✓
10			✓	✓	✓

The randomized block design is very difficult to use if many factors must be considered in "matching" the units. For this reason it is not recommended when, in addition to time, more than two prognostic factors are to be considered. The stratified design is easier to apply, though it is a good rule not to have too many stratification factors and resulting strata.

10.3.4. Balanced Incomplete Block Design

This type of design is used when one wants to compare more than two (k, with $k>2$) treatments, using the blocking technique to control for the time factor (alone or in combination with other factors), but it is not possible to obtain each block of size k in a short enough time window. Therefore, the size of the block (g) will be smaller than k.

Suppose we want to compare five doses of a treatment meant to reduce the symptoms of Raynaud syndrome. In this disease, the weather (a time-related factor) is an extremely important factor, since cold is the trigger for most of the symptoms (paraesthesias and pain to fingers and toes and, in the most severe cases, ulcers and gangrene). Under these conditions, it would necessary to enroll each block of 5 patients within a very tight time window, say within a week, in order to avoid that changes in weather "distort" the comparisons among the treatments. Suppose however that it is realistic to enroll only three patients per week, so that the size of the block (3) would have to be smaller than the number of treatments. Under these circumstances, the **balanced incomplete block design** (BIBD) can be used. In our example it has the structure illustrated in Table 10.3, which has been constructed following the rules provided by fleiss in [39], section 11.1. The three patients forming the first incomplete block are randomly assigned to doses 1, 2 and 3; the three patients of the second block to doses 1, 2 and 4; the three of the third block to doses 1, 2 and 5, and so on.

Table 10.4. Balanced incomplete block design with 3 treatments and two stratification factors, gender and age, using 3 incomplete blocks of size 2

Combination #1 (male, young)	Treatment		
	1	2	3
1	✓	✓	
2	✓		✓
3		✓	✓

...

Combination #6 (female, elderly)			
	1	2	3
1	✓	✓	
2	✓		✓
3		✓	✓

This design is characterized by a fundamental property: in total, each pair of treatments (in our example, each pair of doses of the same treatment) appears the same number of times. This property facilitates the statistical analysis.

The application of this design to an experimental situation in which, in addition to time, other factors must be considered, creates a complex scheme of treatment assignment. Let us go back to the example of seasonal asthma discussed in the previous section. In order to compare the three treatments (fortelukast, montelukast and placebo), we established that patients must be enrolled in blocks of 3, that each block must be made of patients belonging to the same combination of gender and age level (from a total of six possible combinations), and that each block must be enrolled in a short time. Given the nature and the circumstances of our trial, we conclude that one month is the longest acceptable time window for one block to be enrolled, but it is possible to enroll only two patients belonging to the same block each month. Since the size of the block (2) is smaller than the number of treatments (3), we decide to apply the balanced incomplete block design, which for this example has the structure illustrated in Table 10.4.

Therefore, for each of the six combinations, based on gender and age level, three incomplete blocks of two patients each must be considered.

Since these designs are not applied frequently in clinical research, we will stop the discussion here. We refer the interested reader to the above mentioned book by Fleiss [39], illustrating balanced incomplete block designs for up to six treatments and, for a more extensive, but more technical discussion, to the book by Cochran and Cox [24].

10.4. Other Designs with Comparison Between Subjects: Dose-Escalation and Dose-Titration

10.4.1. Dose-Escalation Design

A special form of parallel group design is represented by the controlled **dose-escalation design**, which is used in phase I trials to study the safety of specific dose intervals of new compounds, often with the goal of finding the highest tolerated doses. Generally, as will be discussed in section 12.2.2., data from pre-clinical pharmacology and toxicology studies are used to choose the dose range for such studies.

For our new drug fortelukast, we select the following four doses: 0.1 mg, 1 mg, 5 mg, and 10 mg. The defining feature of this type of study is that we cannot simply randomize the subjects to one of the four doses (or to a random sequence of doses). This is because, at this stage of the development process, we have no experience on the tolerability of the drug in man. Therefore, we can administer a higher dose only after having documented the tolerability of the lower one(s). On the other hand, we want to avoid the bias resulting from a simple non-randomized study in which increasing doses of fortelukast are administered in sequence. In the controlled dose-escalation design, the sample, say 60 healthy volunteers or patients, is divided into four groups of 15 subjects (one group for each dose level). The subjects of the first group are randomized to fortelukast 0.1 mg or placebo with a simple randomized parallel group design, but with uneven randomization, for example with a 4:1 (fortelukast : placebo) ratio, that is to say 12 subjects receive fortelukast and 3 placebo (see section 9.2.2). Naturally, the highest possible level of blinding is applied. The tolerability of the first dose is determined by a comparison between active and placebo, when the 15 subjects of the group have completed the study. If the tolerability profile shown by fortelukast 0.1 mg is acceptable compared to placebo, we can move to the second group of 15 subjects, who are randomized, again with a 4:1 ratio, to fortelukast 1 mg or placebo. If the tolerability is again acceptable, we move to the third group of 15 subjects who receive the third dose of fortelukast or placebo, and so on, until an unacceptable tolerability profile is reached for the active drug, or the highest dose envisaged in the study plan is reached (see Figure 10.1). The decision as to whether or not to move from one dose to the next is not easy and requires a great deal of experience.

This is a parallel group (concurrent) design only when considering each dose and its corresponding placebo, whereas the different doses are studied in sequential groups (therefore with a non-concurrent design), each made up of different subjects.

In this design, the dose effect is confounded with the period effect, generated by changes of the experimental conditions over time. Two types of dose comparisons are possible: one between the groups at the end of the study, pooling together all placebo treated patients; the other between the dose effects that are, in turn, estimated by comparing each dose with its own placebo. The

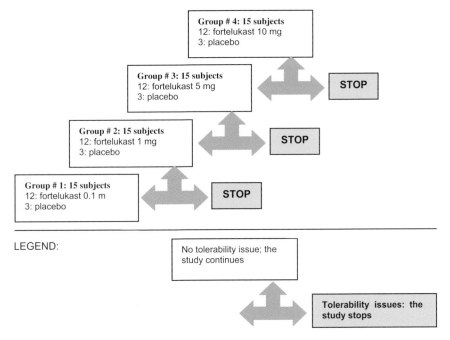

Figure. 10.1. Dose-escalation, placebo controlled design

former analysis ignores the period effect and therefore produces biased estimates of the dose effects if the period effect is not null. The latter analysis produces dose estimates that are "adjusted" for the period effect and therefore unbiased. Unfortunately, this gain in accuracy is at the cost of precision, that is the latter estimates are less precise than the former.

The choice between the two types of analysis must be made in the planning phase because it has an impact on sample size. In general, for each dose, an uneven randomization is used, with a smaller number of patients being assigned to the placebo. However, the choice to have groups of equal size at the end of the study is optimal only if we can assume absence of the period effect and, therefore, plan direct treatment comparisons without adjustment for this effect. Our example, where, if all four doses are tested, we obtain five groups of equal size (12 patients) at the end of the study, implies an analysis without adjustment for the period effect. When the period effect cannot be excluded, the calculation of the sample size must take into account the fact that variability of the comparisons between each dose and its own placebo is increased with an excessively unbalanced allocation at each dose level (for more details see: Senn S (1997), Statistical Issues in Drug Development, John Wiley & Sons, Chichester).

In the example above, we used the simple randomization scheme, but we could also have used, in principle, a stratified randomization, if we were aware of sub-experimental/prognostic factors with a relevant impact on the safety evaluations. However, in making these choices, it is essential to keep the sample size in mind, as stratification carried out on a sample that is too small (in our case 15 subjects, with an unbalanced randomization) can be counterproductive.

In controlled dose-escalation designs, the sample size is generally chosen empirically, based on the availability of volunteers and the number of doses to test, rather than on the typical sample size calculation procedures. Consequently, in this kind of study, only adverse events occurring very frequently can be detected statistically. Therefore, the background noise of random events can play an important role, simulating both positive and negative results, which in fact are only due to chance. Nevertheless, since the purpose of these phase I studies is to eliminate doses that are clearly unacceptable for the patient, that is, to find a "dose ceiling" for later studies, an empirical approach like the one described is generally acceptable. Occasionally such designs are also used in early phase II before the definitive dose finding study.

10.4.2. Dose-Titration Design

A useful design for collecting preliminary data on the dose-response curve of a treatment is the so-called "**dose-titration design**". In this design each subject receives a sequence of increasing doses of a same treatment, generally starting from a very low dose. A higher dose is given if the lower one appears to be well tolerated. This design requires a control group, generally placebo. Patients are assigned through randomization to one of the study treatments. In each group the dose is progressively increased (if the control group receives placebo, this will obviously be a simulation).

The primary comparison is between the dose-response curves of the treatment groups being tested. Therefore, this design belongs to the class of designs with between-subject comparison, even if the different doses are experimented on the same group of subjects. However, it differs from the parallel group design, because it does not fulfill the definition given in section 10.2, according to which in a parallel group design there are as many groups as treatments under comparison and each patient is assigned through randomization to one (and only one) of the treatment groups.

This design can be conducted in two main variants: in the first, called **forced dose-titration**, the dose, if well tolerated, is increased in all patients at preestablished times and regardless of their response to the treatment in terms of efficacy; in the second variant, called **conditional** or **optimized dose-titration**, the dose, if well tolerated, is modified at preestablished times but with guidance from the efficacy response observed in the single patient (for example the dose is increased only if the patient does not obtain a response at least equal to a predetermined threshold).

The dose-titration design has two main advantages:

- It is safer than the dose-ranging designs in which patients are randomized concurrently to the different doses or sequences of doses, with the underlying assumption that a patient can immediately be exposed to the highest dose; consequently, the dose-titration can be applied at a very early phase of the clinical development process.

- The total number of patients required is smaller than in a parallel group design testing the same number of doses.

Along with the above-mentioned advantages, there are several disadvantages:

- These studies are long and complex, because every subject must take several doses, each for a time long enough for the activity of the treatment to manifest itself; as a consequence, more premature discontinuations are to be expected compared to other designs.
- If the response improves with increasing doses, it is impossible to know if this is due to the dose level itself, to the longer exposure to the treatment, or to a cumulative effect of different doses (this disadvantage is especially evident when the response to the treatment is delayed).
- The dose titration design gives little information on the safety of the individual doses, since many adverse events depend on the overall time of exposure to the treatment.
- If used in the conditional dose-titration variant, this design tends to create dose-response curves in the shape of an inverted U, because all patients not responding to the study treatment will be titrated to the higher doses, if no unacceptable toxicity is observed; therefore, at the end of the study most non-responders will end up in the highest dose group. In order to correct this problem, sophisticated statistical analyses are required.

The dose-titration design is generally used for the initial assessment of the activity of new compounds and for the selection of the doses to be used in subsequent trials. It can give a first approximation of the dose-response curve, in terms of both mean curve and distribution of individual curves. Because of the problems mentioned above, the results must be confirmed by studies with a more appropriate design (for example parallel group dose-ranging studies).

We cannot delve any further into this subject, but refer the interested reader to the ICH guideline [59].

10.5. Complete Cross-Over Design

10.5.1. Characteristics

The **cross-over design** is characterized by the fact that each study subject receives more than one study treatment. In the **complete cross-over design** each subject receives, one after the other, all of the study treatments. What changes from subject to subject, is the succession of treatments: each subject is randomized to one of the possible successions of treatments, called **sequences**, and all possible sequences are used. In the simplest situation of just two treatments (A and B), there are two possible sequences (AB and BA). For example, let us consider again a study with fortelukast 5mg/day versus placebo for two weeks, this time in patients with chronic asthma (i.e. with no obvious seasonal pattern). Each patient is randomized to one of the two possible sequences: placebo followed by fortelukast, or fortelukast followed by placebo. With three treatments (A, B and C), there are six possible sequences (ABC, ACB, BAC, BCA, CAB, CBA). With more than three treatments, the possible number of sequences increases according to the formula (10.3) reported in section 10.6. Cross-over designs with many treatments have special problems that will be discussed in section 10.6.2 (incomplete cross-over designs).

Each of the time intervals in which one of the study treatments is administered is called a **period.** Therefore, in the cross-over design with two treatments there are two periods: period 1, in which the group of patients randomized to the sequence AB receives A and the one randomized to the sequence BA receives B; and period 2, in which the first group receives B and the second A. Such design is often referred to as 2×2 cross-over (two treatments and two periods).

It is often not appropriate to start the next treatment immediately after the end of the previous one. For example in the sequence fortelukast/placebo, the effects of the last doses of fortelukast could overlap with the first measurements of the placebo period, distorting the result. The continuation of the effect of one treatment into the following period of a cross-over design is often referred to as "carry-over" effect. In order to eliminate the carry-over effect, it is necessary to introduce an appropriate interval between the end of a treatment and the beginning of the next, called "**wash-out**". Generally, the duration of the wash-out interval is determined by the pharmacokinetic and pharmacodynamic characteristics of the treatments under study (see section 12.1). Obviously, the wash-out has the effect of increasing the duration and complexity of the study for each patient.

The following effects can be studied in a cross-over design:
- Main treatment effect.
- Main period effect.
- Carry-over effect.
- Interaction effect between period and treatment.
- Sequence effect.
- Subject effect.

In this book we will restrict the discussion to a brief explanation of the meaning of these effects, considering a **balanced** 2×2 **cross-over design**, which is a cross-over design with an equal number of patients (in practice, approximately equal) in each of the two sequences. In the unbalanced design, the estimate of the effects listed above must include adjustments for the different size of the groups. For a more detailed discussion of these topics, we refer to the textbooks by Fleiss [39] and Senn [93], the latter entirely dedicated to cross-over designs.

The data of a 2×2 cross-over study can be summarized as illustrated in Table 10.5. In the discussion below we shall assume that the appropriate group indicator is the mean.

Table 10.5. Cross-over study with two treatments and two periods

	Period 1	**Wash-out**	**Period 2**
Sequence: **A → placebo**	Subjects receive treatment A (1)	No treatment	Subjects receive placebo (2)
Sequence: **Placebo → A**	Subjects receive placebo (3)	No treatment	Subjects receive treatment A (4)

Assuming a balanced design and using the number in parenthesis for the group indicator of the corresponding cell, the following applies.

- In the absence of a carry-over effect, within each sequence, the difference between the group indicators of the two periods gives a measure of the treatment effect. Half of the difference between these differences calculated in the two sequences, that is {[(1)-(2)]-[(3)-(4)]}/2, estimates the effect of the treatment (A-placebo) adjusted by the period effect. In the presence of a carry-over effect, this estimate is biased.
- In the absence of a carry-over effect, within each period, the mean of the group indicators of the two treatments gives a measure of the response of the patients in that period. The difference between these means calculated in the two periods, that is [(1)+(3)]/2-[(2)+(4)]/2={[(1)+(3)]-[(2)+(4)]}/2, estimates the period effect. In the presence of a carry-over effect, this estimate is biased.
- Within each sequence, the sum of the group indicators calculated in the two periods gives a measure of the response of the patients in that sequence (to both treatments, in both periods). The difference between these sums calculated in the two sequences, that is [(1)+(2)]-[(3)+(4)], estimates the carry-over effect.

Main treatment effect or simply **treatment effect.** From Table 10.5, relating to a 2×2 cross-over design, one can infer that, within the first sequence, the difference between the group indicators (e.g. mean responses) of period 1 and period 2 measures the difference [A + period 1 - (placebo + period 2)], while the same difference in the second sequence measures the difference [placebo + period 1 - (A + period 2)]. The difference between these two differences gives: 2 A – 2 placebo. Therefore, half of this quantity estimates the effect of treatment A - placebo. This effect is referred to as the treatment effect adjusted by the period effect, meaning that it is not influenced by the period effect (see below). This is because the differences within each sequence are affected to the same extent by the period effect, if any. Therefore, the difference between these differences cannot be influenced by it. This estimate is unbiased only in the absence of a carry-over effect (see below).

Main period effect or simply **period effect.** We shall start with a question: why is it necessary to assign the patients to both sequences AB and BA? Really, there is no interest in the sequence itself. The interest, as usual, is in the difference between the treatments. The reason why we must consider both sequences is that we must know the response to each treatment, both when it is administered as the first and as the second in the sequence, because the response could change due to the period effect. This effect is estimated by the difference between the mean of the responses obtained in one period (for example, the first one) and the mean of the responses obtained in the other period (for example, the second one), pooling the treatments in each period. This estimate is unbiased only in the absence of a carry-over effect (see below). The period effect can be due to the progressive improvement or worsening of the disease under study, to a seasonal or cyclic fluctuation of the disease severity, and to a number of other time related changes, such as changes in the staff conducting the study, the introduction of new concomitant treatments, of new diagnostic instruments, and so on. Such changes are by no means exclusive to the cross-over design and can equally influence the treatment effect in a study with parallel group design, since the patient enrolment often takes a long time to complete. However, in a parallel group design, the influence of these factors is randomly distributed across the treatment groups and can even be eliminated through the randomization in permuted blocks. In the cross-over design, instead, if there were no randomization of the subjects to the different sequences, the influence of any time-related factor would be systematically greater on one treatment than on the other, i.e. would generate a systematic distortion, or bias in the comparison between treatments.

A period effect of low to moderate magnitude is often present. In itself, it does not represent a problem, thanks to the randomization of the subjects to the sequences, which, in turn, allows adjustment of the effect of the treatment for the effect of the period (see above). Suppose that both study treatments A and B are completely ineffective and that they are evaluated in a cross-over design on a disease with slowly progressive deterioration. In the sequence AB the mean effect of A, which happens to be administered in the first period, will tend to be better than the mean effect of B, which happens to be administered in the second period. In the sequence BA, B will be the one showing the best effect, since it happens to be used in the first period. Obviously, in the presence of diseases with progressive improvement, the opposite will occur. In other words, thanks to the randomization of the subjects to the sequences, the period effect does not introduce bias in the comparison between treatments. Returning to the comparison between fortelukast and placebo for the treatment of chronic asthma, let us suppose that the entire study lasts two months: two weeks for patient recruitment, two for the first treatment (first period), two for the wash-out and two for the second treatment (second period); let us also suppose that the end of the first month of the study coincides with the end of the pollen season. The small spontaneous improvement experienced by many asthmatic patients at the end of the pollen season causes a typical period effect. However, the randomization of the patients to the two sequences placebo-fortelukast or fortelukast-placebo ensures that for each of the two treatments about half of the patients are treated in the first period (pollen season ongoing) and the other half in the second period (pollen season over). Therefore in the overall evaluation of the difference between the two treatments, the influence of the period is null or greatly mitigated.

However, when the period effect is extreme, a much bigger problem arises, as illustrated in section 10.5.2.

Carry-over effect. In the cross-over design, in addition to the treatment and the period effects, other effects can potentially occur, among which the carry-over effect and the period by treatment interaction effect (see below). In the 2×2 cross-over design, these two effects cannot be separated (the explanation of why this is the case is outside the boundaries we have set for this book). Commonly, in this design one chooses to estimate the **carry-over effect**, assuming that the interaction effect is nil. The reason for this choice is that the former, as we will see later, is much more problematic than the latter. At the beginning of this section, we defined the carry-over as the continuation of the effect of a treatment into the period following its administration. If the effect of both study treatments were to extend equally into the next period, this phenomenon would not create bias in the estimate of the treatment effect, because both treatments would be equally affected by the persisting effect of the other treatment. However, the possibility of a carry-over which is identical between the two study treatments is extremely unlikely; therefore, the extension of the effect of at least one of the study treatments beyond its administration period, is practically always a problem for the application of the cross-over design. In conclusion, when referring to the carry-over effect, we imply an unequal carry-over across the treatments under comparison. Referring to Table 10.5 relative to the 2×2 cross-over design, one can see that any difference between the sum of the group indicators of the two periods in the first sequence and that in the second sequence cannot be due to the treatments, since all patients took both study treatments. It cannot depend on the period either, since all patients have gone through both periods. However, if the effect of the treatments persists beyond the duration of the period, patients assigned to the first sequence will have a residual effect of treatment A into the second period, while patients assigned to the second sequence will have a residual effect of the placebo into the second period (probably equal to zero). Therefore, any difference between the sums that we are considering will estimate the carry-over effect. As mentioned already, in the presence of this effect, the estimates of the treatment and the period effects are distorted. Therefore, the analysis of a cross-over design starts with the test for the carry-over effect: if the outcome is not statistically significant, treatment and period can be estimated as described above, otherwise the interpretation of these effects becomes very problematic (see below).

Interaction effect between period and treatment. In cross-over designs it is said that there is an **interaction effect** between the period and the treatment when the effect of the treatment is different in different periods. This effect can be studied by treating the cross-over design as a parallel group stratified design, in which the sequences are the groups to which subjects are randomized and the periods are the strata. For simplicity, we describe the period by treatment interaction effect referring to the 2×2 design illustrated in Table 10.5, even if, as said, this effect is never estimated under these circumstances, because it is "sacrificed" to the carry-over effect. Let the disease under study be an intestinal malabsorption syndrome and the primary end-point the frequency of diarrhea episodes. The two study treatments, to be compared through a 2×2 cross-over design, are two enzyme mixtures administered for one month. One study treatment must be stored at room temperature, while the other must be kept refrigerated. The first period takes place in the month of November and the second in the month of December. Unfortunately, during the whole month of November, violent storms cause repeated power black-outs, obviously affecting the refrigeration system. Because of the inappropriate refrigeration, the quality and therapeutic efficacy of the treatment to be stored at low temperature are affected. This is an example of period by treatment interaction: the period has a different impact on the end-point depending on the treatment administered. In fact, the first period (November) has a negative influence on the end-point only for the refrigerated treatment. As for the period effect, the possibility of an interaction effect between period and treatment should not be of particular concern in the planning of a cross-over design.

Sequence effect. The **sequence effect** is defined as the effect of the entire sequence of study treatments on the end-point. It can be studied by treating the cross-over design as a completely randomized parallel group design, where the sequences are the groups to be compared (see Table 10.1) and the end-point, for example, is the mean of the measurements performed at the end of each treatment within each sequence. However, as stated above, the sequence itself is almost never of interest.

Subject effect. The **subject effect** is due to the peculiar characteristics of each individual, influencing the end-point above and beyond any other effect. We will conclude that the subject effect is strong, when all measurements performed on the same subject are similar (correlated) to one another. The estimate of this effect is generally of no interest. It should be noted that the cross-over design stems from the recognition of this effect: in fact, it is in the presence of a relevant subject effect that one has the maximum convenience (in terms of reduced variability) by using a cross-over design.

Generally, in the classical statistical analysis of a 2×2 cross-over design, the treatment, the period, and the carry-over effects are considered. Furthermore, the subject effect is taken into account with specific assumptions to facilitate testing of the carry-over effect.

10.5.2. Advantages and Disadvantages

As mentioned in section 10.1, the advantage of the cross-over approach lies in the smaller sample size that it generally requires compared to the corresponding parallel group design of the same power. The smaller sample size can be explained in part by the fact that in a cross-over design each patient contributes to the sample of more than one treatment and in part by the fact that, generally, the variability of within-subject measurements is lower than that of between-subjects measurements. Making a rough but useful approximation, provided that the other conditions are the same, the sample size of a two treat-ment cross-over design is about four times smaller than the one of the corre-sponding parallel group design (the first halving of the sample size is explain-able mathematically, the second halving occurs, roughly speaking, if the repeat-ed measurements are highly correlated within each subject).

Since access to patients is often a limiting factor in the performance of clini-cal trials, both from a practical/logistical and from a financial perspective, a design such as the cross-over, which "promises to save patients" is extremely attractive. Furthermore, in our experience, the concept of each patient being "his/her own control" is popular among medical researchers and is often con-sidered a "higher quality design". The reasons for such preference are not com-pletely logical, but may have something to do with the fact that a within-patient comparison is conceptually close to what is done in clinical practice.

Unfortunately, in reality, the cross-over design is logistically more complex and methodologically more problematic than the parallel group design.

Logistical aspects. From a logistical point of view, each patient must repeat all of the procedures and measurements dictated by the protocol, as many times as there are treatments to be studied. If, for example, the protocol of the study comparing 5 mg fortelukast and placebo required measurements of PEFR every hour over 12 hours after the first and the last dose of study treatment, in a cross-over design each patient would be asked to spend the entire day at the center four times, against the two times required by the equivalent parallel group design. If there were three treatments, such a request would extend to six whole days. It is clear that one will soon reach a threshold that even the most motivat-ed patient would consider unacceptable. Even more problematic is the fact that the complexity of the procedures of the cross-over design increases the likeli-hood that a patient will initially accept to enter the study and then abandon it prematurely. Premature discontinuations have more serious methodological consequences in a cross-over design than in a parallel group one (see below).

Of course, a cross-over study is not only more complex, but also longer for the individual patient than the equivalent parallel group study. For example, in the comparison between 5 mg fortelukast and placebo, even if the treatments were administered in direct succession without any interruption between the end of one treatment and the beginning of the next, the duration of the study after randomization would be four weeks for each patient, compared to two weeks for the equivalent design in parallel groups. In reality, as already men-tioned, a wash-out interval between the treatments is very often included. By introducing a one-week pause between fortelukast and placebo (or vice versa), the duration of a cross-over study for the individual patient would increase to five weeks. An alternative to the wash-out is to eliminate from the analysis the results of measurements performed during the first days of all treatment peri-ods other than the first. In some cases this is an excellent solution, while in oth-ers it is useless or impossible. Useless, for example, when the remaining days of treatment are insufficient for an appropriate evaluation of the treatment effect.

The solution would have to be an extension of the duration of each treatment, but this would negate the advantage gained by eliminating the wash-out. Impossible, for example, when it is imperative to perform measurements immediately after the beginning of the treatment to find out if tachyphylaxis has occurred (tachyphylaxis is a rapid reduction of the magnitude of the treatment effect after the first doses, a common phenomenon for many drugs acting on receptors).

Methodological aspects. From a methodological point of view, we can point out the following major complications in the cross-over design: premature discontinuations, "extreme" period effect and carry-over effect.

- **Premature discontinuations.** Whatever the experimental design, some patients will decide or be forced to abandon the study before completing it (drop-outs). This phenomenon is problematic and must be addressed at the planning stage, mainly by avoiding excessively complex procedures, by increasing the number of patients randomized to account for the predicted drop-out rate and by determining how to evaluate the patients in the intention-to-treat analysis. A much greater number of premature discontinuations than predicted is always a problem, whatever the experimental design. However, as already mentioned, the problem is more serious in the cross-over design than in the parallel group one. In a cross-over design, a patient abandoning the study before completing the last treatment of the sequence, either must be completely removed from the analysis, or must have all missing measurements "filled in" (imputed) for the entire sequence. If the latter approach is not feasible, the patient is lost. It should be noted that one such drop-out in the cross-over design is equivalent to multiple drop-outs in the parallel group design, as many as the number of study treatments. If replacement of missing values is deemed feasible, the "rescue operation", for example through the "last observation carried forward" procedure (see section 9.4.2), can be both complicated and questionable. In fact, in the cross-over design, it can easily happen that a patient prematurely discontinues from the study before having contributed even one measurement for each study treatment (including the baseline ones). How can we replace the missing values for treatments for which the patient did not achieve a single measurement?

- **Extreme period effect.** By extreme period effect, we mean a situation in which the disease changes so radically during the study that, at some point after the first period, one or more patient eligibility criteria are substantially violated. Whereas a non-extreme period effect is compatible with the cross-over design, thanks to the randomization of patients to the sequences, an extreme period effect renders the cross-over design unfeasible. If, for example, we are evaluating fortelukast versus placebo with the design described above, but in the symptomatic treatment of seasonal allergic rhinitis (SAR) instead of asthma, at the end of the pollen season the majority of patients return to an asymptomatic state, therefore violating the eligibility criteria, which required symptoms of rhinitis. The evaluation of the treatment effects in the second period on asymptomatic patients is clearly useless from a clinical perspective. Worse, it is counterproductive from the perspective of the statistical analysis: in fact, when the two periods are combined in the analysis of the study, any difference between study treatments observed in the first period is "diluted" by the absence of a difference in the second period. An extreme period effect involving a deterioration of the condition (instead of an improvement, as in the example above) will cause the same problem.

Even if we do not consider the extreme situations in which the majority of the patients have either recovered or deceased by the second period of a cross-over study (situations that are actually possible or even likely for some conditions), whenever the clinical features of the disease change so much that the eligibility criteria are violated, the following can occur:

1. Many drugs, even those efficacious on "typical" forms of the disease, have little or no efficacy on very mild or very advanced forms; therefore, the difference between the treatments in the second period is bound to be trivial.

2. Whatever the effect of the treatments, the population under study in the second period is no longer the target population as established in the protocol.

- **Carry-over effect.** The presence of a carry-over effect makes data collected in the periods following the first one useless (or very difficult to interpret). Sometimes, when at the end of a cross-over study, a high drop-out rate or a statistically significant carry-over effect are revealed, only the first period of the study is used and analyzed as if it were a parallel group design. However, even this solution presents many problems. The biggest one is that, almost unavoidably, the sample size becomes insufficient, because the power of a study, planned as a cross-over and then analyzed as parallel group, is reduced to unacceptable levels. Therefore, under such conditions, the study can, at the most, generate hypotheses that will need to be confirmed by other studies.

In summary, the cross-over design, in appearance simple and extremely advantageous, is in reality logistically and methodologically complex, and may present underlying methodological problems that can weaken or invalidate its use.

10.5.3. Conditions of Applicability

In spite of all the limitations discussed in the previous section, the cross-over design is an excellent solution in many situations. It can be used when the following conditions are satisfied:

- The effect of the study treatments manifests early, hence the duration of the treatments can be short.
- The study treatments have reversible effects, that is, they do not modify the clinical picture permanently or for a long time in relation to the duration of the study.

- The disease/condition of interest is relatively stable in the time interval covered by the study, that is, it does not meaningfully improve or worsen spontaneously.
- The study treatments have effects that do not extend to the period following the one during which they are administered. As discussed above, sometimes the carry-over effect can be eliminated by introducing wash-out intervals between the treatment periods. However, the wash-out intervals cannot be too long, especially when the study treatments are many. In some cases, an alternative to the wash-out can be to restrict the evaluation of the effect to just the final measurements for each treatment (see section 10.5.2).

We must remind the reader that the cross-over design has a true advantage with respect to sample size over the parallel group design when the measurements within a subject are highly correlated. Although this requirement is frequently met, this is not always the case: a typical example of within-subject measurements with low correlation are diseases with **"poissez" symptoms**, i.e. symptoms manifesting themselves with intermittent and unpredictable chronology.

Nevertheless, there are numerous classes of drugs for which the above-mentioned requirements are often met, making the use of the cross-over design generally appropriate. These include, among others, pain killers in chronic pain, bronchodilators in obstructive diseases of the airways, and pressure-lowering drugs in hypertension.

The cross-over design is often very useful in phase II studies using pharmaco-dynamic end-points, as opposed to therapeutic end-points used in phase III, which typically require prolonged observation periods (see chapter 12). This design is especially useful in phase II dose-response studies. In such studies, all doses are lower than the maximum tolerated dose, determined in previous studies (see dose-escalation studies, section 10.4.1). Therefore, patients can be randomized to any sequence of doses in a cross-over design. However, since dose-response studies often require many doses (in addition to a placebo and, not infrequently, to an active control), incomplete cross-over designs, covered in the next section, are commonly used. Finally, the cross-over design is indispensable in studies in which the patient is asked to express a preference between two or more treatments or therapeutic regimens, since the patient can express a preference only when he/she has received all of the treatments under comparison.

10.6. Variants of the Cross-Over Design

10.6.1. Variants Based on the Type of Randomization

Simple randomization, randomization in blocks and stratified randomization can all be used in a cross-over design. The more frequently used options are the simple randomization (patients are assigned to the sequences based on a single simple randomization list) and the randomization in blocks (patients are assigned to the different sequences based on a single randomization list in blocks).

Stratification can be used with the limited purpose of balancing the sequences with respect to predefined stratification factors, or with the aim of increasing the efficiency of the design, or when there is an interest in the result in each single stratum. However, it should be noted that the inclusion of stratification factors complicates the statistical analysis.

10.6.2. Incomplete Cross-Over Designs

When two or three treatments are compared (rarely more, see below), it is generally possible to use a complete cross-over design, provided that the requirements illustrated in section 10.5.3 are satisfied. All possible sequences are used and each patient receives, through randomization, one sequence containing all of the treatments under study.

However, there are many situations in which one wants to study more than three treatments, especially in the case of dose-response designs. Cross-over studies with many treatments present two types of methodological problems.

1. As the number of study treatments increases, so do the complexity and duration of the study for each patient. The patients' motivation and ability to adhere to the requirements of the protocol (the so-called compliance) must be extreme in a cross-over study with many treatments. Therefore, the risk of premature discontinuations is high. Furthermore, as the number of study treatments increases, so do the risk of period effects, period by treatment interactions and relevant carry-over effects. For studies with a single treatment administration, the authors managed to test as many as six treatments per patient (naturally, using only some of the possible sequences, see below), whereas for studies with repeated treatment administrations we have rarely gone beyond three treaments.

2. Assuming each treatment is administered only in one period, the number of possible sequences increases with the number of treatments according to the following formula:

$$ns = nt \times (nt - 1) \times (nt - 2) \times \ldots \times 2 \times 1 \qquad (10.3)$$

where ns is the number of possible sequences and nt the number of study treatments. The logical explanation of the formula is the following: assuming that each patient is to receive each treatment in the sequence only once, with nt treatments, there are nt options for the first treatment, $(nt\text{-}1)$ for the second treatment, and so on, until only one treatment remains to be taken. Therefore, if with two treatments there are only two possible sequences, with three there are six, $(ns = 3 \times 2)$, and with four treatments there are already 24 possible sequences $(ns = 4 \times 3 \times 2)$. With six treatments, the possible sequences become 720!

When there are many treatments, it is possible to use the incomplete variants of the cross-over design. There are two main variants of the **incomplete cross-over design**, as described below.

1. Not all of the possible sequences are used, but each patient receives all of the study treatments. In this case, the sequences are complete but not all of them are present.
2. Each patient does not receive all of the study treatments.

First variant of the incomplete cross-over designs (the sequences are complete, but not all are used). If the researcher is reasonably sure that the period effect is irrelevant and that the carry-over effect can be excluded, he/she can simply assign each patient to one of the possible sequences. Under such conditions, there is no need to exercise control on the sequences that are included in the study.

If, on the contrary, the researcher cannot exclude the possibility of a period effect, then he/she must ensure a certain level of balance among the sequences used in the experiment. One way of obtaining such balance is through the **Latin square design.** The distinctive feature of this design is that every treatment appears only once in each row (representing the sequence) and only once in each column (representing the period).

Let us suppose we have three treatments A, B and C. There are two possible Latin square designs that can be obtained with three treatments, as shown in Table 10.6.

The period factor is totally balanced because, in each of the two designs, each treatment is administered only once in each period. To be able to use one of these two designs, we must have a number of patients that is a multiple of three. If we wish to apply both allocation schemes illustrated in Table 10.6 in the same study, the total number of patients must be a multiple of 6.

It should be noted that the Latin square design does not necessarily have to have the time factor (the period) as one of the classification factors. In fact, the Latin square design has a much broader spectrum of applications than the ones for which it has been introduced in this book. This design, useful when dealing with one experimental and two sub-experimental factors, is frequently used in agriculture (the land is divided in a grid pattern, as in a chessboard, with rows and columns representing, for example, different levels of exposure to light and water, respectively) and in laboratory experiments (where the row factor can be for example the litter, and the column the weight of the individual pup). In

Table 10.6. Possible Latin square designs with three treatments (A, B, C) and three periods

		Period	
		123	123
Sequence	1	ABC	ACB
	2	BCA	BAC
	3	CAB	CBA

Table 10.7. Possible Latin square designs with four treatments (A, B, C, D) and four periods (from [93], Table 5.1)

		Period					
		1234	**1234**	**1234**	**1234**	**1234**	**1234**
	1	ABCD	ABDC	ACBD	ADBC	ACDB	ADCB
	2	BADC	BACD	BDAC	BCAD	BDCA	BCDA
	3	CDAB	CDBA	CADB	CBDA	CABD	CBAD
	4	DCBA	DCAB	DBCA	DACB	DBAC	DABA
	1	ABCD	ABDC	ACBD	ADBC	ACDB *	ADCB *
	2	BADC	BACD	BDAC	BCAD	BDCA	BCDA
	3	CDBA	CDAB	CBDA	CADB	CBAD	CADB
Sequence	**4**	DCAB	DCBA	DACB	DBCA	DABC	DBAC
	1	ABCD	ABDC *	ACBD	ADBC *	ACDB	ADCB
	2	BCDA	BCAD	BDCA	BACD	BDAC	BADC
	3	CDAB	CDBA	CADB	CBDA	CABD	CBAD
	4	DABC	DACB	DBAC	DCAB	DBCA	DCBA
	1	ABCD *	ABDC	ACBD *	ADBC	ACDB	#ADCB
	2	BDAC	BDCA	BADC	BCDA	BACD	BCAD
	3	CADB	CABD	CDAB	CBAD	CDBA	CBDA
	4	DCBA	DACAB	DBCA	DACB	DBAC	DABC

* Williams squares. (From: Cross-Over Trials in Clinical Research, Senn S, 1993. Copyright John Wiley & Sons Limited. Reproduced with permission.)

both cases, the experimental factor must have three levels, for example three different seed concentrations per square meter of land or three pharmacological treatments.

With four treatments (A, B, C, and D), 24 Latin squares are possible, that is, 24 sets of four sequences, each forming a Latin square. They are illustrated in Table 10.7.

The six Latin squares marked with * in the figure are called **Williams squares**. These squares have the property that every treatment follows every other treatment only once. In some situations, the designs using the Williams squares can be advantageous, for example in dose-response studies, when it is unknown whether any of the doses has a residual effect at the time of administering the next dose. For example, the $\beta2$-agonist bronchodilators are ideal for cross-over designs, since their action on lung function has a fast onset and is completely reversible. For this type of treatment, the cross-over design is used routinely for dose selection. It is quite common that the study treatments (doses) are administered every third day in order to prevent the carry-over effect, since currently available $\beta2$-agonists have durations of action ranging from 4-6 hours (salbutamol/ albuterol, terbutaline) to 12-15 hours (formoterol, salmeterol), even at very high doses. However, with a new member of this class, it would not be possible to exclude *a priori* an unusual behavior at higher doses, with a carry-over effect much longer than expected. To minimize the impact of such an event, a cross-over design using the Williams Latin squares is advisable. Incidentally, new β2-agonists with very long duration of action actually emerged while this book was being written and are currently in clinical development.

Generally, there is no reason to choose one Latin square over another; therefore, the choice can be made randomly. It is not even required to perform a study based on a single Latin square: the only advantage of using a single Latin square is practical, as the preparation of the study treatment is simpler.

We will not discuss in this book the effects that can be estimated through these designs. We refer the reader interested in this topic to the excellent book on cross-over designs by Stephen Senn [93].

Second variant of the incomplete cross-over designs (incomplete sequences). This type of design is called **incomplete block cross-over design.** In the terminology of cross-over designs, the defining feature of incomplete block designs is the use of incomplete sequences (the single patient does not receive all study treatments), that is to say, the inclusion in the design of more treatments than periods. For example, such a design is applied when one wants to study three treatments, while allowing for two periods only (i.e. each patient is to receive just two of the study treatments) or to study four treatments, but in just three periods (each patient receives only three of the four study treatments). It should be noted that here the expression "blocks" is used as a synonym of "sequences" and therefore has nothing to do with the blocks of the randomization in blocks (such confusion in terminology are unfortunately not rare).

One way of building a cross-over design with four treatments in three periods is to start from any one Latin square block among those reported in Table 10.7 and to eliminate one column. For example, if we consider the first block and eliminate the first column, we obtain the following design:

BCD
ADC
DAB
CBA

Of course, the patients are assigned to the incomplete sequences through randomization. This design maintains some level of balance: each treatment appears in the same number of sequences (in the example, three times), and so does each pair of treatments (in the example, twice); finally, each treatment appears once in each period.

The price to pay for the reduction in the number of treatments per patient is an increase in the number of patients needed to achieve the same power. The smaller the number of treatments per patient with respect to the total number of study treatments, the greater the number of patients needed to achieve the same power, compared to the corresponding complete cross-over design. For more details, we refer again the reader to Senn's textbook [93]. Here it is enough to mention that quite soon the number of patients needed for an incomplete block cross-over design will approach that required for the corresponding parallel group design, which is shorter and simpler for the patients. For example, with six study treatments, an incomplete block cross-over design with sequences of four or five treatments is still advantageous, but one with sequences of three treatments is not.

A vast literature exists on incomplete block designs. We recommend the previously mentioned book by Senn [93] for an approach rich in examples and the books by Cox [27] and Fleiss [39] for a more detailed methodological discussion.

In our experience, the incomplete cross-over design is very useful in many situations, especially in dose-response studies. If used with rigor and common sense, these designs can reduce considerably the sample size compared to the corresponding parallel group design, and at the same time reduce the complexity of the study (and consequently the risk of drop-outs) compared to the corresponding complete cross-over design on the other.

10.7. Other Designs with Within-Subject Comparisons: Simultaneous Treatments and Single Patient Designs

10.7.1. Simultaneous Treatments Design

In ophthalmology, it is often possible to simultaneously apply one treatment to one eye and another treatment to the other eye of each patient (**simultaneous treatments design**), and to analyze the study as a matched-paired design (see section 10.3.3). In dermatology, one can go even further and simultaneously administer to each patient more than two treatments, each applied to a different area of the skin surface and analyze the study as a randomized block design (see again section 10.3.3). For such design to be usable, it is necessary to be sure that all of the study treatments have only local effects. In the presence of a systemic effect (partial or total), each treatment will influence the target area of the other treatments (the other eye or the other skin areas), making the results difficult to interpret. The same applies to the tolerability profile: only the local adverse events can be properly studied with this type of design.

10.7.2. Cross-Over Design on a Single Patient (Or "N of 1" Design)

A very interesting variant of a design with within-subject comparisons is the so-called **"N of 1" design**, in which two or more treatments are repeatedly administered to a single patient, with a random sequence.

Here we report an example of such a design from an article by McLeold et al, published in the Lancet in 1986 [70].

A young patient suffering from a severe form of ulcerative colitis underwent total proctectomy with ileostomy (that is, removal of terminal section of the intestine, followed by suture of the end stump to an surgical opening in the

Table 10.8. "N of 1" design in a patient with ileostomy treated with 10 cycles of double-blind treatment (five cycles of placebo and five of metronidazole), with randomized sequence: total VAS score for abdominal pain in the last week of each treatment cycle (extracted from the table in [70])

Period	1	2	3	4	5	6	7	8	9	10
Treatment	P	M	M	P	M	P	P	M	P	M
VAS score for abdominal pain	214	0	0	285	0	231	483	0	212	0

P, placebo; M, metronidazole.
Abdominal pain was measured daily through VAS (Visual Analogue Scale): min = 0, max = 100 for each day; min = 0, max = 700 for the entire week. (Reprinted from the Lancet, vol 327, McLeod RS et al, Single-patient randomised clinical trial. Use in determining optimum treatment for patient with inflammation of Kock continent ileostomy reservoir, pages 726-728, 1986, with permission from Elservier.)

abdominal wall). About four months after surgery, the patient started to suffer from severe episodes of malaise, with fever and loss of appetite, abdominal pain, flatulence and diarrhea. Such symptoms were attributed to an inflammation of the ileostomy and were treated with 250 mg/day of the antibiotic metronidazole. The antibiotic therapy turned out very efficacious according to the patient and repeated attempts to suspend it were always followed by recurrence of the symptoms. However, multiple endoscopic observations with biopsy of the ileostomy, carried out one week after discontinuation of metronidazole, never revealed any sign of acute inflammation. Therefore, the suspicion arose that the beneficial effect of metronidazole was generic in nature, i.e. was a placebo effect. If this was the case, the continuous use of such drug would have been hard to justify in terms of risk/benefit ratio, given the reports of potential carcinogenicity (i.e. cancer-inducing effect) associated with chronic use of metronidazole.

In agreement with the patient, the doctors decided to address the question of the efficacy of metronidazole through an "N of 1" design.

The patient underwent 10 treatment cycles of 2 weeks each, five with 250 mg/day metronidazole (M) and five with placebo (P) in a double-blind fashion. The order of the treatments was randomized with a balanced randomization in blocks of 10, giving the following sequence: P-M-M-P-M-P-P-M-P-M. The endpoints of the study were discussed with the patient, and those that she considered most important in determining the impact of the disease on her life were chosen. For simplicity, here we concentrate only on one of the end-points of the study, abdominal pain. Once daily the patient assessed the degree of abdominal pain through a visual analogue scale (VAS) of 100 mm, with 0=no pain and 100=unbearable pain. The total score for the last week of each treatment cycle (range from 0 to 700) was selected as the primary end-point. The scores for each treatment are listed in Table 10.8.

From Table 10.8 it is clear that every time metronidazole was administered, the score was 0, whereas every time placebo was administered, the score was higher than 0. In agreement with what any observer would intuitively conclude, an appropriate analysis of these data (see [54] and [70]) allows us to conclude that it is extremely unlikely that the matching between the treatment sequence and the observed sequence of scores could be due to chance.

Based on this study, the researchers concluded that the effect of metronidazole on the patient was real and that its long-term administration was justified, since the real advantages brought by the drug were greater than the potential danger of carcinogenicity.

The restrictions of the "N of 1" design are the same as those of any cross-over design. The "N of 1" design has also several advantages that, in our opinion, should make it more popular in clinical research. These include the following:

- Recruitment is not an issue; therefore such a design is especially suitable for rare diseases, for which the classic rules for sample size calculation are totally useless, since there are not enough patients.
- Unlike any other kind of experimental design, such a design allows conclusions to be drawn for an individual patient: the study treatments, the number of cycles, the duration of each cycle and especially the end-points of the study can all be "tailored" to suit the patient.

10.8. Factorial Designs

10.8.1. Characteristics

The so-called **factorial design** is a very interesting form of experimental design, which allows the effect of more than one experimental factor to be studied simultaneously. When applied to clinical trials, this design allows the individual effects of two or more treatments, as well as the effects of their combinations, to be investigated in the same trial, using a relatively small number of subjects. In the terminology of factorial designs it is common to refer to the study treatments as experimental factors and to their different "modalities" (e.g. presence/absence, different doses, administration schemes, formulations) as levels.

The term factorial design was coined by R.A. Fisher. Surprisingly, there are few articles on the methodology of these designs applied to biomedical research, as opposed to other experimental fields, such as agriculture or industrial production cycles. However, an article by Byar and Piantadosi, published in 1985 in an oncology journal [23], is remarkable for its clarity and simplicity. In writing this section, we have drawn heavily on this article and refer the interested reader to it. Other sources we used are books by Fleiss [39] and by Cochran and Cox [24] and an article by Green et al [53].

In theory, the factorial design can consider any number of experimental factors, each with various levels. However, in clinical applications, it is discouraged to test more than three treatments in the same trial (and, in fact, it rarely happens). We will discuss three variants: one with two treatments, each having two levels, called 2×2 or 2^2, one with two treatments, each of three levels, called 3x3 or 3^2, and one with three treatments, each of two levels, called 2×2×2 or 2^3. We will apply all of these variants to the parallel group design, while for cross-over designs we will only consider the 2^2 variant. Naturally, in factorial designs, placebo and the double-dummy technique can be used to blind study treatments.

Parallel group factorial designs. We will start with the easiest factorial design, the 2^2 **parallel group factorial design.** We want to study the effect of aspirin (A) and a statin (S) in the prevention of myocardial infarction. Each study treatment (factor) has two levels: "Yes" (present) and "No" (absent). Patients are randomized to one of four treatment groups: only aspirin (i.e. aspirin Yes, statin No), only statin (aspirin No, statin Yes), aspirin and statin together (aspirin Yes, statin Yes), placebo that is, neither aspirin nor statin (aspirin No, statin No - we indicate this group with Ø).

If the two factors have more than two levels, for example if aspirin is tested at three dose levels, namely 0, 350, and 700 mg and likewise statin at 0, 100, and 200 mg, the factorial design has a more complex assignment scheme. In this case we have a 3^2 factorial design (that is, two factors, each with three levels), in which the patients are randomized to one of nine groups: only aspirin 350 (A1), only aspirin 700 (A2), only statin 100 (S1), only statin 200 (S2), aspirin 350 and statin 100 (A1S1), aspirin 700 and statin 100 (A2S1), aspirin 350 and statin 200 (A1S2), aspirin 700 and statin 200 (A2S2), placebo, that is, neither aspirin, nor statin (Ø).

Let us turn now to the 2^3 parallel group factorial design. Suppose we add in our prevention study on myocardial infarction a third treatment, carnitine (C), to aspirin (A) and statin (S). With three study treatments, each with two levels, the patients are randomized to one of the following eight groups: only aspirin (A), only statin (S), only carnitine (C), aspirin and statin (AS), aspirin and carnitine (AC), statin and carnitine (SC), all three drugs together (ASC), placebo, i.e. none of the three drugs (Ø).

It should be kept in mind that it is not necessary for all factors to have the same number of levels, although we will not give examples of such cases.

In our example, the end-point is expressed in terms of annual infarction rate (i.e. the annual proportion of myocardial infarctions adjusted by the number of days in which the patient is at risk - see chapter 4), indicated with $\bar{P}$. The data can be summarized as illustrated in Table 10.9 for the 2^2, 3^2 and 2^3 factorial designs, respectively.

The parallel group factorial design allows two types of questions to be addressed:

1. What is the effect of each treatment?
1. What is the combined effect of the treatments, or more precisely, is the effect of one treatment modified by the presence of the other treatment (or treatments)?

Table 10.9. Typical presentation of data for 2^2, 3^2 and 2^3 parallel group factorial designs

2×2 o 2^2 factorial design

	Ø (placebo)	S
Ø (placebo)	$\bar{P}_{\text{Ø}}$	$\bar{P}_{\text{S}}$
A	$\bar{P}_{\text{A}}$	$\bar{P}_{\text{AS}}$

3×3 o 3^2 factorial design

	Ø (placebo)	S1	S2
Ø (placebo)	$\bar{P}_{\text{Ø}}$	$\bar{P}_{\text{S1}}$	$\bar{P}_{\text{S2}}$
A1	$\bar{P}_{\text{A1}}$	$\bar{P}_{\text{A1S1}}$	$\bar{P}_{\text{A1S2}}$
A2	$\bar{P}_{\text{A2}}$	$\bar{P}_{\text{A2S1}}$	$\bar{P}_{\text{A2S2}}$

2×2×2 o 2^3 factorial design

	Ø (placebo)	S
C=absent		
Ø (placebo)	$\bar{P}_{\text{Ø}}$	$\bar{P}_{\text{S}}$
A	$\bar{P}_{\text{A}}$	$\bar{P}_{\text{AS}}$
C=present		
Ø (placebo)	$\bar{P}_{\text{C}}$	$\bar{P}_{\text{SC}}$
A	$\bar{P}_{\text{AC}}$	$\bar{P}_{\text{ASC}}$

The symbols $\bar{P}$ with subscript indicate the annualized rates of myocardial infarction of the corresponding treatment group. For example, $\bar{P}_{\text{ASC}}$ indicates the annualized rate of myocardial infarction in the group treated with the combination of aspirin (A), statin (S) and carnitine (C)

Table 10.10. 2^2 factorial design with two treatments (aspirin and statin), each with two levels (present or absent)

	Ø (placebo)	S (statin)
Ø (placebo)	Patients treated with placebo (1)	Patients treated with statin (2)
A (aspirin)	Patients treated with aspirin (3)	Patients treated with aspirin and statin (4)

Assuming a balanced design and indicating with the number in brackets the group indicator of the corresponding cell, the following applies.

Simple effects: - for A, two simple effects can be estimated, one by [(3)-(1)], when A is administered alone and the other by [(4)-(2)], when A is administered together with S;
   - for S, the two simple effects are estimated by [(2)-(1)], when S is administered alone, and by [(4)-(3)], when S is administered together with A.

Main effects: - for A is estimated by {[(3)-(1)]+[(4)-(2)]}/2
   - for S is estimated by {[(2)-(1)]+[(4)-(3)]}/2

Interaction effect: is estimated by [(4)-(3)]-[(2)-(1)]/2 or by [(3)-(1)]-[(4)-(2)]/2, both expression corresponding to [(4)-(3)-(2)+(1)].

For simplicity, let us consider the 2^2 design and suppose we have an approximately equal number of patients in each group (**balanced factorial design**). Please refer to Table 10.10 as an example of how data from such a design are typically summarized.

The first question can be answered in two different ways. One is by considering the so-called **simple treatment effects**. For treatment A, two simple effects are to be considered: that of A administered without S, obtained by calculating the difference between the groups A and Ø (the differences are between group indicators) and that of A administered together with S, obtained by calculating the difference between the groups AS and S. The same reasoning applies to treatment S (i.e. differences between groups S and Ø, and between AS and A, respectively). The second way to answer the question is by considering the so-called **main treatment effects**. This approach makes sense when the treatments are independent, that is to say the effect of one treatment is the same whether the other is administered or not. This occurs when the answer to the second question is negative, i.e. there is no **interaction effect** between the two treatments. Under these circumstances, considering for example treatment A, each of the two simple effects described above is an estimate of the true effect of A, and therefore it is legitimate to calculate the mean of the two simple effects, which is indeed the main effect (given by [(AS-S) + (A- Ø)]/2). The main effect, being the mean of the two simple effects, is a more precise estimate, which means that it has a smaller variability. Therefore, when there is no interaction, it is convenient to describe the effects of the treatments in terms of their main effects, because they are at the same time more concise and more precise (thus requiring fewer patients, all other conditions being equal, since the variability is smaller). On the other hand, when there is an interaction, the main effects have no meaning in the factorial design (see below).

Referring again to the 2^2 factorial design, the interaction effect can be estimated by the difference between the simple effects of the two factors, that is, the difference between (AS-S) and (A-Ø) or the difference between (AS-A) and (S-Ø). The reader can easily verify that the two differences are algebraically equal (both are equal to AS-A-S+Ø). Since we have only one estimate of the interaction, we do not divide the result by two, as we do when calculating the main effects. Therefore, although we use all of the data, the variance of the estimate of the interaction effect is four times greater than that of the estimate of the main effects (it can be shown algebraically that, if σ^2 is the variance of X, the variance of $2X$ is $4\sigma^2$). Consequently, a sample size that is sufficient to reveal statistically a given main effect will not be sufficient to reveal an interaction effect of equal magnitude.

The reader will have noticed that main effects and interaction effects are found in both the factorial and the stratified designs. Even if formally similar, they have different meanings and implications in the two designs. The difference arises from the fact that in the factorial design we consider the interaction between two or more experimental factors (treatments), whereas in the stratified design we consider the interaction between one or more experimental factors (treatments) and one or more sub-experimental factors. In both designs, the presence of an interaction indicates that the simple effect of one factor is different at different levels (modalities) of another factor. Returning to the 2^2 factorial design with aspirin and statin, let's assume we obtained a significant interaction between the two factors, more precisely, that the effect of A is greater when A is taken together with S compared to A taken alone. Under these circumstances, and assuming the effect is beneficial, any physician would administer AS rather than A alone. Therefore, the researcher, who has control of both factors, will choose to summarize the results of the experiment using the estimates of the simple effects of A and of the interaction between A and S, rather than the estimate of the main effect of A. In a matching stratified design, let's assume the two factors are the treatment (levels: aspirin, placebo) and the study center (a sub-experimental factor with levels: center 1, center 2). Again, we obtain a significant interaction between the two factors, the effect of A (A-placebo) being greater in center 1 than in center 2. In this case, the researcher has no control over the sub-experimental factor (i.e. cannot choose to use treatment A only in center 1) and therefore will choose to summarize the results in terms of the main effect of A (the mean of the effects of A calculated on the two different centers). Such a mean makes sense also in the presence of an interaction, because it reflects the different types of centers contributing to the study population.

Cross-over factorial designs. Factorial designs with treatments assigned in cross-over schemes are used infrequently. An example of a **cross-over** 2^2 **factorial design** can be found in a paper by Brusasco and colleagues [21]. In this study on asthmatic patients, two factors are considered: a "provocation" factor, i.e. an inhaled allergen capable of inducing bronchoconstriction (the so-called late asthmatic reaction) and a "protection" factor, i.e. the inhaled bronchodilator agent formoterol. Both factors have two levels: true allergen and saline solution (placebo allergen) for the first (equivalent to presence or absence of provocation), formoterol and placebo for the second (equivalent to presence or absence of protection).

The four possible combinations are:
- A: provocation with saline solution and protection with placebo.
- B: provocation with saline solution and protection with formoterol.
- C: provocation with allergen and protection with placebo.
- D: provocation with allergen and protection with formoterol.

The primary end-point is the lowest FEV1 (forced expiratory volume in 1 second) value measured between 3 and 8 hours after provocation. Secondary end-points are the FEV1 value measured every hour up to 15 hours and at 24 hours after provocation. There are four study visits and the patients are assigned in a random sequence to one of the four combinations. The visits are separated by an appropriate wash-out period. Since the authors chose not to balance the sequences, they implicitly assumed that there was no meaningful period effect.

On the contrary, had the period effect been considered important, it would have been necessary to ensure some degree of balancing of the sequences, by applying one or more Latin squares (see section 10.6.2). For example, selecting the first Latin square of Table 10.7, a multiple of 4 patients could have been assigned to the following four sequences:

ABCD
BADC
CDAB
DCBA

where A, B, C and D represent the four combinations described above, each to be administered on one of the four visits. Within each group of four patients enrolled in the study, each patient would have been assigned to one of the four sequences.

Whether or not the sequences are balanced, in such a design, the effects typical of a cross-over design can be studied (treatment, period, subject, etcetera-see section 10.5.1) in addition to those typical of a factorial design (individual effects of the experimental factors and interaction effect).

Another example of within-patient factorial design is described in chapter 7 of Senn's book [93].

10.8.2. Advantages and Disadvantages

The factorial design can be useful in two situations:

1. When a primary question concerns the interaction between treatments, in addition to their individual effects.
2. When there is sufficient confidence that the study treatments are independent, that is, have no interaction with one another.

In the first case, the advantage is obvious, but there is a cost to be paid in terms of sample size of the study: this must be such that the interaction effect can be detected statistically, which requires approximately four times more patients than what is required to detect main effects of equal magnitude (see above).

In the second case, the advantage of a single study with a factorial design assessing multiple treatments over separate studies (one for each treatment of interest) is a smaller sample size. This is because all of the patients are utilized to evaluate each of the treatments of interest. The cost is that one can only partially verify the assumption of no interaction. In fact, the small sample size allows to reveal statistically the presence of an interaction only if such interaction is very big, much bigger than the threshold of clinical relevance used for the effects of the individual treatments. To make things worse, in the presence of a small interaction (i.e. not big enough to be detected statistically, given the sample size), the researchers would not only conclude mistakenly that there is no interaction, but would also obtain main treatment effects which are diluted, i.e. smaller than what they really are for some levels of the other experimental factors (see below).

As always, there are complications and open issues not to be underestimated. Three of these are discussed in the above mentioned articles by Byar and Piantadosi [23] and Green, et al. [53].

Multiple comparisons. The "raison d'être" of the factorial design is that of evaluating the effect of two or three treatments at the same time, using a limited number of patients. In the context of the frequentist approach, while for non-factorial designs multiple comparisons require a "penalty" in terms of sample size (see section 4.7), for factorial designs such a penalty is usually not paid. Byar and Piantadosi, in their discussion, do not seem to worry much about this aspect. However, from our point of view, a double standard is being used (favoring the factorial design), and the question remains open.

Potential reduction of the individual treatment effects in the presence of interaction. As discussed above, if a factorial study reveals a statistically significant interaction effect, the results are summarized by reporting the interaction and the simple effects of the individual treatments (as opposed to the main effects). Unfortunately, when the treatment effects are analyzed as simple effects, there is a loss of power, because not all study patients are used, as for the main effects. When the interaction, even though present, is not revealed in the study, i.e. does not reach statistical significance, the problem of the loss of power is more treacherous, because in this case the data are summarized by reporting the result of the interaction test and the main effects of the individual treatments. Under these circumstances, the overall dilution of the main effects, due to the interaction (present but not recognized), remains hidden.

The concepts of statistical and biological interaction between treatments are interconnected but not identical. Statistical interaction is a mathematical phenomenon. Going back once more to our example of the 2^2 factorial study, stating that there is no interaction between A and S is equivalent to stating that, if A improves the effect obtained in the placebo group by the amount Δ then the combination AS improves the effect obtained in the group S by the same amount Δ. Δ can be expressed both in terms of absolute or relative difference. The problem is that the absence of interaction in terms of absolute difference does not necessarily imply the absence of interaction in terms of relative difference and vice versa. For example, let's assume that the rate of myocardial infarction is 0.5 in the placebo group, 0.3 in group A, 0.3 in group S and 0.1 in group AS. Comparing A with placebo and AS with S, one will infer that the same absolute reductions have occurred (because 0.3-0.5 = 0.1-0.3). However, the relative reductions of the rates of myocardial infarction are not the same (because $0.3/0.5 \neq 0.1/0.3$). It is evident that the presence or absence of a statistical interaction depends on the mathematical formulation of the problem. Therefore, statistical interaction cannot coincide with biological interaction. In other words, even if it is likely that a strong biological interaction implies a strong statistical interaction, the lack of biological interaction does not necessarily imply the lack of statistical interaction.

10.8.3. Conditions of Applicability

In addition to the methodological problems reported in the previous section, the factorial design can pose feasibility problems, due to the complications in the conduct and analysis of the study. As discussed by Fleiss [39], when many treatments are tested, the number of eligibility criteria for a patient to enter the study is likely to increase, the rules for dose adjustments become more complex, the adverse events expected from the treatments increase and dealing with such events becomes unavoidably more complex, and so on.

The above mentioned paper by Green and colleagues, reports examples of trials in which the factorial approach worked well, together with examples in which it generated results that were difficult to interpret.

One area in which the factorial design can be very useful is the study of fixed combinations, which are used with increasing frequency in many therapeutic areas. When studying a fixed combination of treatments, one is often interested in both the individual effects and the interactions between the components of the combination. The use of factorial designs for the assessment of fixed-dose combinations is endorsed by the ICH guidelines [59, 62]. In fact these authoritative guidelines recommend a greater use of this design for combinations, beyond the field of antihypertensive agents, where this approach is common. The guidelines also provide useful guidance as to the advantages and limitations of the use of factorial designs in evaluating fixed-dose combinations. Factorial designs are particularly useful to evaluate effectiveness when both agents affect the same variable and to evaluate safety and tolerability when one agent is intended to mitigate the side effects of the other [59]. One dose of each agent can be studied, if the doses are known. In addition, the factorial design is well suited to test multiple doses of each component of a combination. When the factorial design is used to this end, the sample size need not be large enough to distinguish single cells from each other in pair-wise comparisons, because all of the data can be used to derive dose-response relationships for the single agents and the combinations, i.e. a dose-response surface [59]. Interestingly, the guidelines acknowledge that the doses that will eventually be approved for marketing need not be the ones actually tested in the study, but, based on the dose-response surface, may be dose levels in between those studied [59]. The low and high end of the dose spectrum tested in a factorial design require special attention. With regard to the low end, if the tested dose is lower than the recognized effective dose, it is important to have evidence that there is a separation from placebo. The guidelines suggest that this can be accomplished both within the factorial study, by increasing the sample size of the low dose and of the placebo cells to allow a pair-wise comparison(s), or through a separate study of the low dose combination. For the high end of the dose spectrum, it may be necessary to confirm that both components of the combination contribute to the overall effect [59].

10.9. Split-Plot Design

10.9.1. Characteristics

The split-plot technique is frequently used in agricultural, industrial and laboratory experiments, while it is rarely applied to clinical trials. Therefore, we will only briefly introduce the design based on this technique.

The **split-plot design** is potentially useful in two cases. The first is when one would want to use the randomized block design (see section 10.3.3), but the number of treatments (and therefore the size of each block) is too large with respect to the number of experimental units available. The second is when one wishes to randomize groups of units to the different levels of one experimental factor, and then to randomize the individual units of each of these groups to the levels of the other experimental factor, which is administered on top of the former. An example of the first case, applied to the clinical field, will be discussed shortly. An example of the second case could be an experiment on fruit trees, where the effects of different pesticide sprays (first experimental factor) and pruning techniques (second experimental factor) are to be studied: it could be reasonable to treat groups of adjacent plants with the same pesticide and randomize the individual trees of each group to the different pruning techniques.

In the split-plot design, there are two experimental factors: one is called the "sub-plot" treatment (this nomenclature is clearly referred to agricultural experiments; applied to clinical trials, we would use the term sub-group) and is administered to the single experimental units, as defined in chapter 2; the other is called "whole-plot" treatment (in our case, whole group) and is administered to sets of experimental units.

In clinical applications, a modified form is generally used in which the whole-plot factor is not an experimental factor, i.e. a treatment, but rather a sub-experimental factor. To illustrate this design, we shall use an example taken from Fleiss [39]. We want to study the effect of three treatments on the concentration of sodium in the urine, in both males and females. However, there are only 10 subjects available, 5 males and 5 females; therefore, the randomized block design is not applicable (we would need blocks of three males and three females, to whom the three treatments would be administered). As proposed by Fleiss, one feasible option could be to use the design illustrated in Table 10.11. All three experimental treatments are given to each of the 10 subjects, using an independent random sequence for each subject. In this design, the treatment is considered the sub-plot factor, since it is administered to every subject, while gender is considered the whole-plot factor, since it is "applied" to sets of subjects (that is, the level male is "applied" to 5 of the 10 units and the level female to the remaining 5).

This design can be considered the combination of two randomized block designs, one applied to males and one to females. A block is represented by a subject receiving all three treatments.

We assume that each treatment is administered only once and that the study

Table 10.11. Split-plot design with three treatments

| | **Males** | | | | **Females** | | |
| | **(1° level of "whole-plot" factor)** | | | | **(2° level of "whole-plot" factor)** | | |
Subjects	**Tr. 1**	**Tr. 2**	**Tr. 3**	**Subjects**	**Tr. 1**	**Tr. 2**	**Tr. 3**
1	A	C	B	6	C	A	B
2	B	A	C	7	B	C	A
3	C	B	A	8	A	C	B
4	A	C	B	9	A	B	C
5	C	A	B	10	B	A	C

Tr = treatment. The treatment is the "sub-plot" factor (with three levels)

is rigorously planned, in particular, that a wash-out interval of appropriate length is applied at each treatment switch.

The comparisons concerning the whole-plot factor (in our example, the comparison between males and females) are less precise and the corresponding statistical tests less powerful than those concerning the sub-plot factor (in our example, the comparisons among the treatments A, B and C). What causes this increase in variability when testing the whole-plot factor as compared to the sub-plot factor? We shall use the type of reasoning introduced in section 10.1. The residual variance for comparing males and females, i.e. for carrying out a statistical test on the main effect of the whole-plot factor, is based on the variability around the two means of the end-point for males and females, in turn based on the dispersion of the units belonging to all treatment and gender groups around these means. The residual variance for comparing the treatments at the level of the entire experiment, i.e. for carrying out a statistical test on the main effect of the sub-plot factor, is based on the variability around the means of the end-point for the treatments. Since these are computed within each level of the gender factor, the variability around them is obtained as a mean of two separate terms, each computed considering only the units belonging to one level of the gender factor. It is intuitive that the variability term used for the gender comparison is bigger than the variability term used for the treatment comparison, because the latter is computed among units of the same gender, while the former is computed among all units considered together.

The interaction between gender and treatment, i.e. between whole-plot and sub-plot factors, depends on how the differences between the levels of one factor change in the different levels of the other. Since the differences between the levels of the sub-plot factor (treatment) can be calculated within each whole-plot (gender) level, the inference on the interaction is also based on the variation between the means of the levels of the sub-plot factor (treatments), separately for each level of the whole-plot factor (males and females). Therefore, this inference has a precision comparable to that of the main effect of the sub-plot factor.

10.9.2. Conditions of Applicability

The split-plot design should be considered only when one of the following two conditions is met [27]:

- When dealing with a factor that is suitable to be "sacrificed", in the sense that its main effect is not of interest and, therefore, estimates with low precision are acceptable; this factor is included in the design because its interaction with the other factor is of interest (as stated above, such interaction can be precisely estimated).
- When, for practical reasons, it is convenient that one of the factors remains constant inside each block; this situation arises frequently in agriculture.

The split-plot is an example of a design with **confounding.** In jargon, the whole-plot factor is called "confounded". While in epidemiology the term confounding indicates a problem, which causes biased estimates (see section 3.2), in the experimental setting the term confounding indicates an intentional characteristic of the study. This consists of "sacrificing" the comparisons among the levels of the confounded factor (in fact, accepting less precise estimates for this factor) at the advantage of the other factor (in fact, obtaining more precise estimates for this non-confounded factor). There are designs in which the confounded factor is the interaction effect, but these designs are only rarely useful in clinical research.

For a more detailed discussion of the topics introduced in this section we refer the reader to [24], [27] and [39].

10.10. Non-Controlled Designs in Phase II Oncology Studies

As discussed in chapter 12, the clinical development of pharmacological treatments in oncology has some peculiarities, due, on one side, to the seriousness of the disease and, on the other, to the high level of toxicity of many of the experimental compounds (especially the so-called cytotoxic chemotherapic agents).

In this section, we briefly discuss the non-controlled designs, typical of the early phase II development of these compounds. The justification for the use of non-controlled designs has been given in section 8.8.

Non-controlled designs can be:

- Single-stage.
- Multi-stage (two or more stages).

In both variants, the end-point is typically a binary variable, for which success (response) is defined as a reduction of the tumor mass greater than a prefixed percentage of the pre-treatment size. The criteria used to measure the tumor mass, its change over time and the percent reduction qualifying as a response must be recognized by the scientific community (see for example, the so-called RECIST criteria [101]). The end-point (success/failure) has a binomial distribution (see for example [26] or [105]).

In the **single-arm single-stage design**, the simplest, there is only one group of patients treated with the compound under study. We will use the following symbols:

- π = true probability of response (unknown and therefore to be estimated).
- p = statistic for making inference on π.
- p_{obs} = probability (frequency) of response observed in the study, also indicated with $\hat{\pi}$ (that is, $p_{obs} = \hat{\pi}$ is the point estimate of π).
- π_0 = probability of response to the standard therapy or, lacking a standard therapy, a response level considered uninteresting.
- π_1 = probability level representing a clinically significant improvement compared to π_0.

The sample size n of the study is determined so that the statistical test used to verify the hypothesis that π is greater than or equal to π_1, against the null hypothesis that π is less than or equal to π_0, has the desired risk of making a type I error (acceptable risk = α) and type II error (acceptable risk = β) (see chapter 5). Keeping in mind that the primary objective of a phase II study is to select compounds to bring into phase III, in choosing α and β one must consider that the consequence of a type I error is that a phase III trial will be performed on a compound that has no clinical interest, while the consequence of a type II error is that a promising compound will be discarded. The statistical test is performed following the logic discussed in chapter 5 for the unidirectional hypothesis system; therefore, the result of the test is determined by a cutoff, s, with the null hypothesis rejected if the total number of successes is greater than or equal to s and the alternative hypothesis rejected if the total number of successes is smaller than s.

Often, as an alternative to the approach described above, but with a completely equivalent result (see chapter 5), n is chosen so that the confidence interval on π at a given 1-α confidence level (for example 95%) has a predefined width (for example, its lower limit is higher than π_0).

The greatest limit of the single-stage design is that it does not permit the trial to be stopped early if the response rate becomes unacceptably low. This is a serious limit, since the compounds used in oncology are generally very toxic. It is overcome by using **single-arm multi-stage designs.** Schultz et al [92] and Fleming [40] describe a general method for constructing such designs.

At the end of each stage (generically indicated with j) of a multi-stage study, one of three decisions can be made:

1. Terminate the study because of failure (that is, the alternative hypothesis that π is greater than or equal to π_1 is rejected), if the overall number of successes observed on all patients studied up to that point is less than or equal to a pre-established threshold, s_{j1}.
2. Terminate the study because of success (that is, the null hypothesis that π is smaller than or equal to π_0 is rejected), if the overall number of successes is greater than or equal to another preestablished threshold, s_{j2}.
3. Continue the study if the overall number of successes is between s_{j1} and s_{j2} (note that $s_{j1} < s_{j2}$).

If the trial continues to the final stage, say k, then one of the two hypotheses must be rejected, hence $s_{k1} = s_{k2} -1$.

These designs use the sequential approach that will be covered in the next chapter (section 11.2). Briefly, the sample size and the thresholds of each stage are determined in such a way that the overall probabilities α_{study} and β_{study} for the entire study are the desired ones. It is important to note that in multi-stage designs multiple tests are performed and, therefore, the problem of multiplicity of statistical tests, which we have mentioned many times (see in particular section 4.7), is encountered. Thus, if we were to perform each test at each stage at a given level of α, the overall probability of making a type I error in the whole study would be higher than α. Furthermore, in multi-stage designs, there is the additional complexity that the tests are correlated, because they are partially performed on the same data. Therefore, some *ad hoc* adjustment must be made to maintain the type I error of the whole study at the desired level of α_{study} (see section 11.2). This issue must be kept in mind also when calculating the confidence intervals on the probability of response: those constructed for a single-stage design are not valid for a multi-stage one and require an adjustment. The interested reader can consult the article by Atkinson and Brown [6] on this topic.

Two types of design, both in two stages, are widely used: the design proposed by Gehan in 1961 [47] and the one proposed more recently by Simon [95]. In both designs, the study can be terminated in the first stage only in case of failure.

There is a vast literature on these designs, from which we single out the following articles: for a design explicitly considering toxicity, we recommend an article by Bryant and Day [22]; for a three-stage design, one by Ensign et al [34]; for a Bayesian design, those by Thall and Simon [99] and by Thall et al [100]; finally, we recommend the critical revision on phase II designs in oncology by Mariani and Marubini [68].

As outlined in section 8.8, the non-controlled design used in oncology belongs to the before-after treatment family of designs and suffers from all its limitations. For this reason, it is used only for screening purposes (see section 12.3.2).

Summary

There are two main categories of designs for clinical trials: the parallel group design, in which each group receives only one of the study treatments, all groups being treated simultaneously, and the cross-over design, in which each group receives more than one treatment in sequence, but only one of the possible sequences of study treatments.

The experimental designs differ with respect to:
- The level of bias of the estimates.
- The precision of the estimates, i.e. the power of the statistical tests.
- The simplicity of study conduct, data analysis and interpretation of the results.

Two methods can be used to reduce variability without increasing the sample size:

- Grouping of subjects (units) with respect to common characteristics (in strata or blocks).
- Replication of measurements on each subject.

However, the use of these strategies produces the undesired effect of increasing the complexity of the study, at both a practical/operational level and at a conceptual/methodological level. In particular, the use of within-patient comparisons requires that the patients accept a burden of visits and procedures which is often quite heavy, and, from a methodological one, that the researchers accept a considerable increase in the number of assumptions, which may be more or less verifiable. To justify the use of these strategies, these inconveniences must be balanced by relevant "gains" in terms of precision/efficiency and accuracy of the estimates.

Variants of the more frequently used designs exist, which are useful in special situations. A few examples are as follows. In phase I, the controlled dose-escalation designs are frequently used. These designs, in which each patient receives only one dose level, allow the evaluation of higher doses, only once sufficient evidence on the safety of the lower doses has been obtained. Sometimes, for the first assessment of the dose-response curve of a new compound, the dose-titration design is used, in which increasing doses (if well tolerated) are administered to each patient, both in the active and in the control groups, and the entire dose-response curves are compared between groups. In the "N of 1" design, two or more treatments are repeatedly administered to a single patient: this approach is particularly useful in the study of symptomatic treatments of rare diseases or rare variants, for which the common approaches cannot be applied, simply because it is impossible to find the necessary number of patients. The factorial design can be useful for studying two or more treatments simultaneously, when there is interest in both the individual effects and the combined ones.

Some therapeutic areas, such as oncology, present ethical problems of such magnitude that the trial designs must address these concerns first and foremost. Only once these are addressed, the classical methodological criteria for design selection can be used. The multi-stage designs without control group are frequently used in early phase II of the clinical development of such compounds.

11

Study Variants Applicable to More than One Type of Design: Equivalence Studies, Interim Analyses, Adaptive Plans and Repeated Measurements

In this chapter we will cover study variants that can be applied both to designs based on between-subject comparisons and to those based on within-subject comparisons.

We will cover:

- Equivalence and non-inferiority studies.
- Studies with intermediate analyses, referred to as "interim analyses".
- Studies with adaptive (flexible) plans.
- Studies with repeated measurements.

These are not proper experimental designs, that is, are not ways of assigning patients to treatments (see chapters 9 and 10), but study variants that can be applied to different types of design, in order to deal with special types of objectives, end-points and analyses.

11.1. Equivalence and Non-Inferiority Studies

11.1.1. Characteristics

The efficacy and safety of a new treatment can be studied by comparing it with one or more established treatments, where such treatments exist. These comparisons, if rigorously performed, are very useful to position a new treatment in the context of the current best practice. What are its advantages, if any, over the therapeutic standard? Is it worthwhile including it in the hospital formularies? If so, at what level of reimbursement? These are but a few of the fundamental questions that will determine the success or failure of a new treatment on the market. If the scientists in charge of the clinical development of a new treatment do not address such questions through well designed studies, the health care system will in any case return its verdict, which, for several reasons (need to contain costs, attachment to treatments that have gained acceptance through use and time, fear of the unknown) will tend to favor existing treatments. Furthermore, for the more serious diseases, comparisons to active treatments (or presumed active) are frequently preferred, even when the active comparator is not universally acknowledged as a standard by the scientific community. This is because of the considerable ethical problems caused by the use of placebo in serious and life threatening conditions.

The comparison between active treatments can be performed with two different objectives:

- Demonstrate the superiority of the new treatment over the standard (i.e. the one acknowledged as the best by doctors and patients).
- Demonstrate the equivalence or, more frequently, the "non-inferiority" of the new treatment compared to the standard.

Clinical trials with the former objective are called superiority studies. These studies are the object of Chapters 4, 5 and 6. Trials with the latter objective are called **equivalence** or **non-inferiority studies.** The difference between equivalence and non-inferiority is that in equivalence studies the aim is to demonstrate that the new treatment is neither inferior nor superior to the standard one, while in non-inferiority studies the aim is only to demonstrate that the new treatment is not inferior to the standard one (if it is better, it is still not inferior). When the comparison between treatments concerns clinical end-points, non-inferiority studies are most often used, because both equivalence and superiority are typically considered "success". Instead, when the comparison concerns pharmacokinetic or pharmacodynamic end-points (for example, the "area under the curve" of the plasma concentration of the active compound), equivalence studies are often required, since the "superiority" of the new treatment compared to the standard one can be as problematic as its "inferiority". This is especially important in the development of the **generic drugs** (identical copies of marketed drugs, no longer protected by a patent), and of new formulations, therapeutic regimens and routes of administration. In all of these cases, the active principle is the same and the clinical development process is greatly facilitated if one can demonstrate that the key pharmacokinetic and/or pharmacodynamic variables of the new treatment are equivalent, i.e. neither superior, nor inferior, to the standard one.

Although the statistical analysis of equivalence studies differs slightly from that of non-inferiority studies, the methodological and practical issues are very similar in the two types of study. Therefore, from now on, for simplicity we will use the term equivalence to indicate both equivalence and non-inferiority, unless a distinction between the two kinds of study is required. The terms superiority, equivalence and non-inferiority will be used in relation to a single endpoint, typically the primary one. The active comparator will be referred to as "reference" or "standard" treatment. As discussed in Section 2.4, the new treatment (or, if not new, the one which is the main focus of the study) will be referred to as "experimental" treatment.

In clinical research, equivalence studies are performed in the following situations:

- When it is sufficient to demonstrate equivalence in terms of efficacy between the experimental and the reference treatments, having already demonstrated (or having the intention to do so) that the new treatment has other advantages over the standard one, for example that it has a better safety/tolerability profile, it is easier to administer, it is less expensive to manufacture.
- When one wants to develop a therapeutic alternative to the available treatment(s), based on a different active principle and/or a different mechanism of action. It may be an advantage to have several therapeutic options, even if their efficacy and safety are on average about the same. Indeed, the average response may not apply to the individual subject. Some patients may respond better to one treatment than to another; some may be allergic to a particular treatment; some may develop tolerance to one specific compound and so on. Oncology and infectious diseases are therapeutic areas where it is especially useful to have access to multiple products with similar therapeutic value, as this helps to fight the development of resistance.

When considering the option of an equivalence study, three important questions must be asked.

The first question is whether the use of placebo is ethically acceptable. Generally, the answer is negative for serious diseases for which one or more reference treatments have shown efficacy consistently across all major clinical trials. On the other hand, the use of a placebo may be acceptable in non-serious diseases and in those areas where the available therapy shows inconsistent results across major trials. When a placebo is acceptable, the three-arm study, with placebo, experimental and reference treatments, is recommended (the reasons will be discussed below).

The second question concerns the treatment to be chosen as active control. As discussed in Chapter 7, in many therapeutic areas more than one active treatment is available, but no one can unequivocally be considered the standard. Which treatment should be used as the reference in these cases? We refer the reader to chapter 7 and to the specific ICH guideline [62] for a more in depth discussion of this topic.

The third question concerns the main reason for performing an equivalence study. Such a study may have two different objectives:

- Show indirectly superiority over placebo, i.e. use an active comparator because placebo is not acceptable.
- Show that the experimental treatment has no important loss of efficacy compared to the reference active comparator.

For the reasons highlighted at the beginning of this section, many real life clinical trials have the latter objective.

The choices one makes in addressing these three questions have an impact in terms of study design, sample size and methods for the statistical analysis, as outlined in the next sections.

11.1.2. The Statistical Analysis of an Equivalence Study

The choice between the objective of demonstrating superiority and that of demonstrating equivalence has a major impact on the planning of the study, especially when defining the threshold of clinical significance (see section 4.1), calculating the sample size and planning the statistical analysis. A study planned for one objective can hardly be used for the other. We refer the reader to an interesting document on this topic, issued by the Committee for Proprietary Medicinal Products (CPMP) of the European Community [36].

A common mistake made when conducting equivalence studies is that of planning and analyzing them as if they were superiority studies. The mistake resides in the fact that the outcome of the statistical test for superiority is irrelevant for assessing equivalence, whether it is statistically significant or not. A non-significant outcome neither allows the rejection of the null hypothesis of equality between study treatments in the superiority setting, nor allows the acceptance of the same null hypothesis in the equivalence setting because it may not have enough power to detect differences that are outside the threshold of equivalence. On the other side, a statistically significant outcome of such a test does not necessarily imply that the treatments are not equivalent, because the difference between the treatments, even if statistically significant, could be clinically irrelevant and therefore fall within the threshold of equivalence.

In order to verify equivalence between study treatments correctly, it is necessary to set up a system of hypotheses in which the null hypothesis is that the treatments are not equivalent, while the alternative hypothesis is that the treatments are equivalent. In other words, in equivalence studies, the system of hypotheses is inverted compared to superiority studies. The statistical analysis and the sample size calculation must be based on the right system of hypotheses.

Let's assume we are conducting an equivalence study, using means as the group indicators and the absolute difference between treatment means as the signal for an efficacy end-point. The concepts can be extended to relative effects (i.e. the ratio between treatment effects) with only minor changes. Furthermore, let's assume that the experimental and the reference treatments are in reality identical in terms of efficacy. Still, we cannot expect that the study will give a point estimate of this difference equal to zero. In fact, there is a 50% chance that the point estimate will be positive and a 50% chance that it will be negative. Therefore, the point estimate alone does not suffice to show equivalence.

The starting point when planning an equivalence study is the definition of the "delta of clinical non-relevance" or "margin of equivalence" (referred to as Δ, see section 4): this is the greatest difference between the study treatments, in terms of the chosen group indicator, judged not clinically relevant (see section 4.1) and, therefore, compatible with the conclusion of equivalence. Since we are using the difference between treatment means as the signal, the analysis is performed by computing a $(1-\alpha)\%$ confidence interval on the observed mean treatment difference. Equivalence between the treatments is demonstrated if such confidence interval is entirely included between -Δ and +Δ. (not touching the limits). To grasp the sense of this rule, it helps to recall that the confidence interval at the (1- α)% level (for example, at the 95% level) is defined as the set of values of the statistic which includes the true value of the unknown parameter (i.e. the true treatment effect) with a probability equal to (1-α)%. Therefore, when the observed confidence interval on the mean treatment difference is entirely included between -Δ and +Δ, there is a high probability (in fact equal to (1- α)%) that the true value of the parameter (true mean treatment difference) is a clinically irrelevant difference between the treatments.

From this discussion, it should be clear that an equivalence trial aims to demonstrate that the experimental and the reference treatments do not differ by more than a pre-specified small amount (i.e. Δ).

If the trial is a non-inferiority one, the two-sided (1- α)% confidence interval must be replaced with the one-sided (1- α/2)% interval. The limit that matters depends on the direction of the treatment difference. Assuming that the difference is experimental treatment minus reference treatment, when a bigger difference reflects a better outcome for the experimental treatment, we will have to verify that the lower limit of the one-sided (1-α/2)% confidence interval (for example 97.5%) computed on this difference is not touching the -Δ non-inferiority margin. Of course, the opposite applies when the smaller the difference the better the outcome.

If the results of the study are such that the whole confidence interval is located between -Δ and 0 in the former case, or between 0 and +Δ in the latter, without touching the limits, we have shown that the reference treatment is statistically superior to the experimental one (see chapter 5 for the connection between statistical test and confidence interval). However, assuming the Δ has been chosen correctly, this result would not negate the conclusion of non-inferiority of the experimental vs. the reference treatment because, as stated above, the very aim of a non-inferiority trial is that of demonstrating that the experimental treatment is not inferior to the reference one by an amount equal to Δ or bigger.

If it is not possible to accept any degree of inferiority of the experimental treatment as compared to the reference one, the use of a non-inferiority trial may become questionable [38].

11.1.3. Planning and Implementation Problems

Equivalence studies have specific statistical and practical problems compared to superiority studies, which make them difficult to implement, analyze and interpret. In this section and in the next one we will give a brief overview of such problems.

Choice of the equivalence margin. As described above, once the appropriate indicator summarizing the response at a treatment group level and the corrisponding signal have been defined, the planning of an equivalence study begins with the selection of a treatment difference for the chosen signal that is judged *a priori* as clinically irrelevant (see section 4.1). If it is difficult to define *a priori* the smallest clinically relevant difference for a superiority study, due to the considerable subjective component of the choice, then it is even more difficult to define the largest non-clinically relevant difference (i.e. the equivalence margin) for an equivalence study. For a long time there has been no consensus in the scientific and regulatory community in defining the equivalence margin. Recently (January 2006), a guidance document on this topic, under the patronage of the CPMP, has come into effect [38]. The release of this document has been delayed several times because of the complexity of the topic. Clearly, the equivalence margin must be smaller than the difference between the standard treatment and placebo, as observed in previous studies. The problem is to define how much smaller it must be. The new guideline clearly states that "it is not appropriate to define the non-inferiority (equivalence) margin as a [fixed] proportion of the difference between comparator and placebo". The choice of a fixed proportion, say 30%, of the difference between reference treatment and placebo is misleading when the reference has either a large advantage over placebo or a marginal one. In the former case, 30% of the difference between reference and placebo could still be clinically relevant, thus resulting in a too large equivalence margin. In the latter case, since the difference between reference and placebo is barely above the threshold of clinical relevance, 30% of this difference would be too small for an equivalence margin, as it would translate into an enormous sample size that would render impossible the conduction of the equivalence study.

The guideline recognizes the two kinds of objectives for non-inferiority studies reported in the previous section (see last two bullet points of section 11.1.1). In both cases, a systematic review of the literature should be conducted to identify the studies relevant to the comparison of the reference treatment with placebo in the condition being studied.

With regard to the first objective, i.e. to show indirectly superiority over placebo, the guideline reads as follows. "The historical confidence interval compares the reference product with placebo (r – p). The planned trial comparing the test and reference products will also produce a confidence interval (t – r). If these intervals are combined, an indirect confidence interval comparing the test product and placebo can be obtained (t – p). Δ (i.e. the equivalence margin) can be defined as the lower bound of (t – r) that ensures that the lower bound of the indirect confidence interval (t – p) will be above zero. As the comparison is indirect, it might be wise to be conservative and select some value smaller than that suggested by this indirect calculation". Note: the guideline uses the expression "test product" for what we indicate as experimental treatment [38].

As for the second objective, i.e. to show that the experimental treatment has no important loss of efficacy compared to the reference active comparator, the choice of the equivalence margin cannot be based only on historical trials where the reference treatment was compared to placebo. In this case, we must first estimate the equivalence margin as outlined above, but then we may have to reduce it further to ensure that the difference between the two treatments is irrelevant. On this point the guideline reads as follows: "to adequately choose delta, an informed decision must be taken, supported by evidence of what is considered an unimportant difference (between the test and the reference products) in the particular disease area" [38].

The choice of the equivalence margin is complicated further by the typical problems affecting any systematic review of the literature, such as selection and publication bias, inconsistency of effects and of experimental conditions over time and across different studies, etcetera. Such problems are particularly acute when the studies available from the literature are few, and/or undermined by important design issues, and/or inconsistent in their outcomes. The reader is referred to section 11.1.4 and to the above mentioned guideline for a wider discussion of these and other related issues.

Quality of an equivalence study. In superiority studies, the better the quality of the study (appropriate sample size, variability of results kept under control, protocol respected in every part, etc.), the greater the likelihood of detecting a clinically relevant difference between the study treatments, when it exists. Therefore, the researchers have a clear incentive to conduct the study in the best possible way. In equivalence studies, the situation is to some extent reversed, since the goal is to rule out a clinically relevant difference between the study treatments. Since the poorer the quality of the study, the lower the likelihood of detecting differences between treatments, even when they do exist, the researcher has little incentive to conduct the study in the best possible way. In fact, sloppiness does not necessarily increase the likelihood of showing equivalence, because variability also plays a role: when the quality is low, the variability may be high and this reduces the possibility of showing equivalence because the confidence interval on the treatment difference is enlarged. However, the principle that low quality tends to reduce the possibility of catching real treatment differences, i.e. increases the likelihood of showing equivalence, remains valid. Thus, reassurance on the quality on the study conduct is an essential requisite for interpreting correctly an equivalence study showing "positive" results (see also section 11.1.4). Unfortunately, the quality of a trial can be judged only when it is complete.

Sample size. It is a commonly held view that performing equivalence studies is convenient, because they require smaller sample sizes compared to their superiority counterparts (i.e. studies with the same design, objectives and endpoints). Is this true? And why or why not?

To answer these questions, it is helpful to compare the approach to significance testing suitable for equivalence study to that suitable for superiority studies. For this comparison, we will explicitly consider a non-inferiority trial, because in clinical research the non-inferiority approach is more frequently used than the equivalence one. Let us suppose that: (i) the treatment comparison is made in terms of mean difference; (ii) for the end-point of interest the higher the result, the better the patient's condition; (iii) the non-inferiority margin is 10 (for example, 10 meters of walking distance on a treadmill). Under these circumstances, to prove non-inferiority, the one-sided 97.5% confidence interval computed on the treatment mean difference (experimental treatment – reference treatment) should lie entirely above -10. Instead, to prove superiority of the experimental treatment over the reference one, the same confidence interval would have to be placed completely above 0. In fact, we know from chapter 5 that this is equivalent to obtaining a statistically significant result at the 2.5% significance level with a one-sided test. Now, let's assume that the results of our study give an estimate of the treatment mean difference of 2 (for example, 2 meters on the treadmill) and a lower limit of the one-sided 97.5% confidence interval computed on this difference of -5. With such results, we would be able to show non-inferiority, but not superiority, of the experimental treatment vs. the reference one. Clearly, given the observed treatment mean difference of 2, we can find another confidence interval at a lower confidence level (for example at the 85% level) that is completely placed above 0. In other words, we can demonstrate superiority at a higher significance level (in the example at the 15% level) than conventionally required (5%). Therefore, we can equate running a non-inferiority study to running a superiority study at a less stringent significance level. This, in turn, implies that the sample size needed for a non-inferiority study is indeed smaller than the one needed for the corresponding superiority study.

The above conclusion, however, only applies when the non-inferiority study and its superiority counterpart are conducted under identical experimental conditions, which include a non-inferiority margin in the former study identical to the threshold of clinical significance (superiority margin) in the latter. But this cannot be the case. Would it be realistic to plan a superiority study when expecting a clinically irrelevant treatment difference? Going back to our example, would any researcher plan a superiority study, if expecting a treatment difference as small as 2 meters of walking distance on a treadmill? And if such a study were conducted, would the scientific community be willing to judge one of the two treatments superior to the other, given such a small clinical advantage? The experimental conditions under which non-inferiority studies are planned usually require *per se* big sample sizes, much bigger than those usually required under the experimental conditions suitable for conducting superiority studies. The reason can be summarized as follows: all other conditions being the same, the treatment differences on which the sample size calculation is based are smaller in a non-inferiority study than in a superiority study. In fact, by definition, the non-inferiority margin is lower than the threshold of clinical significance and, while in a superiority study we bet on treatment differences bigger than the threshold of clinical significance, in a non-inferiority study we bet on treatment differences smaller than the non-inferiority margin. From chapter 6, we know that, all other conditions being equal, the lower the expected treatment differences, the bigger the sample size.

In conclusion, the right answer to the questions about sample size is as follows: it is true that equivalence studies require less patients than superiority studies under the same experimental conditions, but the experimental conditions cannot be the same. Indeed, an equivalence study is conducted when no clinically significant difference is expected between the treatments under comparison. In such conditions the sample size of an equivalence study is usually very large. The corresponding superiority study would be both unfeasible (or extremely difficult to conduct) and not meaningful.

Superiority for one end-point and non-inferiority for another. Suppose we have a study in which we wish to prove non-inferiority between the two study treatments in terms of efficacy, and, at the same time, prove that the experimental treatment is superior to the active control in terms of safety. In such cases, sample sizes can be calculated by applying the non-inferiority criterion to the primary efficacy end-point and the superiority criterion to the primary safety end-point. The actual sample size of the study will be the bigger between the two.

11.1.4. Analysis and Interpretation Problems

As an introduction to the discussion on the interpretation of results of equivalence studies it is worth introducing the concept of **assay sensitivity.** This is "a property of a clinical trial defined as the ability to distinguish an effective treatment from a less effective or ineffective treatment" [62]. This property is relevant to both superiority and equivalence trials. However, in the former it can be measured directly, whereas in the latter it can be detected only indirectly. In fact, if a superiority study lacks assay sensitivity, it will fail to show superiority of the experimental treatment over the control. Likewise, if a superiority study does show superiority of the experimental treatment over the control, i.e. efficacy of the experimental treatment, this is a proof that the study has adequate assay sensitivity. On the contrary, if an equivalence study lacks assay sensitivity, the two treatments under comparison could still result equivalent because both are ineffective. In these circumstances, the conclusion on the efficacy of the experimental treatment would be wrong.

How can one verify the presence of assay sensitivity in equivalence trials and, therefore, be sure that the absence of a relevant difference between the two treatments under comparison means that the experimental treatment is efficacious? As stated before, this can only be done indirectly, by examining elements that are external to the trial itself, which in some cases can be assessed only after study completion. These are:

- Confirm that adequately designed trials conducted in the past on the reference treatment consistently showed that this was efficacious.
- Show that the equivalence study is similar to the above mentioned confirmatory studies on the reference treatment in the way it is planned and implemented (treatment duration, end-points, study population, allowed previous and concomitant medications, etcetera).
- Confirm that the trial conduct was of high quality (good compliance, low drop-out rate, etcetera).

In this way, one should theoretically obtain for the active control results similar to those obtained in the previous superiority studies vs. placebo and, under such conditions, one should be able to judge whether the treatments under comparison in the equivalence study are both efficacious or both non-efficacious. Unfortunately, this reasoning is theoretical and has many weak points.

First of all, what happens when the historical results for the reference treatment differ from study to study, i.e. cannot consistently support the conclusion that the reference is superior to placebo? If the differences between these results cannot be explained convincingly by differences in study design or conduct, the assay sensitivity cannot be confirmed for the equivalence studies using the reference treatment in question. Depression, anxiety, dementia, seasonal allergies are examples of diseases where well-conducted clinical trials have historically given very variable results and it was not possible to relate this variability to known trial characteristics. Therefore, these are medical conditions in which the use of equivalence studies may be problematic.

Second, it is common in real life that the trials providing confirmatory evidence of the efficacy of the active control have been conducted according to protocols which would not be considered adequate today, because of progresses in the clinical practice and/or clinical trial methodology.

Third, the comparison between the results of the confirmatory superiority studies vs. placebo and those of the equivalence study has all the weakness of a comparison with a historical control, which ultimately makes it impossible to guarantee it is bias-free (see chapter 8).

Because of these problems, whenever possible, it is recommended to include a placebo arm in equivalence studies, i.e. conduct a three-arm equivalence study with an experimental treatment, a reference (standard) treatment, and a placebo. When the placebo arm is included in an equivalence study, most of the problems discussed in the previous sections disappear: a) the efficacy of the two treatments presumed active (experimental and reference) can be tested by direct comparison with placebo; b) the motivation for researchers to produce good quality data is ensured, since a failure in the demonstration of efficacy in the comparison with placebo would automatically result in the failure of the entire study, whether or not equivalence is achieved; c) the choices of the clinical significant difference and the non-inferiority margin would validate each other. With a placebo arm, the assay sensitivity of the equivalence study can be measured directly, i.e. the study has its own internal validity, meaning that it allows valid comparative conclusions to be drawn (see chapter 4). For these reasons, the three-arm study is considered the "gold standard" design for equivalence studies (see guideline ICH [62]). However, as discussed at the beginning of this chapter, researchers often resort to equivalence studies vs. active comparator because the use of placebo is considered unethical. In these cases, the "gold standard" design is not applicable. Thus, the indirect demonstration of the superiority of the experimental treatments over placebo, i.e. the demonstration of their efficacy in equivalence studies, may be problematic.

Before closing this section, we would like to make a final remark on the sta-

tistical analysis of safety and tolerability end-points in placebo-controlled studies in which the primary objective is to prove superiority of the experimental
treatment over placebo in terms of efficacy. As pointed out in section 4.2.2, comparative trials versus placebo typically have the objective of demonstrating
equivalence for safety and tolerability end-points. Because of this, and because
of the issue of multiple comparisons (see section 4.7), significance tests conducted as illustrated in chapter 5 are inappropriate for the analysis of safety and
tolerability end-points. Such analyses should test equivalence between the
groups under comparison, based on confidence intervals. In any case, a study
designed to demonstrate superiority over placebo in terms of efficacy will almost
inevitably be too small for definitive conclusions on safety and tolerability to be
reached.

11.2. Studies with Interim Analyses and Sequential Designs

Several months to several years elapse between the time the first patient is
enrolled in a clinical study and the time the researchers gather to examine the
final results (a moment full of excitement and tension!). During this long wait,
many questions concerning the final outcome assail the researchers (at least
those who have the overall responsibility for the study). If the new treatment
were clearly better than the control, it would be reprehensible to deny it for
such a long time to the patients assigned to the placebo or to a less effective
active control (such patients could have died or irreversibly deteriorated before
gaining access to the new treatment). Vice versa, if the new treatment were
harmful, it would be reprehensible to wait until the end of the study before dis-
continuing it from those patients who had the misfortune of receiving it. Finally,
if the new treatment were totally ineffective, it would be just as reprehensible
to wait until the end of the study, if treatments of proven efficacy (even if partially proven) exist. In addition, in all of the situations mentioned above, having
the information and taking action before the end of the study, would translate
into great savings in financial and human resources.

Therefore, it is absolutely natural and legitimate from a medical, ethical and
logistical point of view that the researchers may want to "have a look" at the data
while the study is still ongoing. However, it is imperative that such "looks" be justified by good reasons (simple curiosity not being one of them) and be rigorously planned before the start of the study. If this does not happen, as we shall see,
such "looks" will irreparably compromise the study. In fact, unjustified "looks"
render the study methodologically and statistically unreliable and ethically unacceptable, since they do not enhance the protection of patients. Ironically, they
also greatly increase the logistical complexity and the cost of the study.

11.2.1. Definitions and Classification

An analysis of data while the study is still ongoing is defined **interim analysis.** An experimental design allowing for one or more interim analyses on groups of patients enrolled sequentially is referred to as a **group sequential design.** In oncology trials, for example, it is not uncommon to allow for two or three interim analyses, each performed when a predefined proportion of patients reaches the end-point or the longest treatment (or follow-up) duration allowed by the protocol.

Suppose we plan to compare a new chemotherapeutic agent with the standard treatment, using tumor mass reduction after two months of treatment as the end-point and 90 patients as the sample size for the final analysis. We decide to use a group sequential design with two interim analyses, to be conducted every time a new group of 30 patients completes the two month treatment (thus, the two analyses are to include 30, and 60 patients, respectively). If the predefined criteria for early closure of the study for proven efficacy or proven lack of efficacy are not met in any of the two interim analyses (see below), the final analysis is performed on all 90 patients constituting the entire sample.

When a new analysis is performed every time a new patient or pair of patients (one for each treatment, see below) reaches the primary evaluation time point, the design is referred to as **pure sequential design.** The corresponding intermediate analyses are called **sequential analyses.** Once again, the objective of each new analysis is to decide whether or not to continue the study, based on predefined criteria. In the oncology and cardiovascular fields, for example, these types of designs are often used to monitor the mortality of the treatment groups being compared.   For the sake of simplicity, in this section we will call both types of studies **sequential designs** and the corresponding analyses interim or intermediate analyses.

The potential objectives of interim analyses go beyond that of interrupting the study because of demonstrated efficacy (better than expected) or lack of efficacy (worse than expected). We can divide them into two large categories: "decision making" and "administrative".

Most of the **interim analyses** are planned with a **decision making** intent, that is, with the aim of deciding whether to interrupt or to modify the study.

The premature interruption of a study can occur for the following three reasons.

- Safety/tolerability: the study is stopped when safety or tolerability problems concerning one or more study treatments emerge.
- Efficacy: the study is stopped when it "becomes evident" that one of the treatments under comparison is more efficacious than the other(s).
- Lack of efficacy: the study is stopped when the possibility of demonstrating, in the remaining part of the study, that one of the treatments is more efficacious than the other(s) "becomes very unlikely".

Analyses conducted when the study is still ongoing for the purpose of modifying it, "if needed", in terms of sample size or design, are the basis of the so-called adaptive (or flexible) designs, discussed in section 11.3.

The expressions "becomes evident", "becomes very unlikely", "if needed" are in quotation marks to highlight that, in each case, it is imperative to predefine the rules that will guide the decision as to whether to stop the study, to modify it or let it proceed unchanged. The rules will differ from case to case, but, in all cases, must be predefined. Interim analyses always have a cost in terms of overall sample size, which will differ depending on the type of objective. We will come back to this important issue in section 11.2.5.

Administrative interim analyses, constituting the second category of interim analyses, are not aimed at making decisions on whether to interrupt or modify the study, but at making decisions external to the study itself, generally concerning safety issues or issues related to the planning of other studies.

For example, suppose that during the health authority review of the registration dossier of a new antibiotic, the reviewer notices a slight tendency toward low levels of serum potassium in the group receiving the antibiotic, but not in that receiving placebo. In this situation, before deciding whether or not to include warnings or restrictions in the package insert, the reviewer may be very interested in knowing if this trend is confirmed in the ongoing clinical studies (at least in the bigger ones), without having to wait until these studies are finished.

An interim analysis that does not allow for the possibility of interrupting or modifying a study is often (inappropriately) called "administrative interim analysis". Historically, the term 'administrative' implied that there would be no penalties in terms of sample size on the study on which the analysis was conducted. Recent papers by FDA officials have made clear that this approach is not acceptable [73, 91]. All interim analyses, including the administrative ones, will have an impact on the overall sample size, with only one exception: analyses that do not call for any comparative testing of differences between treatments, i.e. do not require unblinding of the study. Whenever an unplanned administrative analysis requiring unblinding is decided, its rationale and methods, including those to be used for the assessment and protection of the overall type I error, should be documented in a formal protocol amendment.

In summary, an interim analysis is an analysis of the data performed while the study is still ongoing for one of the two fundamental reasons: first, to decide whether or not to stop or modify the study based on predefined criteria (decision making objective); second, to extract information from data accumulated thus far for reasons external to the study (administrative objective). The various types of interim analyses are summarized in Figure 11.1.

The remainder of this section will focus on interim analyses aimed at deciding whether to interrupt an ongoing study; section 11.3 will be dedicated to the interim analyses aimed at deciding whether to modify an ongoing study.

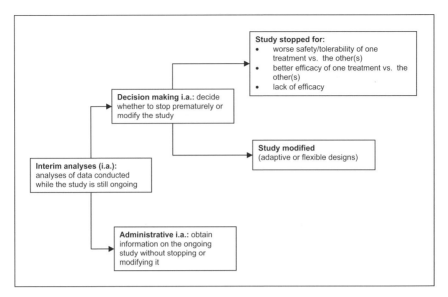

Figure 11.1. Classification of interim analyses based on their objective

11.2.2. Conditions of Applicability

Whatever the objective of an interim analysis, it is important to determine whether it is possible to conduct such an analysis at all. To this end, two important questions should be asked:

1. Is the duration of the study (recruitment + treatment) compatible with an interim analysis? Although an interim analysis can be compared to a snapshot of a specific moment of an ongoing study, the process leading to such snapshot is long and elaborate. It requires the preparation of the database, the analysis of the data and the interpretation of the results (see below). In many cases, the duration of the above mentioned process is comparable to or even longer than that of the remainder of the study. This of course negates the very reason for conducting an interim analysis. It is only in studies with very long duration of recruitment, compared to the duration of treatment, that interim analyses can actually be useful in protecting patients, or in avoiding waste of resources, or even, simply, in obtaining useful information before the end of the study. An interim analysis that is completed a few weeks before the end of the study basically leads to nothing else than a considerable waste of resources. In forecasting the time required for the interim analysis compared to that of the study, the researcher must keep in mind the almost unavoidable delays due to the complexity of data collection, analysis and interpretation of the results.

2. Are the end-points suitable for an interim analysis? In many cases the answer is "no". The most typical case is when the primary end-point is the occurence of an event that, on average, is expected months or years after the beginning

of the study. In this case, it is very unlikely that an interim analysis performed when the majority of patients have only recently entered the study will yield useful results. When the primary end-point does not lend itself to an interim analysis, a secondary or surrogate end-point could theoretically be used (see section 4.9). However, this in turn brings other kinds of problems: these will be discussed in section 11.2.3.

Even when the conclusion is that it is technically possible to perform an interim analysis, it is still necessary to question whether it is appropriate to carry it out. Are the benefits of such a procedure actually higher than the costs and risks? The answer depends on the objectives one wants to pursue with such analysis.

Concerning the possibility of ***stopping a study prematurely for demonstrated efficacy***, one should keep in mind the context in which the study is performed and its objective. Ideally, once it is proven that one treatment is more efficacious than the other(s), the study should be immediately interrupted and all patients transferred to the best treatment. However, this can only occur, in a relatively simple and rapid way, if the treatment in question is already on the market, for example, in the case of a study demonstrating the superiority of a new cocktail of anticancer or antiviral drugs, already available individually, in the therapy of Hodgkin's lymphoma or in HIV infection, respectively, or in the case of a study demonstrating the efficacy of a well known inhaled corticosteroid, such as budesonide, in mild forms of asthma. However, the new treatment is often still in the experimental phase, that is, it has not been approved by the health authority. In such cases, the results of one interim analysis from one study are rarely sufficient to warrant immediate approval. This may occur, but only under exceptional circumstances. It is more likely, instead, that a conflict will arise between the health authority on one side, requesting more studies before approval, and the pharmaceutical industry and the patients' associations on the other side, requesting immediate approval. These kinds of conflicts will often interfere heavily with the timely completion of the clinical development program. Paradoxically, the premature interruption of a study, which aims at making the best treatment quickly available to the small group of patients enrolled in it, ends up delaying the marketing authorization and hence the access to the treatment by all patients. Furthermore, before registration, if the study treatment is a drug, it is often produced in small quantities, sufficient to treat only a small number of patients for a limited period of time. Finally, one should keep in mind that the objective of many clinical trials does not immediately translate into a therapeutic benefit, but does so only in the context of a development program consisting of many studies. In fact, the premature interruption of a study for proven efficacy can prevent reaching reasonable evidence of safety and tolerability, because this may require a longer observation period and/or a greater number of patients.

Concerning the possibility of ***stopping a study prematurely for non-efficacy*** in order to save resources, one should be realistic about the savings that are truly attainable, in terms of both human and financial resources. "Liberating" patients from the burden and risk (even if small) associated with their participation in the study is definitely a valid reason to stop the study when efficacy cannot be demonstrated. However, the time at which the decision is actually made must be carefully considered, because, if too late in the study, the advantage for the patients may be more apparent than real. From a financial point of view, one should consider that payments to investigators are generally not uniformly distributed over the course of the study and most of the fees may already have been paid when the study is stopped. Furthermore, in many contracts, researchers have the right to be paid in full if the study is interrupted for reasons unrelated to their performance. Finally, a study stopped prematurely cannot be "discarded" as if it never happened: the analysis must be completed and the results reported and published. The savings in terms of cost, time and energy for the researcher may be relative.

Despite all of the above, we are not implying that interim analyses should always be avoided. On the contrary, in many circumstances they are extremely useful or even imperative from an ethical, medical and practical point of view. However, as in many other areas of research, it is dangerous to generalize, and every study must be evaluated in its own context. Among the interim analyses with decision making objectives, those aimed at stopping a study for safety or tolerability concerns are the least problematic.

Once it is established that an interim analysis with decision making objectives is appropriate, it should be planned to the smallest detail, before starting the study. Planning for such an analysis while the study is ongoing is discouraged, because it would generally endanger the credibility of results. Nevertheless, if a study has just started, the inclusion of a decision making interim analysis through a protocol amendment may still be possible without jeopardizing the study. However, such a change must be agreed upon with the health authority and/or ethics committees.

On the other hand, administrative interim analyses may well be unplanned at the time the protocol is written. The need to perform one or more analyses of this type may surface after the start of a study, generally due to an unexpected problem affecting another study or to a specific request from a regulatory authority. In such cases, the inclusion of an interim analysis in the research plan after the study has begun is legitimate. Nevertheless, the planning of the analysis must be completed and documented by means of an appropriate protocol amendment before the randomization code is opened.

11.2.3. Choice of the End-Points

It is almost never useful to extend the interim analysis to all the end-points of a study. Instead, one should select a limited number of end-points, based on the aims of the analysis and their nature (as discussed above, some are not suitable for interim analyses). A delicate issue arises when a secondary efficacy end-point, but not the primary one, is suitable for the interim analysis. This, for example, is common in oncology, when survival time is the primary end-point and tumor size a secondary one. As mentioned above, the median survival time can be so long that it makes an interim analysis impossible, while the tumor mass reduction tends to occur more rapidly and therefore can be analyzed sooner. The problem is that the secondary end-point is rarely a good surrogate (see section 4.9) of the primary one. In our example, reduction of tumor mass is not a good surrogate of survival time. If our interim analysis were to demonstrate that a new anticancer treatment is significantly better than the standard treatment in reducing tumor mass, would we be willing to stop our study in which the survival time is the primary end-point? Moreover, if we were to do so, would the regulatory authorities be willing to approve the drug based on such a result? If the correlation between tumor mass and survival time were so strong to allow the stoppage of a survival study based on an early reduction in tumor mass, why did we embark on such a costly and long type of study in the first place? The use of a secondary end-point for an interim analysis aimed at deciding whether to interrupt a study on the basis of proven efficacy (or lack of efficacy) is very problematic and generally unjustified. As always, there could be exceptions, but the authors can find no supporting examples. The situation is different for administrative interim analyses: it can be very useful to perform an interim analysis on a secondary end-point of a study, in order to help the planning of another study in which one wants to make that end-point the primary one.

11.2.4. Data Management Issues

Before an interim analysis can begin, the database must be completed, validated and "locked". To this end, all data must be collected from the centers and checked for completeness and plausibility. First of all, the database must be checked for data entry errors (e.g. via a double entry of each individual datum). Missing and questionable data must be queried with investigators, and "clean" data loaded in the database. Thereafter, the database must be properly validated and quality controlled. Such procedures go beyond the aim of this book, but the reader will appreciate that they require considerable time, personnel, IT support and money. Electronic data capture systems (see section 12.4) make things only slightly better.

It is true that data must be collected, checked and loaded into the database in any case for the final analysis. However, in preparing the database for one or more interim analyses, times are often shorter compared to those allowed for the final analysis and some procedures must be repeated at every analysis, for example the quality control procedures for the database "locking", those for the analysis itself and the writing of reports. In addition, it is desirable that data management for interim analyses be coordinated by groups independent of the study sponsor (see section 11.2.6). Finally, the fact that all activities related to the preparation of the database for an interim analysis must be performed while the study is ongoing should not be underestimated. The time and effort of physicians, CRAs (Clinical Research Associates), statisticians and data managers will have to split between the issues related to the ongoing study and those related to the interim analysis. This creates frequent episodes of internal conflict that, if not properly managed, end up damaging the interim analysis, as well as the study as whole.

A few years ago, a young doctor working with one of us was in the middle of the "data cleaning" process for an interim analysis when he received a message indicating that a serious adverse event had occurred the day before. The event needed immediate attention, both to follow its evolution and to check if similar events (even if not serious) had occurred in the study or in other studies testing the same experimental treatment. However, arrangements had already been made for a meeting with external experts to evaluate the results of the interim analysis and time was tight for the database lock. Somewhat intimidated by pressure from within the company and by the reputation of some of the experts, the young doctor favored the interim analysis. Unfortunately, the health authority, concerned by the adverse event in question, decided to put on hold, not only the specific study, but also the entire research program, while awaiting a satisfactory assessment of the potential safety signal. Many months were needed to restart the program.

11.2.5. Statistical Issues and Decision Making Criteria

When there is one or more interim analyses in a study, the problem of multiple comparisons arises, intuitively similar to that discussed in section 4.7, but with the additional complexity that each new test is conducted on a dataset that includes the datasets used in the previous tests, i.e. there is an obvious correlation among the datasets analyzed sequentially. The statistical methodology of interim analyses goes beyond the scope of this book. We will only emphasize the basic concept that the inclusion of multiple "looks" with a decision making purpose in the study design comes at a "cost" in both logistical and statistical terms. The magnitude of this "cost" depends on the number and objective of the "looks" and the type of design.

Let us first consider the interim analyses conducted with the aim of prematurely interrupting a study for proven efficacy. In these cases, the "cost" is the need to lower the threshold of statistical significance for each analysis, including the final one. The reason for this should be clear by now.

When the data are analyzed repeatedly in search of a statistically significant difference, the probability of finding one by chance, i.e. in the absence of a real difference between the treatments, is higher compared to when only one test is performed at the end of the study. In other words, the overall probability of making a type I error (erroneously concluding that the experimental treatment is efficacious) increases as the number of statistical tests increases. We use the expression **nominal significance level** to indicate the probability of making a type I error in a single test, and the expression **real significance level** to indicate the overall probability of making this type of error when multiple tests are performed, each at the established nominal significance level. Suppose we perform five interim analyses, each at a nominal significance level of 0.05. The overall probability that at least one of the tests will show a statistically significant difference by chance is no longer 0.05, but 0.14 (i.e. the latter is the real significance level – see [79]). To keep the real significance level as low as 0.05, a nominal significance level lower than 0.05 is required for each individual test. In other words, we must lower the threshold not to be exceeded in each intermediate analysis and in the final analysis, in order to be able to claim that the corresponding result is statistically significant.

As stated in section 4.7, the methods for determining the nominal significance level to be used in each analysis are called α **adjustment** methods. It is important to point out that the α adjustment methods required for the interim analyses, even though conceptually similar to those used for multiple comparisons, have specific features to account for the fact that the sequential analyses are repeated on progressively accumulating data, and that are therefore correlated. For example, the famous **Bonferroni's method**, in which the nominal α is set equal to the real α divided by the number of tests to be performed, cannot be applied to interim analyses, since it is too conservative. This is because it requires that the comparisons are independent, an assumption that is definitely violated in the case of interim analyses. Generally, having decided the alternative hypothesis, the number of interim analyses and the real α and β levels, the α adjustment methods for interim analyses provide the "optimal" levels of nominal significance, which minimize the average number of patients when the alternative hypothesis is true. This does not mean that, by using designs with interim analyses, one would necessarily use fewer patients compared to the same designs allowing for the final analysis only (i.e. designs with a fixed sample). On the contrary, since the significance level of the single test is lower than 0.05, in order to maintain a given power of the study, the total sample size must be greater than that of a study with an identical design, but with only the final analysis to be carried out at a significance level of 0.05. In conclusion, even though one of the fundamental reasons for applying sequential designs is to reduce sample size compared to that required by an equivalent design with a fixed sample, in reality this goal is only achieved when one of the interim analyses yields a significant result before enrolment is complete. Vice versa, a larger sample is required when none of the interim analyses produces a statistically significant result.

The simplest α adjustment method is the one described in Pocock's textbook. The nominal significance level is kept constant for each interim analysis and for the final one; all of the sequential groups have the same size. Such method makes no "optimization" attempt, but is easy to understand and to apply. It should be noted that, even though the significance level is the same for each interim analysis, the earlier the analysis occurs in the course of the study, the smaller is the sample size available for it. Thus, in order to be able to stop the study prematurely, the earlier the analysis, the bigger the treatment difference and/or the smaller the variability should be, as compared to what was originally expected.

More complex methods "spend" the overall level of significance unevenly across the different interim analyses. Generally, lower (more stringent) significance levels are used in the earlier analyses, whereas a higher significance level, closer to 0.05, is allowed for the later analyses. With these methods, the likelihood of closing a study prematurely on the grounds of efficacy in the early interim analyses is very low (this occurrence requires a truly exceptional result). A well-known method belonging to this category is that of O'Brien and Fleming [72].

Returning to the simplest method, if we assign the classical value of 0.05 to the real significance threshold and choose to perform four interim analyses in addition to the final one, the threshold for declaring each of the five comparisons significant (i.e. the nominal significance level) decreases to 0.016 (see [79]). The implication of this is that, in case none of the intermediate comparisons reaches statistical significance at the 0.016 level, a final analysis yielding for example a p-value of 0.03, which would be statistically significant in the absence of interim analyses, would have to be declared not statistically significant in our example, due to the four interim analyses introduced in the design. The possibility of these tricky results must be kept in mind when planning sequential designs and must be accepted if it occurs. If the probabilistic framework behind sequential designs is not fully understood, even the most principled of researchers will be tempted to forget about the interim analyses when confronted with such a result.

In pure sequential designs, the adjustment of the significance level is generally carried out by building the so-called **decision making barriers.** Pocock [79] and Armitage and Berry [3] clearly lay out the simplest form of **continuous sequential design**, referred to as **paired preference design.** Briefly, such design is applicable when two treatments are compared and the selected end-point allows the "winner" between two patients, each receiving one of the study treatments, to be declared. The patients are enrolled in the study in pairs, with one patient of each pair randomized to A and the other to B. When a pair completes the treatment, the researcher must express a preference for A or B, based on the outcome of the predefined end-point. As the preferences accumulate, they are registered in a graph where the number of patients examined is reported on the horizontal axis and the number of preferences in favor of A or B is reported on the vertical axis. The plot, drawn on graph paper, is marked off with boundaries, one establishing the superiority of A, another the superiority of B and a third determining the end of the study without evidence that one treatment is better than the other (see Figure 11.2). These designs can be open (no predefined maximum number of preferences) or closed (maximum number of preferences predefined). The one illustrated in Figure 11.2 is an example of a closed design, as it has central boundaries (those leading to stopping the study without a definitive conclusion).

The boundaries can only be reached at specific points, but are drawn as continuous lines for simplicity. Their position is calculated based on the characteristics of the distribution of the end-point (in our case, binomial), the threshold of clinical significance and the levels for type I and II errors chosen for the

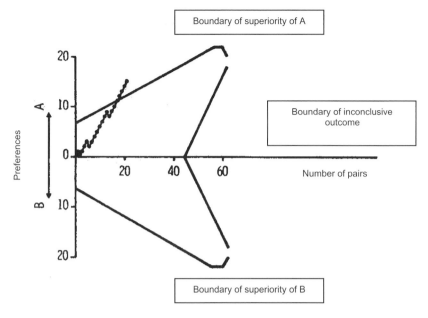

Figure 11.2. Example of a closed sequential continuous design. The bold, dotted line represents the sequence of preferences. In this example, the study was interrupted because of superiority of treatment A. (From: Clinical Trials. A practical Approach, Pocock SJ, 1983. Copyright John Wiley & Sons Limited. Reproduced with permission.)

study. For example, in Figure 11.2, the boundaries are positioned based on the following statistical specifications:

- The region of rejection of the null hypothesis corresponds to a real α of 5%, with a bi-directional alternative hypothesis (under the null hypothesis, the probability of reaching one of the two external barriers is 0.025).
- The probability (power) of statistically detecting a difference between the treatments, if one of the two is preferred in 75% of cases, is set at 95%.
- The maximum number of preferences is 62.

The starting point is the origin 0 (the crossing of the horizontal and vertical axes). For each preference in favor of A, one moves one square up and to the right; for each preference in favor of B one moves one square down and to the right. Gradually, as new pairs of patients complete the study and new preferences are expressed, the preference curve grows, approaching one of the boundaries. The study is interrupted when the preference curve crosses one of them. The result plotted in Figure 11.2 is from a true study conducted in the early '60s on patients with acute leukemia; A was the experimental treatment and B was placebo. The sequence of preferences, of which three favor B and 15 favor A, led to the interruption of the study with a statistically significant result in favor of treatment A (the preferences beyond the superiority boundary represent pairs of patients who were enrolled before the study was stopped).

Interim analyses carried out with the aim of prematurely interrupting a study for lack of efficacy are based on the so-called **conditional power,** i.e. the probability that, given the results observed so far, superiority of one of the treatments under comparison will be demonstrated, once the entire predetermined sample of patients completes the study. The study is terminated if, considering reasonable hypotheses about the difference between treatments, this power (probability) is lower than a preestablished threshold, called **futility index**. If this is not the case, the study is to continue until the entire sample is completed. The "cost" of the interim analyses is only logistical in this case, that is, no adjustment of α is required. The interested reader can consult articles by Halperin et al [55] for the methodology and by Lachin et al [64] for a practical example.

Interim analyses conducted with the aim of modifying the design of a study are the basis of the so-called adaptive designs, which are covered in section 11.3.

Three important points remain to be made before closing this section. The first is that regulatory circumstances must be thoroughly assessed when deciding whether to start a sequential design. In pivotal registration studies, it is imperative to confirm with the appropriate regulatory authorities that the study, if stopped prematurely on the grounds of efficacy, would still be acceptable for registration, in terms of both efficacy and safety/tolerability. If there is any doubt, it is better not to plan for an interim analysis. The second point is that, to legitimize the decisions based on a decision making interim analysis, the analysis plan and the criteria for deciding whether or not to interrupt the study must be defined before the start of the study (see above). The third point is that it is advisable to conduct the interim analyses and make decisions without knowing to which study treatment each group corresponds (the groups are to be identified as A, B, C, etc). Only once the decision to stop the study has been made, should one proceed to unmask the treatments.

11.2.6. Conflict of Interest and Confidentiality Issues

Ideally, the experts performing the interim analysis and deciding whether to interrupt or continue the study are external to all other procedures related to the study, including the database preparation. This group of independent experts is commonly called the **data monitoring board.** In practice, it is not always possible to have such a committee completely independent from the sponsor of the study, for logistical and/or financial reasons. Nevertheless, an effort must be made to ensure that the separation of roles be maintained at least for some key figures, such as the person in charge of data management, the head statistician and the president of the decision making committee (generally an independent researcher with long standing experience in the therapeutic area of the study). In our opinion, when this is not possible, the appropriateness of interim analysis must be reconsidered.

Once the results of an interim analysis become available, the problem of disclosure arises. Clearly, if the decision is made to stop the study, the researchers must be informed of the reason. However, it is essential that, before the start of .the study, all researchers agree that the decision of the committee charged with evaluating the interim analysis is final. If, instead, the decision is to continue the study, in our opinion it is important that the knowledge of results be strictly limited to the decision making committee. In fact, if the committee's decision is that the study is to continue in spite of a clear trend in favor of (or against) the new treatment, because the outcome is below the predefined statistical or clinical threshold, a researcher aware of such a trend may be influenced in the selection of patients, or may even want to transfer all of his/her patients to the "best" treatment, ignoring the decision of the committee. Even more problematic would be the decision to publish the results of an interim analysis while the study is still ongoing. If the final results were to contradict those of the interim analysis (by then in the public domain), the publication of the final results would be much more difficult, especially if the final results are "worse" than the interim ones.

In spite of all of the complexities discussed here, there are many cases in which interim analyses are very useful and must be carried out. However, we believe that the performance of interim analyses with suboptimal rationale and/or preparation is still too common in the practice of clinical research.

11.3. Adaptive (Flexible) Designs

The so-called **adaptive designs** or plans are designs which envisage interim analyses with the aim of modifying the study while it is ongoing. These are also known as **flexible designs.**

We warn the reader that the terminology is all but standard, since this is a relatively new area. The broader definition of adaptive or flexible designs includes designs with the aim of modifying the study without interrupting it, as well as the sequential designs, i.e. those with the aim of prematurely closing the study for proven efficacy or, vice versa, because efficacy can no longer be proven. The stricter definition only includes designs of the first type. The broader definition is used more and more and recent methods integrate design changes and early shopping rules. It should be noted that sometimes the term "adaptive plan" is used with a completely different meaning, i.e. to indicate designs with adaptive randomization (see section 9.2.3).

In this section we will focus on adaptive designs with the aim of modifying a study without interrupting it.

These designs make sense when, at the time a study is being planned, the researchers lack some key information, necessary for a "fixed" (i.e. completely predefined) design. Therefore, the study is planned with the available information and, at the same time, interim analyses are planned. Based on the outcome of the interim analyses, changes to the design are made, where appropriate.

Changes can concern the most diverse aspects of the study including the following:

- Sample size (for example, the size of all treatment groups is increased evenly or unevenly; in the latter case changing the ratio of patient allocation to the treatments).
- Choice of doses (for example, groups receiving ineffective doses are closed and/or groups receiving new doses are added).
- Choice of primary and/or secondary end-points.
- Decision making criteria (for example, future interim analyses are added or removed, or their temporal sequence is modified).
- Objective of the trial (for example, the objective of showing non-inferiority is changed to that of showing superiority of the experimental treatment over the reference one).

Obviously, there is a price to pay for this flexibility. If the changes determined by the interim analyses are not explicitly taken into account when analyzing the data and interpreting the results, the overall level of the type I and II errors can be seriously inaccurate and/or the estimates of the effects can be distorted. Adaptive designs must allow changes to be made without compromising the levels of the type I and II errors, so as to obtain unbiased estimates of the effects of interest.

A unique "recipe" for the application of these designs does not exist: the methods depend strictly on the type of changes that one wants to make.

The following general guidelines must be followed:

- The forms of "flexibility" of interest must be specified before beginning the study (even if the protocol will be "adapted" in stages).
- Many of the problems pointed out for sequential designs extend also to adaptive designs, for example, the operational and confidentiality issues are the same.
- The contribution of statisticians specializing in planning and analyzing these designs is essential.

Acceptability of adaptive designs for pivotal phase III studies (see chapter 12) is problematic. The biggest stumbling block is that, after the modification determined by interim analyses, the study is no longer the one initially planned. Consequently, the pooling of the results of the two phases (the one before and the one after the modifications) is conceptually similar to the pooling of results from two separate studies (meta-analysis). This procedure is not acceptable as definitive proof of efficacy, unless special experimental conditions exist (see again chapter 12). The adaptive design approach is especially promising for studies combining different phases of clinical development (for example, phases I and II, or phases II and III – see chapter 12). A practical example can be found in Zeymer et al [108]. In oncology, adaptive designs are adopted with increasing frequency for ethical reasons. In the experimental conditions that are often encountered in this therapeutic area (end stage disease, at times rare, without therapeutic options), it is easier to accept the drawbacks of these designs and the attitude of the regulatory authority is more flexible.

On the topic of adaptive (flexible) designs, we recommend articles by Bauer and Kohne [8] and Posh et al [81]. For the application of this approach to flexible determination of the sample size, we recommend articles by Gould [51] and by Frieder and Kieser [46]. The field of adaptive designs is extremely active and every year a great deal of new papers appears in the literature.

11.4. Studies with Repeated Measurements

So far we have focused our interest only on the scenario in which the primary comparison between the study treatments is made at a single evaluation time point. However, very often the end-point is measured repeatedly throughout the treatment period and at the end of it, the objective of the study being to use the entire set of measurements to compare the study treatments

A typical example is that of studies on pain killers. Suppose we plan to compare two treatments for the symptomatic control of chronic cervical pain due to arthritis by means of a parallel group study, with one month treatment duration, and pain assessment at baseline, the end of each week of treatment, and end of study. Under these conditions, the researchers are not likely to be satisfied with a "snapshot" of the situation as seen at a single visit. Instead, it is common practice to compare the effects of the two treatments on pain level over the entire course of the study. These kinds of studies are known as **studies with repeated measurements**, also known as **longitudinal data.**

The complexity of such studies lies mainly in the statistical analysis. Indeed, it is quite common to find in the medical literature studies with repeated measurement analyzed with the wrong statistical approach. There are two major problems:

- By definition, there are multiple sets of data to compare (in our example, five sets of data for each treatment at the five evaluation times, ten in total); therefore, if the comparison between treatments is performed separately at each time point, a problem of multiple comparisons will arise.
- The data sets are not independent, since evaluations repeated on the same subject are correlated; this must be kept in mind when trying to combine evaluations obtained at different time points on the same group of patients.

One way of dealing with repeated measurements on the same patient is that of combining them into one summary measurement, which becomes the efficacy end-point. An example is the **area under the curve** (**AUC**), i.e. the area of the region which is delimited by the line-plot of the various observations at the top and by the X axis, from the first to the last visit, at the bottom. This area is generally calculated by dividing the whole region in many trapezia: each has the height equal to the interval between two consecutive visits and the two bases (minor and major) equal to the measurements of the efficacy variable taken at these two visits. Provided that this end-point has a clinical meaning, from a statistical point of view it has the advantage of smaller variability, as compared with the variability of the same variable assessed at a single time point.

However, by combining the repeated measurements as described above, we have no information about the trend of the responses over time. If such a time trend is deemed an important objective of the trial, we should use all the different measurements as a multivariate efficacy end-point. One way of analyzing parallel group designs with repeated measurements treated as a multivariate end-point is to consider the design as a split-plot (see section 10.9), where the plot is the subject, the whole-plot factor is the treatment, the sub-plot factor is the time, and the visits at which the measurements are made are the levels of the sub-plot factor. However, the design involving repeated measurements differs from the split-plot one in that in the former, the times of observation must follow, by definition, a strict temporal sequence, while in the latter the order of the levels of the sub-plot factor is typically random. In general, in trials with longitudinal data, the measurements made at visits close together are more highly correlated than those further apart. On the contrary, one of the main assumptions for the analysis of split-plot designs is that all pairs of observations have the same correlation. An analysis of longitudinal data that ignores this difference is almost certainly invalid and it is mandatory that the analysis used for the split-plot designs be adjusted in order to render it appropriate for the analysis of designs with repeated measurements.

For readers interested in this topic, we recommend references [4] and [39].

Summary

In this chapter we considered variants of study designs, classified according to type of objective, end-point, and modality of analysis. These variants can be applied both to designs with between-subject comparisons (typically, parallel group designs) and to those with within-subject comparisons (typically, crossover designs).

In equivalence and non-inferiority studies, the objective is to demonstrate that two or more treatments do not differ in a clinically relevant manner. In these studies the usual hypothesis testing, aimed at demonstrating the superiority of one treatment over the other by rejecting the null hypothesis of no difference between treatments, loses its meaning, since the inability to reject such null hypothesis does not imply equivalence (or non-inferiority), and, likewise, the rejection of such null hypothesis does not imply the absence of equivalence (or inferiority). A common mistake is to plan and analyze an equivalence/non-inferiority study as if it were a superiority one. Instead, specific methods must be used for defining the delta on which to base the sample size calculation (in the case of equivalence/non-inferiority studies, this delta is called the margin of equivalence/non-inferiority), analyzing the data and interpreting the results.

Sequential designs, characterized by one or more interim analyses, have the objective of obtaining information on the results before the conclusion of the study. In interim analyses conducted for decision making purposes, such information, though obviously incomplete, can lead to the premature interruption of the study, if it indicates with a "sufficient degree of certainty" either that the experimental treatment has unacceptable safety/tolerability problems, or that it is more efficacious than the control, or that it can no longer be superior to the control in the final analysis, whatever the response of the remaining patients.

For the interim analysis to be valid, the decision making criteria must be defined before the start of the study; likewise, all the analysis procedures must also be defined *a priori*, preferably before the start of the study and certainly before the disclosure of the randomization code. Furthermore, it is highly desirable that those responsible for the interim analyses and decision making are not involved in the study in any other way. One should keep in mind that interim analyses are complex, costly and lengthy, and that generally several months elapse from the start of the database preparation to the decision on whether or not to continue the study. Therefore, interim analyses are to be considered only for studies of long duration and with appropriate support in terms of staff and IT. Finally, the regulatory circumstances and availability of the study treatments must be considered when deciding whether to embark in a sequential design. When the study in question is intended to provide pivotal evidence for registration, it is imperative to discuss with the relevant regulatory authorities if the study will still be considered acceptable for registration in case of early interruption for achieved efficacy. If there are doubts, it is better not to perform interim analyses. Regarding the treatments, it is necessary to make sure that it is feasible to transfer all patients to the best treatment in the case of premature interruption of the study for proven efficacy. For new treatments in the pre-registration phase, this is often completely impossible, since they are manufactured on a very small scale, in which case it is best to avoid efficacy interim analyses.

Interim analyses that are conducted for decision making external to the study (e.g. planning of a different study) are called administrative analyses. They also carry a sample size penalty for the study they are conducted on, unless no unblinding is required.

Adaptive (flexible) designs allow changes to be made to the study plan while the study is ongoing, without compromising the level of the type I and II errors. Adaptive designs are particularly attractive when key information required for the planning of a "fixed" design study is lacking. However, they are generally difficult to conduct and are only accepted by the regulatory authorities as pivotal phase III studies under special conditions.

In studies with repeated measurements, the objective is that of comparing the trends between treatments in a pre-specified time interval and not just the treatment responses at given time points; therefore, the assessment of results is based on multiple evaluations repeated over time on the same subjects.

All of these variants have numerous implications that must be kept in mind when planning and performing the study and when analyzing the results. If used without considering these implications, serious errors may occur leading to completely unreliable results.

12

The Drug Development Process and the Phases of Clinical Research

The reader should be aware of two semantic conventions we adopted in this chapter: first, the terms "research" and "development" are used interchangeably; second, the term "drug", which technically only applies to compounds with proven efficacy and effectiveness, is also used to indicate compounds undergoing the development process, for which, by definition, efficacy and effectiveness have not be proven.

12.1. Overview of the Preclinical Development Process

Clinical experiments begin when a treatment is administered for the first time to a human being ("first in man"). In the case of pharmacological treatments, which are the focus of this chapter, the start of clinical research and development (R&D) is preceded by many years of preclinical R&D. The preclinical development process is outside the scope of this book. However, we believe it is important for the clinical researcher to recognize the great amount of knowledge and work required to bring a drug to the stage of clinical experimentation. The preclinical development of a drug involves hundreds of people, who bring with them a wide variety of top level professional skills.

Broadly speaking, the preclinical development process includes the areas described in this section, which interact with one another on an ongoing basis.

Screening. Generally, the development of a drug starts with the **screening** of thousands of molecules, using one or more biological assays that have a predictive value on the disease under study. Each molecule undergoing screening usually represents a small variation of a basic molecular structure. The basic structures can be completely unknown in their pharmacological potential (**random screening**) or can be based on previous knowledge (**guided screening**). In the case of guided screening, the starting compound can belong to at least three categories.

1. A drug of demonstrated efficacy in the specific therapeutic area. For example, many benzodiazepines used in the therapy of anxiety were developed starting from the basic structure of diazepam (Valium®), which was itself discovered through random screening.

2. A drug used in other therapeutic areas for which clinical observations suggest potential novel uses. Minoxidil, for example, was developed as an antihypertensive. The observation that it often caused hypertrichosis (i.e. excessive hair growth) prompted the development of a topical formulation against male and female baldness.

3. A molecular structure guided by the knowledge of the structure and function of its target, usually a receptor or mediator. For example, omalizumab (Xolair®) is a "humanized" monoclonal antibody (i.e. an antibody with an amino acid sequence about 95% human and 5% murine) targeted against immunoglobulins E (IgE), which has been developed for the treatment of allergic asthma. Omalizumab has been "designed" based on a very detailed knowledge of the structure and antigenic properties of the human IgE.

Molecules for mass rapid screening are traditionally generated by chemical synthesis. However, increasingly common are the so-called **biotechnological products**, generated by cell lines modified to produce great quantities of a single protein. Monoclonal antibodies, such as omalizumab, are an example of great therapeutic success.

At the end of the screening process, a small number of compounds are selected, based on their efficacy in the selected biological assays. Naturally, the development of good biological assays is of crucial importance for an effective screening process: the higher the predictive value of a biological assay in a given therapeutic area, the more effective the screening.

Choice of the "lead compound". At the end of a screening campaign one hopes to obtain a certain number of molecules that, at the same time, are simple to synthesize (in fact or potentially), have physico-chemical characteristics compatible with the predicted function, and demonstrate pharmacological activity in the selected biological assays. Unfortunately, this is not always the case and screening campaigns that do not yield a single acceptable candidate are not rare. When candidates are obtained, preclinical researchers must choose a very restricted number of "champions" to promote to more advanced stages of development. Generally, a **lead compound** is selected, along with a small number of **back-up compounds** (two to five), to be used if the lead compound runs into unexpected problems (as often happens). The choice of the lead compound always results from a compromise. To draw an analogy from the world of sports, the lead compound is comparable to a decathlete: such an athlete must perform satisfactorily in all ten disciplines, rather than be exceptionally good in some, but totally inadequate in others.

Synthesis and physico-chemical characterization of the lead compound. For a molecule to have the potential to become a drug, not only must it be pharmacologically active in the chosen biological models, but it must also lend itself to being produced in large quantities at acceptable costs and have physico-chemical characteristics compatible with the expected function. Initially, the synthetic process may be very laborious and require many steps. However, it is necessary to simplify it as much as possible, both by reducing the number of steps, and by substituting the more complex steps with simpler ones. Optimization of the synthesis of the active compound requires years of research and often continues long after clinical development has begun. In any case, from the beginning, it is generally possible to estimate the feasibility of an acceptable simplification of the synthetic pathway and discard molecules that will be too difficult to synthesize. Furthermore, a detailed characterization of the physico-chemical properties of the most promising molecules (solubility in water and lipids, pH, etcetera) makes it possible to discard *a priori* those that are incompatible with either interaction with the molecular target or use in living organisms.

Pharmaceutical formulation. The confusion between the **active compound** (drug substance) and the **drug product** or **pharmaceutical product** is a mistake commonly made by "outsiders". The drug product contains the active (or presumed active) compound, a series of **excipients** (pharmacologically inert substances) such as lactose, fructose, starch, etcetera, and a **delivery system.** Examples of delivery systems include capsules for oral administration; syringes for intermittent parenteral injection; pumps for continuous parenteral injection; inhalers for inhalation of powders, solutions or suspensions; patches for transdermal administration, etcetera. An optimal combination of active compound, excipients and delivery system into a drug product, i.e. the achievement of an optimal **pharmaceutical formulation**, is often one of the most complex steps in the preclinical development of a drug. As with the synthetic process, the optimization of the pharmaceutical formulation requires many years of work and, almost always, continues well into the stage of clinical experimentation. As a consequence, early clinical trials are generally conducted with the so-called **service formulation**, i.e. a formulation that is easier to make compared to the **final formulation** (for example, a solution to drink instead of a capsule, or a nebulizer instead of a portable inhaler). However, one should make sure that the service formulation is not too different from the final one, since the formulation can dramatically modify the effects of a drug (both desirable and undesirable). In any case, the phase II dose-response studies and the phase III pivotal studies (see below) should be performed using the final drug product, identical to the one that will be commercialized ("final market image"). In practice, this does not always happen, because the race against time and competitors is ferocious, and it does happen that pivotal trials are carried out with formulations that are similar, but not identical, to the final market image. Such an approach is generally discouraged. Even when it is acceptable from a clinical point of view, it is dangerous from the regulatory one (even when discussed with the authorities in the planning stage). Often further **studies** will be required, which will have to show **bioequivalence** (that is, that different formulations of the same active compound are equivalent in their pharmacokinetic profile, see below), or pharmacodynamic equivalence, or even therapeutic equivalence (see below and chapter 11). These additional studies can take more time than the time saved by starting the pivotal studies without the final formulation, and provide no guarantee of a result that supports equivalence between service and final formulation. The worst potential outcome is that the pivotal studies must be repeated.

Scale-up of production and quality control. Initially, both the drug substance and the drug product are produced "manually". This is obviously extremely laborious and yields very small quantities, which can be measured, in the case of the active compound, in the order of grams (or milligrams). As the preclinical process progresses, and more departments need access to the active compound, production must be transferred to dedicated laboratories, capable of scaling-up to much larger quantities, in the order of kilograms (sometimes referred to as "kilo-labs"). Naturally, we are still far from the amounts required for the market. Production on the scale needed for the market requires automated processes with the appropriate infrastructure, often in sterile environments. Even if the decision regarding the investments for mass production is made later in the development process, the design and testing of the machinery must start "at risk" very early. In fact, often, such machines can not simply be purchased off the shelf, but must undergo more or less radical modifications compared to the commercially available products, in order to meet unique manufacturing requirements of a given drug. Not infrequently, nothing suitable is available from the market and the machinery must be designed and built almost "from scratch". Going back to the investment decision for the manufacturing equipment and facilities, it is an extremely complex and risky one. If the decision is made too soon, one may end up with entire buildings full of equipment ready for a drug that will never come. The "recycling" of such investments is possible, but it is generally partial, causing large financial losses. On the other hand, if the decision is made too late, one risks not being ready for the market. The drug is approved, the medical community is ready for it, but the "launch" must be delayed by six months or one year because supplies are not ready. Both types of mistakes can potentially bring entire companies to their knees. Finally, we must mention briefly the quality control procedures, aimed at guaranteeing that the processes, the analytical methods and the products satisfy the predefined quality standards. Quality control procedures must be in place right from the beginning of preclinical experimentation. In fact, drug batches of inappropriate quality can invalidate the results of experiments in practically every preclinical area, from formulation development, to pharmacokinetics and toxicology (see below).

Toxicology. The lead compound, once selected, must undergo a long sequence of **toxicology studies** in various animal species, starting with single dose acute toxicology tests and continuing with multiple dose tests, the duration of which depends on the expected duration of treatment in the clinical setting (drugs to be taken for a lifetime require much longer toxicology investigations than drugs to be taken for short periods of time). Toxicology includes also **teratogenicity studies** (investigating the potential of causing birth defects), **carcinogenicity studies** (investigating the potential of causing cancer), and **fertility studies**. The toxicology research program continues well after the start of clinical trials. However, specific toxicology studies must be completed before the start of each phase of clinical development. Detailed national and international guidelines regulate the chronology and duration of toxicology investigations and their relationship to the phases of clinical development and to the duration of clinical trials.

Preclinical pharmacology: pharmacokinetics and pharmacodynamics. The pharmacokinetic and pharmacodynamic characteristics of the lead compound are studied intensely in animal models before clinical experimentation begins. As a reminder, **pharmacokinetics** is the branch of pharmacology that studies what the body does to the drug (absorption, distribution, metabolism and excretion – ADME), while **pharmacodynamics** studies what the drug does to the organs and systems of the body. Preclinical pharmacology studies can be "**ex-vivo**", i.e. conducted on isolated biological systems such as cell lines or blood, and "**in-vivo**", i.e. conducted on intact, living animals.

Promotion of a potential drug to clinical research. From this brief overview one can understand how significant an event the promotion of a potential drug to clinical experimentation is to the hundreds of preclinical researchers involved in the process. It is also a rare event. It has been calculated that the ratio between the number of molecules undergoing initial mass screening and the number of molecules promoted to clinical experimentation is on the order of 250,000 to 1 [87]. All other molecules are lost along the way, the majority during the early phase of screening, but some at advanced stages, after much work and hope have been invested in them.

12.2. The Phases of Clinical Development

12.2.1. Introduction

The preclinical research "champions" are the "newborns" of clinical research. They must undergo another cycle of experimentation, just as complex as and much more expensive than the previous one, this time on the human species.

The term "clinical" is used to mean "on human subjects". Clinical experimentation takes place in phases, from small studies on few subjects, strictly selected and closely followed, to very large studies in patients with heterogeneous characteristics and in a context similar to clinical practice. By convention, clinical drug development is divided into four phases, indicated with roman numerals I to IV, which will be discussed in the following paragraphs. However, it is important to point out that the succession of phases, as well as the content of each phase, are flexible and change from project to project.

As the clinical experimentation proceeds and the degree of certainty surrounding the therapeutic potential of a new compound increases, experiments proceed in parallel in many non-clinical areas, from toxicology to production, becoming more complex and ambitious, in preparation for the more advanced clinical phases and eventually for commercialization.

12.2.2. Phase I

Phase I is the phase of clinical experimentation which starts with the first administration of the drug to humans. Traditionally it is carried out on healthy volunteers. The complexity of the meaning of "healthy" was discussed in chapter 6 (section 6.1.1).

Two are the main objectives of phase I:
- Obtain indications on the safety and tolerability of the drug over a wide range of doses.
- Study the pharmacokinetic properties of the drug in man.

If the phase I studies are performed on patients, instead of healthy volunteers (see below), a third objective is added:
- Obtain preliminary pharmacodynamic indications.

In a typical first phase I study ("first in man"), a sequence of increasing single doses is used. The selection of the dose range to test in the initial studies in man is a difficult choice, loaded with downstream consequences on the drug development process. Generally, the outcome of animal toxicology tests on the most sensitive species is used as a starting point. Often (although not always), these experiments allow the so-called **maximum tolerated dose** or "non-toxic effect level" (NTEL) to be determined. It is the highest dose that can be administered to the animal without observing undesired effects considered unacceptable. The maximum tolerated dose in the animal is then converted to a dose considered equivalent in man, allowing for the different weight and/or body surface (and sometimes other variables). The highest dose used in phase I studies is, generally, a fraction of the human dose corresponding to the maximum tolerated dose in the most sensitive relevant animal species (relevant in the sense that the metabolic processes under study are similar to those in man). Once the highest dose is established, four to five fractions are selected (with the help of dose-response curves in animals, whenever possible), to complete the dose range to be tested in the first phase I study. The starting dose (the lowest one) is always much lower than the highest one. The entire dose selection process for human trials relies on the predictive value of the maximum tolerated dose in the chosen animal model. If the projected maximum tolerated dose in man is very different from the true (and unknown) one, the entire range of doses tested in man would be too low or too high. If too low, the drug will be less efficacious, if too high, more toxic, compared to its true potential. In both cases, often, it will not progress to phase II. In our experience, basing the choice of the dose range to test in phase I exclusively on animal data is often unsatisfactory and establishes a kind of "original sin" that is carried throughout the clinical development process. In our opinion, in some situations it would be scientifically and ethically preferable not to rely heavily on animal data for predicting doses in man, especially when it is known that the available animal models are not predictive (not an uncommon scenario). In these cases, one should find the courage to rely almost entirely on the human species. When the animal model does not work, the risk of testing completely wrong dose ranges (possibly too high!) in phase I is high. One could instead start with a very low dose (the order of magnitude of which could still be obtained from limited animal toxicology experiments), and then very carefully increase it, in numerous steps, the number depending on the compound under development. The advantage of not having to rely on extrapolations made from other species is clear.

Once the dose range is selected, each dose is first studied as a single administration. The subjects are divided into groups and the experimentation starts with the group assigned to the lowest dose. Often the dose escalation randomized design is used, as illustrated in chapter 10 (section 10.4.1). In phase I studies, the subjects are kept under very close observation, repeatedly questioned regarding the onset of undesired signs or symptoms and required to undergo numerous laboratory and instrumental investigations, the nature and chronology of which depend on the characteristics of the drug and the target disease. Furthermore, the volunteers undergo repeated sampling of biological fluids, in order to build the pharmacokinetic profile of the drug under investigation. If the researchers are satisfied with the safety and tolerability of the first dose, they move to the dose immediately above it, then to the third dose and so on. The study ends when either a dose presenting side effects considered unacceptable, or the highest dose is reached. We wish to point out, once again, that the decision on whether to move to the next dose, or not, i.e. stop the study, is only occasionally obvious; more frequently, it is not obvious at all. Such a decision relies heavily on the subjective judgment and experience of the researchers.

The doses considered safe and well tolerated in the single dose study are then tested in one or more multiple-dose studies (i.e. with repeated dosing), the duration of which depends on both the toxicology data available at the time the study starts (often the limiting factor) and the type of disease under study. The same dose-escalation design is used, although often with a narrower range of doses (a higher starting dose and/or a lower final dose), based on the results of the previous single dose study.

If more than one therapeutic regimen is considered (for example, once and twice daily regimens), phase I may require more than one multiple dose study. Furthermore, quite frequently, ancillary pharmacokinetic studies are performed, for example, comparing administration in a fasting state with that following a meal, or studies testing the pharmacokinetic interaction of the experimental drug with drugs that are likely to be administered concomitantly. However, more often, such "special" studies are performed in phase II or III (see below).

As mentioned at the beginning of this section, generally phase I is performed on healthy volunteers. The use of healthy volunteers in phase I, instead of patients suffering from the disease under study, is based on three assumptions.

- Methodological: it is assumed that adverse events are less frequent in healthy volunteers than in patients, making it easier to establish a causal link between the drug and the observed adverse events.
- Ethical: it is assumed that in the early stages, the human testing of a drug is ethically more acceptable in healthy subjects than in sick subjects.
- Logistical: it is assumed that for these kinds of studies it is easier and faster to recruit healthy volunteers than patients.

In our opinion, the only truly valid assumption is the last, the logistical one. It is indeed very difficult in the relatively restricted pool of patients with a specific condition, to find those who have the time and the inclination to submit themselves to the intensive investigations required for a phase I study (even if the subject is paid). On the contrary, in the much larger pool of the general "healthy" population, it is relatively easy to find subjects willing to volunteer for this type of study. On the other hand, the methodological and ethical arguments are both difficult to support. From the methodological point of view, investigations on subjects treated with placebo have demonstrated that healthy volunteers suffer from all sorts of adverse events unrelated to study drug, to an extent similar to placebo-treated patients. From the ethical point of view, one should remember that, because of the intense monitoring, the risk of serious adverse events in phase I studies is very low, despite some well known episodes of catastrophic outcome of phase I studies. Furthermore, in oncology, where drugs are very toxic, the opposite ethical argument is used, and phase I studies for anticancer drugs are traditionally performed in terminally ill patients.

12.2.3. Phase II

Phase II is performed on patients affected by the disease under study. Generally, the patient selection criteria for phase II are more restrictive compared to phase III, in the sense that subjects with serious or atypical forms of the disease and those with concomitant diseases or laboratory abnormalities are generally excluded. Such an approach has advantages and disadvantages: on the one hand, the drug is tested under the best conditions for demonstrating a pharmacodynamic effect and a dose-response relationship (see below), since subjects with serious or atypical form of the disease, or with multiple diseases are often the most resistant to therapy; on the other hand, the ability of phase II studies to predict the true therapeutic value of the drug is limited by this choice.

The main objectives of phase II are the following:

- Prove that the drug is active on relevant pharmacodynamic end-points.
- Select the dose (or doses) and the frequency of administration for phase III.
- Obtain safety and tolerability data.

Sometimes phase II is sub-divided into two "sub-phases".

- Phase IIa aimed at proof of concept.
- Phase IIb aimed at dose selection (referred to as dose-finding or dose-ranging).

The **proof of concept studies (phase IIa)** are particularly useful when dealing with an innovative compound. Their aim is to confirm in man the basic biological and pharmacodynamic concepts concerning the mechanism of action of the new drug. Such concept, before phase II, is based only on "proofs" on in vitro and animal models, generally with service formulations.

In a proof of concept study, the drug is put in the best conditions to show efficacy.

- The sample is rigorously selected, in that only subjects with a "pure", text book-like clinical picture are included, while subjects with severe, atypical or mixed forms, as well as those with concomitant diseases, are excluded.
- The chosen dose is the highest that can be administered based on phase I results (unless there are reasons to believe that a lower dose might be more efficacious).
- The chosen pharmacodynamic model is validated and accepted, for example diastolic blood pressure for antihypertensive drugs or lung function after metacholine challenge for antiasthma drugs. This third criterion is generally the most difficult to achieve, sometimes because a valid and recognized pharmacodynamic model does not exist, but more often because researchers cannot resist the temptation of using new models, which they believe to be better than the established ones. By doing so, the new drug and the new model are tested at the same time. If the results of the study are disappointing, one will never know whether to attribute them to the failure of new drug or of the new model.
- The selected center is highly specialized in performing studies of this kind.

Proof of concept studies are generally small and complex. They are of high strategic importance, because, if the concept is not proven, the development of the drug is stopped. Naturally, the criteria to decide whether or not to continue development must be established before knowing the results. The great advantage of this approach is that, if a drug does not show a sufficient pharmacodynamic action, it is possible to discontinue its clinical development when the investments (in terms of both time and resources) are still relatively limited, i.e. before entering the long and extremely costly phase IIb and – even more – phase III studies. The disadvantage is that the future of the drug depends entirely on a small pharmacodynamic study, especially on the adequacy of the pharmacodynamic model and the competence and skills of the investigators.

As for the dose selection, unfortunately, quite often, preclinical results cannot be easily transferred to the living human and to the formulation of the drug chosen for the clinical trials (which once again casts serious doubts on the usefulness of many animal experiments). Studies for the choice of the dose, commonly called **dose-finding** or **dose-ranging** (**phase IIb**), have the main objective of selecting the dose or the doses and the frequency of administration to be tested in phase III. Secondary objectives of such studies are to obtain information on the pharmacodynamic and sometimes therapeutic activity of the drug. When phase IIa is not carried out, they also serve as the proof of concept. Such studies have special methodological and practical problems that cannot be discussed in this book. We refer the interested reader to the ICH guideline [59] and to the previously cited articles by Ruberg [85, 86].

Traditionally, a number of so-called "special" studies, the objective of which is to investigate the action of the drug in "special" conditions or subgroups of patients, are also assigned to phase II. These include:

- Studies in elderly patients.
- Studies comparing different races.
- Studies in patients with hepatic or renal insufficiency.
- Studies evaluating interactions between the new drug and other drugs of common use in the disease under study.
- Studies evaluating interactions between the new drug and food and/or water.

These "special" studies are defined phase II studies because the treatment duration is relatively short and the end-points are of pharmacokinetic and/or pharmacodynamic nature. However, chronologically they are usually carried out during phase III, once the "concept" has been validated and the dose selected.

12.2.4. Phase III

Phase III has two key goals:

- To demonstrate the therapeutic efficacy of the drug in a representative sample of the population at which the treatment is targeted, generally by means of at least two well designed and adequately performed independent studies (see section 12.2.5).
- To demonstrate the safety and tolerability of the drug in a sufficiently large sample of the population at which the drug is targeted, by means of studies of sufficiently long duration, compared to the intended duration of the treatment in clinical practice.

The "therapeutic" efficacy is different from the "pharmacodynamic" efficacy demonstrated in phase II. For example, in the treatment of osteoporosis, bone density is a pharmacodynamic variable from which the end-points commonly used in phase II are derived. In fact, bone density is a "biomarker" of the process of bone weakening (see section 4.9). An end-point of therapeutic importance, in this case, could be the incidence of bone fractures. A drug capable of increasing density of the femoral or vertebral bone (or of slowing down its spontaneous decrease) shows promise with regard to reducing the frequency of fractures in elderly patients (such fractures are one of the main causes of morbidity, deterioration of quality of life and mortality in this population). If the pharmacodynamic end-point were a perfect surrogate (that is, highly correlated to the clinical end-point and capable of completely capturing the net effect of a treatment on the same clinical end-point - see again section 4.9), there would be no need to demonstrate the efficacy of the drug on the clinical end-point. Unfortunately, this rarely happens. For example, as illustrated in section 4.9, bone density does not capture a sufficient proportion of the net effect of treatments on the incidence fractures to allow its use as a primary end-point in phase III (the probability of suffering a fracture also depends on the three-dimensional microscopic architecture of the bone and on factors that have nothing to do with bone, such as the subject's balance and muscular strength). For this reason, in the majority of cases, phase III studies must use clinical end-points (see also section 4.2.2).

As usual, there are exceptions.

- In some cases pharmacodynamic end-points are accepted as clinically relevant in pivotal phase III studies. Diastolic blood pressure for antihypertensive drugs and forced expiratory volume in 1 second (FEV1) for bronchodilators are two examples. Such situations are often a combination of science and tradition. Diastolic pressure and FEV1 are surrogates with "acceptable" predictive value for clinical endpoints (a low FEV1 is predictive of shortness of breath; a high diastolic pressure is predictive of cardio- and cerebrovascular events), but, most importantly, have been used for registration purposes for decades.

- There are serious diseases for which no cure is available, where it is appropriate to approve a drug and make it available to patients based on efficacy demonstrated exclusively on pharmacodynamic end-points, instead of waiting for the conclusions of studies on clinical end-points, normally requiring many years. A typical example is represented by the antiretroviral drugs in the treatment of AIDS, already mentioned in section 4.9. It is important for patients and doctors to be aware that unpleasant surprises may occur once the studies on the clinical end-points are completed. For example, survival studies with zidovudine (AZT) mono-therapy in AIDS, completed many years after registration of the drug (based on efficacy demonstrated on a single surrogate end-point), gave relatively disappointing results.

Phase III has a "confirmatory" role not only for efficacy, but also for safety and tolerability of the treatment. The number of patients treated and the treatment duration must be such that it can be concluded that the drug is sufficiently safe and well tolerated to be approved and made available to doctors and patients. This is another very complex area that will be covered only briefly here.

The duration of the treatment depends on the disease being studied: at one end of the spectrum are treatments designated to be used only occasionally for one or few days, for example anesthetics or some antibiotics; at the opposite end are treatments that must be taken for a lifetime (at times starting from childhood), such as inhaled corticosteroids in the treatment of asthma. The duration of phase III studies for treatments designated to be administered for many years or for a lifetime, generally ranges from 1 to 3 years. This treatment duration may seem very brief for therapies lasting 30-40 years or longer (as in the case of chronic diseases). However, postponing for many years the introduction of an efficacious treatment is just as problematic at multiple levels.

- Methodological: longitudinal studies lasting many years are very difficult, if not impossible, to perform and, unless one treats a substantial part of the entire population, a rare adverse event due to the experimental drug will not be separable from the background noise resulting from biological variability.
- Ethical: patients would be left without a potentially important therapeutic option for years, in order to increase the degree of comfort concerning long term safety and tolerability.
- Commercial: without revenues, there are very few companies or institutions that can sustain studies of such duration.

With increasing frequency, health authorities deal with this kind of dilemma by imposing studies to test long-term safety (both experimental and observational), after the introduction of the drug on the market (i.e. in phase IV, see below).

A typical phase III database includes between 2000 and 5000 patients treated with the experimental drug, as well as patients treated with placebo and active controls. Sometimes, however, the numbers are considerably higher.

Finally, more and more frequently, it is required to demonstrate the impact of the new treatment on health care and social resources. No health care system, including those of the richest countries, can sustain an indiscriminate influx of high cost new treatments. For a new treatment to be "reimbursed" by public and private health insurance funds, it must bring cost savings in other areas. For example, a new drug can decrease the duration of hospitalization or of days in intensive care units, allow home assistance to replace hospitalization, reduce the amount of social service support needed, decrease the quantity and number of concomitant drugs, decrease the number of days missed at work or school, and so on. The science that studies the socio-economic impact of treatments and other health care solutions is called pharmaco-economics. Socio-economic studies and socio-economic end-points (see section 4.9) included in clinical studies are now an integral part of clinical development in phases III and IV. An increasing number of regulatory and reimbursement authorities require such studies for every new treatment, in order to establish the market price, determine the level of reimbursement, or even as a condition for obtaining regulatory approval.

12.2.5. Registration Dossier

The approval of a new drug by regulatory authorities is the main goal, though not the only one (see below), of a development program.

The large phase III pivotal studies have the role of providing conclusive proof of the safety, tolerability and efficacy of the new drug in a given disease and population. However, all the data generated on the drug must be summarized and discussed in a logical and comprehensive way in the **registration dossier**, to be submitted to the regulatory authorities as the basis of the request for approval. The dossier is divided into various sections, each corresponding to a development area:

- Physico-chemical characteristics and pharmaceutical formulation.
- Delivery device (if applicable).
- Production and quality control.
- Toxicology.
- Pharmacology.
- Pharmacokinetics.
- Clinical evidence.

In its entirety, a registration dossier is an impressively large and complex document (hundreds of thousands of pages or the electronic equivalent).

Concerning the clinical evidence, for each registration typically two independent phase III studies are needed; each appropriately designed and powered to prove the primary objectives. There are, however, numerous exceptions to this rule. For example, when one of the pivotal studies does not provide straightforward results, it may be necessary to perform one or more additional pivotal studies. On the other hand, for dossiers that expand the population of an original dossier, for example to pediatric or geriatric patients, one phase III pivotal study is generally sufficient. On the topic of a single pivotal study see also section 12.4.

As mentioned above, not only the pivotal studies, but all available clinical data, those generated by the company or institution (referred to as the sponsor) and those generated by third parties and published in the literature, must be summarized and discussed in a series of "integrated" documents, the detailed structure of which is determined by the regulatory authorities such as the **Food and Drug Administration (FDA)** in United States, the **European Medicines Agency (EMEA)** in the European Community, the **Ministry of Health Labor and Welfare (MHLW)** in Japan, and other national authorities.

The last 15 years have seen a large international effort to harmonize the requirements and standards of many aspects of the development and approval process and registration documents for both pharmacological and non-pharmacological treatments. Such effort became tangible with the joint approval of the documents of the **International Conference on Harmonization (ICH)** (see the ICH web-site: www.ich.org). These are consolidated guidelines that must be followed in the clinical development process and in the preparation of the registration dossiers in all the three regions covered by the ICH: Europe, Japan, United States.

With regard to the registration dossier, the ICH process culminated with the approval of the "**Common Technical Document**" (**CTD**). The CTD is the common format of the registration dossier recommended by EMEA, FDA and MHLW. It is organized in five modules, each composed of several sections. The structure of the CTD is summarized in Table 12.1.

The clinical overviews of the CTD replace the integrated documents specific to individual regulatory authorities such as:

- FDA's Integrated Summary of Efficacy and Integrated Summary of Safety.
- EMEA's Expert Report and Clinical Data Summary of Results and Statistical Analysis.

In practice, in spite of the great advancements in the harmonization process, regional differences abound, both in format and content, particularly for Japan. Furthermore, it is important to keep in mind that the ICH guidelines are intended as true guidelines, as opposed to rigid bureaucratic impositions: if there is a good scientific reason (for example, an uncertain safety profile) or administrative reason, it is absolutely legitimate for a regulatory authority to request a registration dossier different from that called for by the ICH guidelines.

In order to keep within the boundaries of this book, it is impossible to do justice to the complex issues raised by the integrated documents. All we can do is to touch upon four key points.

Pooling of the databases. The integration of the results implies the pooling of the databases of multiple studies into one or more common **integrated databases**, from which analyses and evaluations on the entire population studied or on sub-groups of the population are carried out. This is done in the assessment of efficacy, for example, for special groups, such as the elderly or subjects with renal or hepatic failure, and, even more, in the assessment of safe-

Table 12.1.   Structure of the Common Technical Document (CTD)

Module	Title
1	Regional administrative information and overall table of contents
2	Overviews:
	2.1 Table of contents
	2.2 Introduction
	2.3 Overview of quality
	2.3S Active compound
	2.3P Pharmaceutical product
	2.4 Preclinical overviews
	2.5 Clinical overviews
	2.5.1 Rationale for the development of the product
	2.5.2 Biopharmaceutical overview
	2.5.3 Clinical pharmacology overview
	2.5.4 Efficacy overview
	2.5.5 Safety overview
	2.5.6 Conclusions on benefits and risks
	2.5.7 Bibliography
	2.6 Written and tabulated preclinical summary
	2.7 Clinical summary
3	Quality
4	Non-clinical study reports
5	Clinical study reports

ty and tolerability. In the assesment of safety, data on adverse events and laboratory tests of all available studies, or most of them, must be "pooled" into integrated databases, on which sub-group analysis by age, sex, dose, etcetera, are performed. The merger of databases coming from different studies requires detailed planning at the beginning of the project. The more complete the harmonization of procedures and programming conventions of the individual studies constituting the clinical development program, the easier the final pooling. Vice versa, the lack of such harmonization will necessitate an extenuating ad hoc programming effort at the end of the development process, which will inevitably require a number of arbitrary assumptions and coding decisions, in order to harmonize the data collected in the different studies. In some cases, this can reduce the reliability of the integrated database.

Integrated reports. The **integrated reports** of efficacy and safety must not be an endless series of summaries – all given the same importance - of the results from the various studies. Instead, a convincing overview requires strict prioritization, where more space is given to the results of pivotal studies, as well as an intense effort of transparency in the critical discussion of results: the negative aspects of the pharmacological and clinical profile of the new drug must be identified and discussed, never minimized or, even worse, hidden. There is no drug (or treatment of any nature), which does not have negative aspects in the efficacy profile and potentially serious side effects. The aim of an integrated report must be to demonstrate that the balance between positive and negative aspects of the treatment under study (the so-called **benefit/risk ratio**) is, all things considered, favorable for the majority of patients and for the healthcare system. An integrated report attempting to show that there are no problems and that everything is positive becomes a marketing operation, as naïve as it is counterproductive, which renders the review by and the interaction with regulatory authorities much longer, more complex and convoluted.   ·

Meta-analysis. It is almost always useful to perform proper **meta-analyses**, that is, analyses on the integrated databases. Glass [49] gave the original definition: "the meta-analysis is the statistical analysis of a large collection of results from individual trials for the purpose of integrating the findings". In the clinical-regulatory context, the definition can be found in the above mentioned ICH guideline [61]: "the formal evaluation of the quantitative evidence from two or more trials bearing on the same question". On the efficacy front, a meta-analysis cannot be considered a substitute for phase III pivotal trials, each of which must be designed so as to reach its objectives "in its own right" (there are rare exceptions to this rule – see [37]). Nevertheless, meta-analyses are generally recognized as a useful instruments for:

a. Summarizing clinical results (the estimate of the treatment effect made on large databases, such as the integrated ones, is more precise than that obtained from individual studies).

b. Evaluating apparently conflicting results from individual studies.

c. Performing sub-group analyses.

d. Evaluating secondary end-points.

e. Evaluating the value of potential surrogate end-points (see section 4.9).

For items c, d and e, in general, individual clinical studies do not have enough power to reach reliable conclusions.

Naturally, meta-analyses are more valuable if planned prospectively, that is, before knowing the results of the studies. On the safety and tolerability front, the role of meta-analysis is even more crucial. Generally, individual studies are undersized in the context of statistically detecting infrequent adverse events (for example, at an 80% power, approximately 1600 patients are needed to observe at least one patient reporting an adverse event with 0.1% probability of occurrence). A meta-analysis performed on integrated databases is therefore indispensable when formally submitting one or more rare events to statistical analysis. Clearly, for the meta-analysis to make sense, the integrated studies must have a certain degree of similarity with regard to design, patient selection, time of exposure to treatment, adverse event definition and detection methods, etcetera. On the topic of meta-analysis, we recommend the book by Hedges and Olkin [56].

Summary of product characteristics. The summaries of the product characteristics, which are added to each commercial package of the drug, are probably the most important integrated documents. Great attention must be paid to them, in both format and content. In these documents, the disease and the type of patients for which the use of the treatment is permitted are described, together with the clinical advantages and disadvantages, contraindications and precautions, the main pharmacokinetic, pharmacodynamic and toxicological characteristics, the modality of use and the permitted dosages. In many countries two versions are required. One, known as the **Package Insert** (PI) in the United States and **Summary of Product Characteristics** (SPC) in Europe, is addressed to the doctors; the other, the **Patient Information Sheet** is tailored for the patients. The latter uses simpler language and is more difficult to prepare. These documents have, first and foremost, a crucial medical value, being the only documents available to both the doctor and the patient as a guide to the correct use of the treatment. Then, they have legal value, in case of legal proceedings of any kind. Finally, they determine the limits of the advertising campaigns and, therefore, have an enormous value for the marketing departments: the addition or omission of just one word in the package insert can allow or preclude highly efficient advertisement in the campaign against competitors and ultimately determine the commercial success of the new treatment.

12.2.6. Phase IV

Clinical experiments on a new treatment are far from over when it is approved and introduced onto the market. Despite the marketing authorization by a health authority, outstanding questions always outnumber the answers.

The expression **phase IV** is used to indicate the set of clinical studies performed after the approval of a new drug within the approved indication(s) and restrictions imposed by the Summary of Product Characteristics.

It is important to stress the fact that studies performed after approval, but on different indications or outside of the restrictions imposed by the SPC (for example, new dose strengths or regimens, special populations, use with contraindicated concomitant medications) are not phase IV studies. They are phase I to III studies, generally part of a new development process, which requires new pivotal studies and a new registration dossier, in order to obtain approval for a broader population or range of concomitant medications, a new indication or dosage, etcetera.

Sometimes, a distinction is made between studies performed after submission of the registration dossier, but before approval by regulatory authorities, referred to as phase IIIb studies, and studies performed entirely after approval, the proper phase IV studies. Others use the term phase IV to indicate both of these categories. In this book, we will adopt the latter definition.

Phase IV studies can have many different aims, among which are the following:

- Comparisons between the new treatment and frequently used current treatments (in phase II and III, a maximum of one or two active controls are tested, if at all, not rarely the only comparison being with the placebo).
- Pharmaco-economic assessments, intended to extend the information obtained in phase III.
- Safety assessments via clinical trials and/or **pharmaco-vigilance studies**; the latter are large observational studies aimed at evaluating the safety of the new treatment on samples of patients much larger than those used in phase III and in a context much closer to the reality of clinical practice. Such studies are particularly useful for evaluating rare and/or delayed adverse events, i.e. events appearing only after prolonged exposure to treatment, which generally cannot be quantified in the preregistration phase; an example is the assessment of the Churg-Strauss syndrome associated with leukotriene antagonists.
- Pharmacodynamic assessments.
- Assessments on subgroups of the patient population for which the treatment has been approved, for example, patients more seriously affected or more at risk.

Since the drug is available on the market, phase IV studies can be performed more easily by independent research groups, that is, not linked directly or indirectly to the pharmaceutical company producing the drug (and sponsor of the entire preregistration development process). This is a very positive situation, because it allows for independent verification of the efficacy and safety of a new drug. On the other hand, we must warn against uncritical acceptance of data generated by independent groups that contrast the conclusions of studies performed by the sponsor. Unfortunately, not rarely, the independent studies are underpowered and methodologically more problematic compared to those performed by pharmaceutical sponsors; furthermore, sometimes the so-called independent studies are only independent in respect of the company sponsoring a given product, but they are not at all independent in respect of other companies or the interests of the organization or research group who conducted the study. Therefore, we urge the reader to base his/her judgment on the quality of the study and of the publication, not on the affiliation of the authors or on a claimed absence of conflicts of interest.

12.2.7. Project Management

In this section, we wish to emphasize the importance of **project management.** In any project of the complexity, duration and cost of a clinical development program, the presence of one or more project managers of proven experience is absolutely vital. Among the functions of project management, the following are of the greatest importance for the success of the project.

- Coordination of the temporal sequence of activities performed in different departments. For example, a clinical trial cannot start if the preclinical toxicology studies of the required duration have not been completed and if the drug has not been shipped to the research centers.

- Coordination of the enormous quantity of scientific information generated over years of preclinical and clinical development. For example, suppose that in the course of the clinical development of a new beta-agonist, the results of pharmacology experiments show that the new drug has a smaller effect on the QT interval of the electrocardiogram compared to established drugs of the same class. Such an observation can translate into a major clinical and commercial advantage for the new drug, provided that it is recognized, brought to the attention of the clinical researchers, and tested in properly planned clinical trials.

- Management of unexpected negative events, both scientific and non-scientific. Over the course of the development process, the occurrence of negative events, from cost overruns, to the failure of a production cycle of the active component, to a possible side effect of the drug, is not an exception but an absolute certainty. Such events must be faced in a calm, transparent and decisive fashion, without falling into the two extremes of defeatism or denial.

- Finally, an efficient project manager must be prepared for the difficult task of recommending the interruption of the development of a drug when necessary, avoiding the mistake of dragging a project with no future into the late stages of development. The discontinuation of a "doomed" project, before the start of phase III, translates into a big advantage for the researchers and for the sponsor company, since it allows the funds and resources to be transferred to other projects. At any given time, there are always more projects proposed than are sustainable by the available financial and human resources.

12.3. The Phases of Clinical Development for Oncology Compounds

The contents of the previous sections reflect the traditional clinical development process, which applies to most pharmacological treatments. As already mentioned (see section 8.8 and 10.10), the development of oncology products is different, especially for phases I and II.

In general terms, oncology treatments can be grouped into two categories: cytotoxic and non-cytotoxic. Compounds of the former group are characterized by a mechanism of action that "kills" the cells, preferably, but not exclusively, the cancer cells. Those of the latter group, which includes, among others, cytostatic drugs, hormones, hormone modulators and vaccines, act by blocking, or more often delaying, the proliferation of tumor cells. Historically, cytotoxic compounds were developed first, and, over the course of years, the clinical development model in oncology has been tailored to such compounds. The classification in phases is the same for oncology products as for products developed in other therapeutic areas, but the objectives and designs of the studies included in each phase have many peculiarities.

12.3.1. Phase I

The primary objective of **phase I in oncology** is to identify the dose to be recommended for phase II studies. The basic assumption is that the higher the dose, the greater the efficacy. Since cytotoxic compounds typically show toxicity already at therapeutic (or even sub-therapeutic) doses, and almost always show a dose dependent increase in toxicity, the dose recommended for phase II is usually the highest dose associated with an acceptable level of toxicity. To identify this dose, a dose-escalation design is used (see chapter 10). Dose-escalation continues, in subsequent small cohorts of different patients, until an unacceptable toxicity level is reached, i.e. a toxicity so serious and/or severe, as to preclude any further dose increment. The medical adverse events (and the relevant seriousness/severity criteria) defining the **dose limiting toxicity** (DLT) for an individual patient must be defined before the start of the study. The threshold for an unacceptable percentage of patients with DLT at any given dose must also be established in the planning stage. A dose reaching this threshold frequency of patients with DLT will determine the end of the study. The next lower dose in the tested sequence is referred to as the maximum tolerated dose (MTD). The MTD is the dose recommended for phase II. Sometimes, the cohort receiving the MTD is enlarged, before recommending the MTD for phase II.

Because of the considerable toxicity of cytotoxic compounds, it is paramount that the risk to and the suffering of the enrolled patients be minimized. Usually this objective is achieved with phase I studies that:
- Use a very low starting dose, conventionally, about 1/10 or less of the human dose equivalent to the lethal dose in 10% of animals of the most sensitive animal species (the so-called LD10).

- Enroll patients in small cohorts (generally of three subjects).
- Adopt a cautious dose-escalation strategy. The sequence of doses is determined in different ways: a classic method consists of increasing the doses with decreasing relative increments. For example, the sequential increments are 100%, 65%, 50%, 40% and 30-35% of the previous dose (modified Fibonacci method). Recently, a number of alternative designs has been proposed, mainly with the goal of limiting the exposure of patients to sub-therapeutic doses and reaching the recommended dose as quickly as possible. On this topic the reader can refer to Eisenhauer et al [33].

Phase I studies can test a single compound or combinations of compounds. Typically, phase I studies enroll patients with different forms of cancer (although sometimes only with the cancer of interest) and in advanced or terminal stage.

12.3.2. Phase II

There are two principal objectives of **phase II** studies **in oncology**: confirming the pharmacodynamic action (activity) and obtaining a preliminary quantification of the clinical effect (efficacy). Activity is often measured as a yes/no response, where "yes" is generally defined as the combined frequency of two types of positive result: partial response (a reduction of the tumor mass of at least 30% to 50% as compared to the baseline condition) and complete response (a 100% reduction, i.e. disappearance of the tumor mass). Clearly, this end-point is appropriate only for solid tumors with measurable mass. It is conventionally used in phase II for many types of tumor, even if its value as a surrogate marker of survival is generally limited. Phase II studies are tumor-specific and frequently use "multi-stage" designs with no control group, of the type described in section 10.10. The rationale for the use of designs without a control group is given in section 8.8.

When the experimental treatment appears sufficiently active according to preestablished criteria, sometimes it proceeds to phase III but other times it is further experimented in randomized phase II trials, with or without control arms. These studies use typical phase II end-points, such as the tumor mass modification, and may or may not be fully comparative, i.e. they can be performed with sample sizes and early stopping rules that are traditionally used for non-randomized studies. The reader interested in this topic is referred to a paper by Simon et al (Simon R, Wittes RE, and Ellenberg SS (1985), Randomized Phase II Clinical Trials. Cancer Treat Rep 69:1375-1381).

12.3.3. Phase III

As for all other therapeutic areas, one primary objective of **phase III in oncology** is that of demonstrating the clinical efficacy of the new treatment. This is achieved through randomized trials with active control (the standard treatment for the disease under study). Generally, the primary end-point is linked to survival, often complemented by quality of life and pharmaco-economic data. The assessment of safety and tolerability is the other key objective of phase III studies in oncology. Again, this is the same as for other therapeutic areas. However, in oncology, one generally considers acceptable safety profiles that, as for the nature of the adverse events, their frequency, seriousness and severity, would instead be considered unacceptable in other areas.

Because of the seriousness of the oncologic conditions, and the absence of therapies capable of modifying their natural course, regulatory agencies often allow "shortened" development plans in order to facilitate registration. For example, the FDA allows the so-called "**Treatment IND**" [44], a set of regulations aimed at making treatments for very serious diseases available to patients not included in clinical trials before the development of such treatments has been fully completed, when there are no other therapeutic options. The sponsor is of course still required to carry out the pivotal trials to prove efficacy and safety. Another example, again adopted by FDA, is the so-called "**Subpart H**" [42], a set of regulations aimed at accelerating the development, evaluation and commercialization of products for the treatment of patients with life-threatening or seriously debilitating diseases.

These regulations are not limited to oncology treatments. For example, several AIDS treatments have achieved rapid registration in this way.

If the cancer under study is rare, it is possible to ask for "**Orphan Drug Status**" [45]. A compound given this status benefits from both shorter development plans, and longer patent protection.

The development of non-cytotoxic compounds is more recent. Sometimes the same development model used for cytotoxic compounds has been used for these compounds. Such an approach is limited by the fact that the assumptions that justify its use are not generally fulfilled.

1. The assumptions that the efficacy is proportional to the dose and that the dose is proportional to the toxicity are often wrong for non-cytotoxic agents. Therefore, the oncology phase I approach reported above is not justified, whereas the classic phase I designs are acceptable (see section 10.4.1), perhaps without the use of the placebo.

2. It may not be ideal to use the reduction of tumor mass as an end-point, because the mechanism of action is not that of "killing" the cancer cells; this makes the application of multi-stage phase II oncology studies very difficult, as they are based on binary end-points and require relatively short evaluation times. With non-cytotoxic compounds, end-points such as "time of stable disease" and "time to progression" are often used, and tested through classical randomized, controlled clinical trials.

Unfortunately, many non-cytotoxic compounds are still inadequately developed using the standard oncology development plan. It will be some time before the technical weaknesses of this approach are broadly recognized, hopefully leading to new, more appropriate solutions and new guidelines.

12.4. Accelerating Clinical Development

The time and costs of the clinical development process for new drugs are pro-hibitive. Therefore, in recent years, a faster, cheaper development has been a key objective in the pharmaceutical world (not only pharmaceutical companies, but also regulatory organizations and universities). The mean duration of clinical development has shifted from more than 7 years in 1993-1995 to about 5 years in 1999-2001, with considerable variations from one therapeutic area to another (Tufts Center for the Study of Drug Development, [2002], Impact Report 4). However, a reduction of development times is not always mirrored by a reduction in costs. In fact, in many areas costs are steadily increasing. It is clear that a reduction of costs is a priority for the future of research. However, here we will focus on the time factor.

Many methods have been proposed to accelerate clinical development. Clearly, there is no magic solution and no method is universally applicable. We shall briefly discuss some of the most promising approaches.

1. Avoid the repetition of studies, especially phase III studies, which are the longest and most expensive. For this purpose, it is very important to concentrate efforts on the initial part of the clinical development program, mainly on phase II. As mentioned above, this phase aims at validating the basic biological concept and at identifying the optimal dose to be used in phase III pivotal studies. If the dose selection is wrong, the phase III studies will fail and, at best, will have to be repeated. Useful methods to avoid unpleasant surprises include meta-analyses (see section 12.2.5) performed on the data that the sponsor collects over time on the new treatment, and **simulations**, a set of statistical techniques aimed at evaluating the consequences of a variety of assumptions, i.e. at answering "what happens if...?" questions. Typical uses of simulation include the following:

   - Evaluation of the power or other proprieties of statistical tests on variation of the assumptions made on the signal, the sample size, the drop-out rate, etcetera.
   - Detection of bias, generated by statistical models not suitable to describe the experimental conditions of interest, by missing data or by other violations of the protocol.
   - Comparison of alternative study designs.
   - Evaluation of the consequences of different decision making rules in determining the success or failure of a study or an entire study program.

   An example of an application of simulation can be found in the article by Green and O'Sullivan [53].

2. Use strategies that combine different phases of development, mainly phase II and III. One way of reaching this objective is to carry out the studies of different phases in parallel or with partial overlap, rather than in sequence, as in the traditional development programs. For this purpose it may be helpful to include interim analyses in the phase II studies, with the objective of obtaining the information required for the planning of phase III studies (see

section 11.2). Another strategy is that of adopting adaptive designs (see section 11.3). Although generally still reluctant to accept such "shortcuts" for registration, FDA, EMEA and other regulatory authorities are moving in this direction, appreciating that an untenable development burden will result in a loss not only for the pharmaceutical companies, but for public health and society as a whole. Interesting changes in the development model can be expected in the next decade or so.

3. Make full use of the special regulatory options made available for the very purpose of accelerating the clinical development of life saving and essential drugs. Prominent among these are the "Treatment IND", the "Subpart H" and the "Orphan Drug Status" regulations reported in the section on oncology studies, which, however, are by no means exclusive to that therapeutic area. Recently, situations for which it is acceptable to obtain registration with a single pivotal study have been contemplated (see below).

4. Adopt technological innovations. For example, "**electronic data capture**" (**EDC**) is a technological platform allowing the entry of data into the central database directly at the study centers, or from the measurement instruments, without the intermediate step of the traditional paper case report forms (CRFs). EDC allows a considerable reduction in the time taken between the end of the study ("Last Patient Last Visit", LPLV) and database lock. Another example is the use of "**computerized registration dossiers**" (that is, directly submitted in electronic format), which reduces the revision time required by regulatory authorities.

5. Improve the professional qualifications and organizational skills of the teams responsible for planning and performing clinical trials. For example, the systematic use of project management techniques reduces waste and optimizes time by facilitating coordination across different functions.

With reference to the use of just one pivotal trial as the basis for requesting approval of a new drug, two documents must be considered [37, 43], one by EMEA, the other by FDA. Basically, such a model is viable when the primary endpoint is based on mortality or serious and irreversible morbidity (the treatment can be aimed at either prevention or cure). In order to be a candidate for the single pivotal study option in a registration dossier, the trial must be very large (and multi-center) and have a well-balanced distribution of the sample across the centers. Results must be persuasive overall and show excellent internal consistency, i.e. must be consistent across centers, across end-points and across relevant subgroups. Finally, the study should not have "grey areas" in the planning, performance or analysis. From a statistical point of view, "persuasive result" means that the p-value (two-sided) must be lower than 0.001, instead of 0.05, as conventionally required. There are three key reasons for moving the significance threshold to 0.001. First, "evidence" obtained in this way can be considered equivalent to that obtained from two independent studies, each performed at the level 0.05. Second, the probability of reproducing the results in a subsequent study is high (around 90%). Third, the confidence interval on the parameter of interest is narrow and far from zero (Robert O'Neil, personal communication, 2003).

As mentioned above, in clinical development, time savings are not necessarily mirrored by cost savings. Indeed, in many areas of clinical research, costs are becoming increasingly prohibitive, especially for small to middle size companies and for almost all public research organizations. It is easy to predict that, in the coming years, much effort will be devoted to further reducing both the time and the costs of the development of new drugs. Naturally, in cases of clinical and regulatory success, reduction of the development time will lead to earlier availability of the new treatment on the market, which, in cases of commercial success, will translate into a relevant financial benefit for the sponsor.

Summary

Clinical experiments are preceded by many years of preclinical development. In broad terms, the preclinical development process can be summarized in a sequence of seven large areas:

1. Screening of thousands of active compounds by means of biological assays.
2. Choice of the lead compound.
3. Synthesis and physico-chemical characterization of the lead compound.
4. Formulation of the drug product, consisting of the drug substance, excipients and delivery system.
5. Scale-up of production and quality control.
6. Toxicology.
7. Preclinical pharmacology, composed of pharmacokinetics (which studies what the body does to the drug: absorption, distribution, metabolism and excretion – ADME), and pharmacodynamics (which studies what the drug does to the different organs and body systems).

Conventionally, the clinical development of drugs is divided into four phases.

As the clinical experimentation proceeds and the level of confidence on the therapeutic potential of a new compound grows, experimentation also proceeds in many non-clinical areas, from toxicology to production, becoming increasingly complex, in preparation for the more advanced clinical phases and finally for commercialization.

Phase I begins with the first administration of the drug to man. The two objectives of phase I are:

a) To obtain indications on the safety and tolerability of the drug over a wide range of doses.
b) To study the pharmacokinetics of the drug in man.

If phase I studies are performed on patients, instead of healthy volunteers, a third objective is added.

c) To obtain preliminary pharmacodynamic indications.

Phase II is carried out on selected groups of patients suffering from the disease of interest, although patients with atypical forms and concomitant diseases are excluded. The main objectives of phase II are:

a) To demonstrate that the drug is active on the relevant pharmacodynamic end-points.
b) To select the dose (or doses) and frequency of administration for phase III.
c) To obtain safety and tolerability data.

Sometimes phase II is itself divided into two "sub-phases": IIa, for proof of concept; IIb, for dose-finding.

The aim of phase III is to demonstrate the therapeutic efficacy, safety and tolerability of the drug in a representative sample of the target population, with studies of sufficiently long duration relative to the treatment in clinical practice. The large phase III pivotal studies are to provide decisive proof in the registration dossier.

All data generated on the drug, from the preclinical stage to phase III (or even phase IV, when it has already been approved in other countries), must be summarized and discussed in a logical and comprehensive manner in the registration dossier, which is submitted to health authorities as the basis for the request of approval.

Clinical experimentation of a new treatment continues after its approval by health authorities and launch onto the market. Despite the approval, there are always many questions awaiting answers. Phase IV studies provide some of the answers. The expression "phase IV" is used to indicate clinical studies performed after the approval of a new drug and within the approved indications and restrictions imposed by the summary of product characteristics (also known as package insert).

The so-called cytotoxic drugs used in oncology have many peculiarities in their clinical development, mainly concerning phase I and II. These differences are determined mostly by the toxicity of these compounds, even at therapeutic or sub-therapeutic doses, combined with the life threatening nature of the diseases in question.

The search for methods and strategies to reduce the time and costs of clinical development is one of the central themes of methodological research.

Appendix

Areas under the Standard Normal Curve

Areas under the Standard Normal Curve

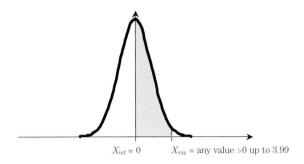

$X_{inf} = 0$ $X_{sup} =$ any value >0 up to 3.99

X_{sup}	0	1	2	3	4	5	6	7	8	9
0.0	0.0000	0.0040	0.0080	0.0120	0.0160	0.0199	0.0239	0.0279	0.0319	0.0359
0.1	0.0398	0.0438	0.0478	0.0517	0.0557	0.0596	0.0636	0.0675	0.0714	0.0754
0.2	0.0793	0.0832	0.0871	0.0910	0.0948	0.0987	0.1026	0.1064	0.1103	0.1141
0.3	0.1179	0.1217	0.1255	0.1293	0.1331	0.1368	0.1406	0.1443	0.1480	0.1517
0.4	0.1554	0.1591	0.1628	0.1664	0.1700	0.1736	0.1772	0.1808	0.1844	0.1879
0.5	0.1915	0.1950	0.1985	0.2019	0.2054	0.2088	0.2123	0.2157	0.2190	0.2224
0.6	0.2258	0.2291	0.2324	0.2357	0.2389	0.2422	0.2454	0.2486	0.2518	0.2549
0.7	0.2580	0.2612	0.2642	0.2673	0.2704	0.2734	0.2764	0.2794	0.2823	0.2852
0.8	0.2881	0.2910	0.2939	0.2967	0.2996	0.3023	0.3051	0.3078	0.3106	0.3133
0.9	0.3159	0.3186	0.3212	0.3238	0.3264	0.3289	0.3315	0.3340	0.3365	0.3389
1.0	0.3413	0.3438	0.3461	0.3485	0.3508	0.3531	0.3554	0.3577	0.3599	0.3621
1.1	0.3643	0.3665	0.3686	0.3708	0.3729	0.3749	0.3770	0.3790	0.3810	0.3830
1.2	0.3849	0.3869	0.3888	0.3907	0.3925	0.3944	0.3962	0.3980	0.3997	0.4015
1.3	0.4032	0.4049	0.4066	0.4082	0.4099	0.4115	0.4131	0.4147	0.4162	0.4177
1.4	0.4192	0.4207	0.4222	0.4236	0.4251	0.4265	0.4279	0.4292	0.4306	0.4319
1.5	0.4332	0.4345	0.4357	0.4370	0.4382	0.4394	0.4406	0.4418	0.4429	0.4441
1.6	0.4452	0.4463	0.4474	0.4484	0.4495	0.4505	0.4515	0.4525	0.4535	0.4545
1.7	0.4554	0.4564	0.4573	0.4582	0.4591	0.4599	0.4608	0.4616	0.4625	0.4633
1.8	0.4641	0.4649	0.4656	0.4664	0.4671	0.4678	0.4686	0.4693	0.4699	0.4706
1.9	0.4713	0.4719	0.4726	0.4732	0.4738	0.4744	0.4750	0.4756	0.4761	0.4767
2.0	0.4772	0.4778	0.4783	0.4788	0.4793	0.4798	0.4803	0.4808	0.4812	0.4817
2.1	0.4821	0.4826	0.4830	0.4834	0.4838	0.4842	0.4846	0.4850	0.4854	0.4857
2.2	0.4861	0.4864	0.4868	0.4871	0.4875	0.4878	0.4881	0.4884	0.4887	0.4890
2.3	0.4893	0.4896	0.4898	0.4901	0.4904	0.4906	0.4909	0.4911	0.4913	0.4916
2.4	0.4918	0.4920	0.4922	0.4925	0.4927	0.4929	0.4931	0.4932	0.4934	0.4936
3.0	0.4987	0.4987	0.4987	0.4988	0.4988	0.4989	0.4989	0.4989	0.4990	0.4990
3.1	0.4990	0.4991	0.4991	0.4991	0.4992	0.4992	0.4992	0.4992	0.4993	0.4993
3.2	0.4993	0.4993	0.4994	0.4994	0.4994	0.4994	0.4994	0.4995	0.4995	0.4995
3.3	0.4995	0.4995	0.4995	0.4996	0.4996	0.4996	0.4996	0.4996	0.4996	0.4997
3.4	0.4997	0.4997	0.4997	0.4997	0.4997	0.4997	0.4997	0.4997	0.4997	0.4998
3.5	0.4998	0.4998	0.4998	0.4998	0.4998	0.4998	0.4998	0.4998	0.4998	0.4998
3.6	0.4998	0.4998	0.4999	0.4999	0.4999	0.4999	0.4999	0.4999	0.4999	0.4999
3.7	0.4999	0.4999	0.4999	0.4999	0.4999	0.4999	0.4999	0.4999	0.4999	0.4999
3.8	0.4999	0.4999	0.4999	0.4999	0.4999	0.4999	0.4999	0.4999	0.4999	0.4999
3.9	0.5000	0.5000	0.5000	0.5000	0.5000	0.5000	0.5000	0.5000	0.5000	0.5000

(*) Areas of the sections from 0 to any positive value up to 3.99

References

1. ALLATH Collaborative Research Group (2002) Major outcomes in high-risk hypertensive patients randomized to angiotensin-converting enzyme inhibitor or calcium channel blockers vs. diuretics. JAMA 288: 2981-2997
2. Altman DG (1994) The scandal of poor medical research. BMJ 308, 283-284
3. Armitage P, Berry G (1987) Statistical methods in medical research. Blackwell Scientific Publications, Oxford.
4. Armitage P, Colton T (1998) Encyclopaedia of biostatistics. John Wiley & Sons, New York
5. Ast DB, Schlesinger ER (1956) The conclusion of a ten-year study of water fluoridation. Am J Public Health, 46: 265-271
6. Atkinson EN, Brown BW (1985) Confidence limits for probability of response in multistage clinical trials. Biometrics 41: 741-744
7. Azzalini A (1996) Statistical inference based on the likelihood. Chapman and Hall.
8. Bauer P, Kohne K (1994) Evaluation of experiments with adaptive interim analyses. Biometrics 50: 1029-1041
9. Beecher GH (1955) The powerful placebo. JAMA 159: 1602-1606
10. Bergner M, Bobbitt R, Carter W, Gibson B (1981) The sickness impact profile: development and final revision of a health status measure. Med Care 19: 787-805
11. Bero L, Remmie D (1995) The Cochran Collaboration: preparing, maintaining and disseminating systematic reviews of the effects of health care. JAMA 274: 1935-1938
12. Berry DA (1996) Statistics. A Bayesian perspective. Duxbury Press, Pacific Grove, CA
13. Biomarkers Definition Working Group (2001) Biomarkers and surrogate end-points in clinical trials: proposed definitions and conceptual framework. Clin Pharmacol Ther 69: 89-95
14. Bland JM, Altman DG (1986) Statistical methods for assessing agreement between two methods of clinical measurements. Lancet i: 307-310
15. Bland JM, Altman DG (1994) Regression towards the mean. BMJ 308:1499
16. Bland JM, Altman DG (1994) Some examples of regression towards the mean. BMJ 309:780

17. Bolton S (1990) Pharmaceutical statistics. Practical and clinical applications, 2nd edition. Marcel Dekker, New York/Basel
18. Box GEP, Tiao GC (1973) Bayesian inference in statistical analysis. Addison Wesley, Boston
19. Brown BW (1980) Statistical controversies in the design of clinical trials - some personal views. Control Clin Trials 1: 13-27
20. Brown DJ (2003) ICH E9 guideline. Statistical principles for clinical trials: a case study. Response to Phillips A and Haudiquet V. Stat Med 22: 13-17
21. Brusasco V, Crimi E, Gherson G, Nardelli R, Oldani V, Francucci B, Della Cioppa G, Senn S & Fabbri LM (2002) Actions other than smooth muscle relaxation may play a role in the protective effects of formoterol on the allergen-induced late asthmatic reaction. Pulm Pharmacol Ther 15: 399-406
22. Bryant J, Day R (1995) Incorporating toxicity considerations into the design of two-stage phase II clinical trials. Biometrics 51: 1372-1383
23. Byar DP, Piantadosi SP (1985) Factorial designs for randomized clinical trials. Cancer Treat Rep 69: 1055-1062
24. Cochran WG, Cox GM (1957) Experimental Designs, 2nd edition. John Wiley & Sons, New York
25. Colburn WA (2003) Biomarkers in drug discovery and development: from target identification through drug marketing. J Clin Pharmacol 43: 329-341
26. Colton T (1974) Statistics in medicine. Little Brown and Company.
27. Cox DR (1958) Planning of experiments. John Wiley & Sons, New York
28. Crane J, Pearce N, Flatt A, Burgess C, Jackson R, Kwong T, Ball M, Beasley R (1989) Prescribed fenoterol and death from asthma in New Zealand, 1981-1983: a case control study. Lancet i: 917-922
29. Dall'Aglio G (1987) Calcolo delle probabilità. Zanichelli, Bologna
30. Daniel WW (1987) Biostatistics: a foundation for analysis in the health sciences, 5th edition. John Wiley & Sons, New York
31. Davey Smith G, Ebrahim S (2002) Data dredging, bias or confounding. They can all get you into the BMJ and the Friday papers. BMJ 325: 1437-1438
32. Ederer F (1972) Serum cholesterol changes: effects of diet and regression toward the mean. J Chronic Dis 25: 277-289
33. Eisenhauer EA, O'Dwyer PJ, Christian M, Humphrey JS (2000) Phase I clinical trial design in cancer drug development. J Clin Oncol 18: 684-692
34. Ensign LG, Gehan EA, Kamen DS, Thall PF (1994) An optimal three-stage design for phase II clinical trials. Stat Med 13: 1727-1736
35. European Agency for Evaluation of Medicinal Products (EMEA) (1997) Note for guidance on medicinal products in the treatment of Alzheimer's Disease (CPMP/EWP/553/95).In www. emea.eu.int/index/indexh1.htm (see: Guidance Documents /Efficacy / Approved Guidelines)
36. European Agency for Evaluation of Medicinal Products (EMEA) (2000) Points to consider on switching between superiority and non-inferiority (CPMP/EWP/482/99). In www.emea.eu.int/index/indexh1.htm
37. European Agency for Evaluation of Medicinal Products (EMEA) (2001) Points to consider on application with: 1. meta-analysis; 2. one pivotal study (CPMP/EWP/2330/99). In www. emea.eu.int/index/indexh1.htm
38. European Agency for Evaluation of Medicinal Products (EMEA) (2006) Guideline on the choice of the non-inferiority margin (EMEA/CPMP/EWP/2158/99). In www. emea.eu.int/index/indexh1.htm
39. Fleiss JL (1986) The design and analysis of clinical experiments. John Wiley & Sons, New York
40. Fleming TR (1982) One sample multiple testing procedure for phase II clinical trials. Biometrics 38: 143-151
41. Fletcher AE, Gore SM, Jones D R, Fitzpatrick R, Spiegelhalter DJ, Cox DR (1992)

Quality of life measures in health care II: design, analysis and interpretation. BMJ 305: 1145-1148

42. Food and Drug Administration (FDA) Application for FDA approval to market a new drug (Part 314): Accelerated approval of new drugs for serious or life-threatening illnesses (Subpart H). In www.accessdata.fda.gov/scripts/cdrh/cfdocs/cfcfr/CFRSearch.cfm?CFRPart=314

43. Food and Drug Administration (FDA), Center for Drug Evaluation and Research (CDER) (1998) Guidance for industry: providing clinical evidence of effectiveness for human drugs and biological products. In www.fda.gov/cder/guidance/1397fnl.pdf

44. Food and Drug Administration (FDA) Investigational new drug application (Part 312): Treatment use of an investigational new drug (Subpart B-312.34). In www.accessdata.fda.gov/scripts/cdrh/cfdocs/cfcfr/CFRSearch.cfm?CFRPart=312

45. Food and Drug Administration (FDA). Orphan Drugs (Part 316). In www.accessdata.fda.gov/scripts/cdrh/cfdocs/cfcfr/CFRSearch.cfm?CFRPart=316

46. Friede T, Kieser M (2001) A comparison of methods for adaptive sample size adjustement. Stat Med 20:3861-3874

47. Gehan EA (1961) The determination of the number of patients required in a follow-up trial of a new chemotherapeutic agent. J Chronic Dis 13: 346-353

48. Gillings D, Kock G (1991) The application of the principle of intention-to-treat to the analysis of clinical trials. Drug Inform J; 25: 411-424

49. Glass GV (1976) Primary, secondary and meta-analysis of research. Educational Res 5: 3-8

50. Gould AL (1980) A new approach to the analysis of clinical drug trials with withdrawals. Biometrics: 36: 721-727

51. Gould AL (2001) Sample size re-estimation: recent developments and practical considerations. Statistics Med 20:2625-2643

52. Gould AL (2002) Substantial evidence of effect. J Biopharm Statist 12: 53-77

53. Green S, Liu PY, O'Sullivan J (2002) Factorial design considerations. J Clin Oncol 20: 3424-3430

54. Guyatt GH, Heyting AH, Jaeschke R, Adachi JD, Roberts RS (1990) N of 1 trials for investigating new drugs. Control Clin Trials 11: 88-100

55. Halperin M, Gordon KK, Ware JH, Johnson NJ, DeMets DL (1982) An aid to data monitoring in long-term clinical trials. Control Clin Trials 3: 311-323

56. Hedges LV, Olkin I (1985) Statistical methods for meta-analysis. Academic Press, New York

57. Hennekens CH, Buring JE (1987) Epidemiology in medicine. Little Brown and Company, Boston/Toronto

58. Hunt SM, McEwen J, McKenna SP (1986) Measuring health status. Croom-Helm, London

59. International Conference on Harmonization (ICH) ICH Topic E4: Note for guidance on dose response information to support drug registration (CPMP/ICH/378/95). In www.ich.org

60. International Conference on Harmonization (ICH) ICH Topic E6: Note for guidance on Good Clinical Practice (CPMP/ICH/135/95). In www.ich.org.

61. International Conference on Harmonization (ICH) ICH Topic E9: Note for Guidance on Statistical Principles for Clinical Trials (CPMP/ICH/363/96). In www.ich.org

62. International Conference on Harmonization (ICH) ICH Topic E10: Note for guidance on choice of control group in clinical trials (CPMP/ICH/364/96). In www.ich.org.

63. Kalish LA, Begg CB (1985) Treatment allocation methods in clinical trials: a review. Statistics Med 4: 129-144

64. Lachin JM, Shu-Ping L, the Lupus Nephritis Collaborative Study Group (1992) Termination of a clinical trial with no treatment group differences: the Lupus Nephritis Collaborative Study. Control Clin Trials 13: 62-79

65. Lange S (2001) The all randomized/full analysis set (ICH E9) - May patients be ex-

cluded from the analysis?" Drug Inform J 35: 881-891

66. Liberman R (1962) An analysis of the placebo phenomenon. J Chronic Dis 15: 761-783

67. Lilienfeld AM, Lilienfeld DE (1980) Foundations of epidemiology, 2nd edition. Oxford University Press, Oxford

68. Mariani L, Marubini E (1996) Design and analysis of phase II cancer trials: a review of statistical methods and guidelines for medical researchers. International J Review 64: 61-88

69. Marubini E, Valsecchi MG (1995) Analysing survival data from clinical trials and observational studies. John Wiley & Sons, New York

70. McLeod RS, Taylor DW, Cohen Z, Cullen JB (1986) Single-patient randomised clinical trial. Use in determining optimum treatment for patient with inflammation of Kock continent ileostomy reservoir. Lancet i: 726-728

71. Miettinen OS (1985) Theoretical epidemiology. Principles of occurrence research in medicine. John Wiley & Sons, New York

72. O'Brien PC, Fleming TR (1979) A multiple testing procedure for clinical trials. Biometrics 35: 549-556

73. O'Neill R (2002) Regulatory perspectives on data monitoring. Statistics Med 21:2831-2842.

74. Parmar MKB, Spiegelhalter DJ, Freedman LS (1994) The CHART trials design and monitoring. Statistics Med 13: 1297-1312

75. Phillips A, Haudiquet V (2003) ICH E9 guideline. Statistical principles for clinical trials: a case study. Statistics Med 22: 1-11

76. Piccinato L (1996) Metodi per le decisioni statistiche. Springer-Verlag Italy, Milan

77. Piccinato L (2001) Il concetto statistico di evidenza. Rapporto Tecnico Interno n° 8, Dipartimento di Statistica, Probabilità e Statistiche Applicate. In http://pow2.sta.uniroma1.it)

78. Pocock SJ, Highes MD, Lee RJ (1987) Statistical problems in the reporting of clinical trials: a survey of three medical journals. NEJM 317: 426-432

79. Pocock SJ (1983) Clinical trials. A practical Approach. John Whiley & Sons, New York.

80. Pompilj G, Dall'Aglio G (1959) Analisi degli esperimenti. Boringhieri, Torino

81. Posh M, Bauer P, Brannath W (2003) Issues in designing flexible trials. Statistics Med 22: 953-969

82. Powe NR, Griffiths RI (1995) The clinical-economic trial: promise, problems, and challenges. Control Clin Trials 16: 377-394

83. Prentice R (1989) Surrogate end-points in clinical trials: definition and operational criteria. Statistics Med 8: 431-440

84. Riggs BL, Hodgson SF, O'Fallon WM, Chao EJ, Wahner HW, Muhs JM, Cedel SL, Melton LJ (1990) Effect of fluoride treatment on the fracture rates in postmenopausal women with osteoporosis. NEJM 322: 802-809

85. Ruberg SJ (1995) Dose response studies. I. Some design consideration. J Biopharm Statist 5: 1-14

86. Ruberg SJ (1995) Dose response studies. II. Analysis and interpretation. J Biopharm Stat 5: 15-42

87. Rubin AA (Editor) (1978) New drugs: discovery and development. Marcel Dekker, New York/Basel

88. Sackett DL (1979) Bias in analytical research. J Chronic Dis 32: 51-63

89. Sackett DL, Richardson WS, Rosenberg WMC, Haynes RB (1997) Evidence Based Medicine: How to practise and teach EBM. Churchill Livingstone, Edinburgh

90. Sackett DL, Rosenberg WMC, Gray JAM, Richardson WS (1996) Evidence based medicine: what it is and what it isn't. BMJ 312: 71-72

91. Sankoh AJ (1999). Interim analyses: an update of an FDA reviewer's experience and perspective. Drug Inform J 33:165-176

92. Schultz JR, Nichol FR, Elfring GL, Weed SD (1973) Multiple stage procedures for drug screening. Biometrics 29: 293-300
93. Senn S (1993) Cross-over trials in Clinical Research. John Wiley & Sons, New York
94. Shirtcliffe P, Weatherall M, Beasley R (2002) An inverse correlation between estimated tubercolosis notification rate and asthma symptoms. Respirology 7:153
95. Simon R (1989) Optimal two-stage designs for phase II clinical trials. Control Clin Trials 10: 1-10
96. Spiegelhalter DJ, Freedman LS, Parmar MKB (1994) Bayesian approaches to randomised trials. JR Stat Soc 157: 357-416
97. Speigelhalter DJ, Abrams KR, Myles JP. (2004) Bayesian approaches to clinical trials and heath-care evaluation. John Wiley & Sons
98. Tan SB, Dear KBG, Bruzzi P, Machin D (2003) Strategy for randomized clinical trials in rare cancers. BMJ 327: 47-49
99. Thall PF, Simon R (1994) A Bayesian approach to establishing sample size and monitoring criteria for phase II clinical trials. Control Clin Trials 15: 463-481
100. Thall PF, Simon RM, Estey EH (1995) Bayesian sequential monitoring designs for single-arm clinical trials with multiple outcomes. Statistics Med 14: 357-379
101. Therasse P, Arbuck SG, Eisenhauer EA, Wanders J, Kaplan RS, Rubinstein L, Verweij J, van Glabbeke M, van Oosterom AT, Christian MC, Gwyther SG (2000) New guidelines to evaluate the response to treatment in solid tumors. J Natl Cancer Inst 92; 205-216
102. Ware J, Sherbourne CD (1992) The MOS 36-item short form health survey (SF-36). I. Conceptual framework and item selection. Med Care 30: 473-483
103. Webster's New World Dictionary, Third College Edition (1988), Simon & Shuster, New York
104. Wei LJ, Durham S (1978) The randomized play-the-winner rule in medical trials. JASA 73: 840-843
105. Wonnacott TH, Wonnacott RJ (1990) Introductory Statistics, 5th edition. Wiley and Sons, New York.
106. World Medical Association Declaration of Helsinki: Ethical Principles of Medical Research involving Human Subjects. In www.wma.net/e/policy/b3.htm
107. Yudkin PL, Stratton IM (1996) How to deal with regression to the mean in intervention studies. Lancet 347: 241-243
108. Zeymer U, Suryapranata H, Monassier JP, Opolski G, Davies J, Rasmanis G, Linssen G, Tebbe U, Schrôder R, Tiemann R, Maching T, Neuhaus KL, Monassier JP (2001) The Na+/H+ exchange inhibitor eniporide as an adjunct to early reperfusion therapy for acute myocardial infarction. J Am Coll Cardiol 38: 1644-1651

Analytical Index

Printed in December 2006